Sleep Disorders and Neurological Disease

NEUROLOGICAL DISEASE AND THERAPY

Series Editor

William C. Koller

Department of Neurology
University of Kansas Medical Center
Kansas City, Kansas

1. Handbook of Parkinson's Disease, *edited by William C. Koller*
2. Medical Therapy of Acute Stroke, *edited by Mark Fisher*
3. Familial Alzheimer's Disease: Molecular Genetics and Clinical Perspectives, *edited by Gary D. Miner, Ralph W. Richter, John P. Blass, Jimmie L. Valentine, and Linda A. Winters-Miner*
4. Alzheimer's Disease: Treatment and Long-Term Management, *edited by Jeffrey L. Cummings and Bruce L. Miller*
5. Therapy of Parkinson's Disease, *edited by William C. Koller and George Paulson*
6. Handbook of Sleep Disorders, *edited by Michael J. Thorpy*
7. Epilepsy and Sudden Death, *edited by Claire M. Lathers and Paul L. Schraeder*
8. Handbook of Multiple Sclerosis, *edited by Stuart D. Cook*
9. Memory Disorders: Research and Clinical Practice, *edited by Takehiko Yanagihara and Ronald C. Petersen*
10. The Medical Treatment of Epilepsy, *edited by Stanley R. Resor, Jr., and Henn Kutt*
11. Cognitive Disorders: Pathophysiology and Treatment, *edited by Leon J. Thal, Walter H. Moos, and Elkan R. Gamzu*
12. Handbook of Amyotrophic Lateral Sclerosis, *edited by Richard Alan Smith*
13. Handbook of Parkinson's Disease: Second Edition, Revised and Expanded, *edited by William C. Koller*
14. Handbook of Pediatric Epilepsy, *edited by Jerome V. Murphy and Fereydoun Dehkharghani*
15. Handbook of Tourette's Syndrome and Related Tic and Behavioral Disorders, *edited by Roger Kurlan*
16. Handbook of Cerebellar Diseases, *edited by Richard Lechtenberg*
17. Handbook of Cerebrovascular Diseases, *edited by Harold P. Adams, Jr.*
18. Parkinsonian Syndromes, *edited by Matthew B. Stern and William C. Koller*
19. Handbook of Head and Spine Trauma, *edited by Jonathan Greenberg*
20. Brain Tumors: A Comprehensive Text, *edited by Robert A. Morantz and John W. Walsh*

21. Monoamine Oxidase Inhibitors in Neurological Diseases, *edited by Abraham Lieberman, C. Warren Olanow, Moussa B. H. Youdim, and Keith Tipton*
22. Handbook of Dementing Illnesses, *edited by John C. Morris*
23. Handbook of Myasthenia Gravis and Myasthenic Syndromes, *edited by Robert P. Lisak*
24. Handbook of Neurorehabilitation, *edited by David C. Good and James R. Couch, Jr.*
25. Therapy with Botulinum Toxin, *edited by Joseph Jankovic and Mark Hallett*
26. Principles of Neurotoxicology, *edited by Louis W. Chang*
27. Handbook of Neurovirology, *edited by Robert R. McKendall and William G. Stroop*
28. Handbook of Neuro-Urology, *edited by David N. Rushton*
29. Handbook of Neuroepidemiology, *edited by Philip B. Gorelick and Milton Alter*
30. Handbook of Tremor Disorders, *edited by Leslie J. Findley and William C. Koller*
31. Neuro-Ophthalmological Disorders: Diagnostic Work-Up and Management, *edited by Ronald J. Tusa and Steven A. Newman*
32. Handbook of Olfaction and Gustation, *edited by Richard L. Doty*
33. Handbook of Neurological Speech and Language Disorders, *edited by Howard S. Kirshner*
34. Therapy of Parkinson's Disease: Second Edition, Revised and Expanded, *edited by William C. Koller and George Paulson*
35. Evaluation and Management of Gait Disorders, *edited by Barney S. Spivack*
36. Handbook of Neurotoxicology, *edited by Louis W. Chang and Robert S. Dyer*
37. Neurological Complications of Cancer, *edited by Ronald G. Wiley*
38. Handbook of Autonomic Nervous System Dysfunction, *edited by Amos D. Korczyn*
39. Handbook of Dystonia, *edited by Joseph King Ching Tsui and Donald B. Calne*
40. Etiology of Parkinson's Disease, *edited by Jonas H. Ellenberg, William C. Koller, and J. William Langston*
41. Practical Neurology of the Elderly, *edited by Jacob I. Sage and Margery H. Mark*
42. Handbook of Muscle Disease, *edited by Russell J. M. Lane*
43. Handbook of Multiple Sclerosis: Second Edition, Revised and Expanded, *edited by Stuart D. Cook*
44. Central Nervous System Infectious Diseases and Therapy, *edited by Karen L. Roos*
45. Subarachnoid Hemorrhage: Clinical Management, *edited by Takehiko Yanagihara, David G. Piepgras, and John L. D. Atkinson*

46. Neurology Practice Guidelines, *edited by Richard Lechtenberg and Henry S. Schutta*
47. Spinal Cord Diseases: Diagnosis and Treatment, *edited by Gordon L. Engler, Jonathan Cole, and W. Louis Merton*
48. Management of Acute Stroke, *edited by Ashfaq Shuaib and Larry B. Goldstein*
49. Sleep Disorders and Neurological Disease, *edited by Antonio Culebras*

Additional Volumes in Preparation

Sleep Disorders and Neurological Disease

edited by

Antonio Culebras
Department of Veterans Affairs Medical Center
Syracuse, New York

MARCEL DEKKER, INC. NEW YORK • BASEL

ISBN: 0-8247-7605-4

This book is printed on acid-free paper.

Headquarters
Marcel Dekker, Inc.
270 Madison Avenue, New York, NY 10016
tel: 212-696-9000; fax: 212-685-4540

Eastern Hemisphere Distribution
Marcel Dekker AG
Hutgasse 4, Postfach 812, CH-4001 Basel, Switzerland
tel: 41-61-261-8482; fax: 41-61-261-8896

World Wide Web
http://www.dekker.com

The publisher offers discounts on this book when ordered in bulk quantities. For more information, write to Special Sales/Professional Marketing at the headquarters address above.

Current printing (last digit):
10 9 8 7 6 5 4 3

PRINTED IN THE UNITED STATES OF AMERICA

Foreword

Sleep is a topic that holds great fascination. While the British never seem to get bored of discussions about their weather, Americans are equally prepared to discourse to almost anyone about their own sleep patterns. Even the most rigorous scientists have their own anecdotal evidence for the success of some strategy to contend with life's major challenges to sleep, including jet lag, shiftwork, and young children and other noisy housemates.

Neurologists are asked to see large numbers of patients with sleep disorders and the subspecialty of neurosomnology—neurological sleep medicine—has developed rapidly over the past three decades. Patients with sleep disorders often develop respiratory problems, and one of the commonest of the sleep disorders, sleep apnea, can result from airway obstruction and causes neurological symptoms. Thus, pulmonologists are appropriately involved in the care of some patients with sleep disorders. However, the vast majority of causes of sleep apnea and other sleep disorders are neurological. Similarly, psychiatric diseases cause sleep disorders and sleep disorders cause psychological dysfunction, but the evaluation of patients requires sophisticated neurological and neurophysiological assessment of the type best coordinated by a clinical neuroscientist. It is thus extremely welcome and timely to have Antonio Culebras' volume on sleep disorders and neurological disease. Not many multiauthored texts are a good read. This one is. Most of the chapters start with either an illustrative case or the history of the topic. They then proceed to the clinical importance and on to pathophysiology and treatment. The chapters are so well written that the nonneurologist will find them easy reading. Yet they contain all that neurologists and most that sleep specialists need to know, including a synopsis of relevant, current neuroscience and extensive recent literature citations.

It is an honor to be asked to write the Foreword to a major new book. Since I am not an expert in sleep medicine, I feel I must justify agreeing to do so. First, as a specialist in neuromuscular disease and an internist/neurologist, I have seen a wide spectrum of clinical medicine and have always had an amateur's interest in sleep disorders. Second, since 1996 I have edited the journal *Neurology* and have seen a large number of papers on sleep disorders. I have increased the number of articles on sleep published by *Neurology*, inviting editorials on several papers and otherwise highlighting this important subspecialty area.

It is a major undertaking to embark on the task of conceiving a text, developing its content, cajoling authors, editing chapters, and finally completing a multiauthored volume that covers an entire field. Antonio Culebras has most definitely been up to the task. Why should he have been the one to do the job? First, he has himself contributed substantially to the clinical investigation of sleep disorders for over 30 years. He was, in fact, one of the first to begin to characterize sleep disorders in neuromuscular diseases. Second, he has a career as a broadly based clinical neurologist, expert in CNS disorders—particularly stroke—as well as ''peripheral'' neurology. Finally, he has had high-profile leadership in the international affairs of American neurology and has fostered intellectual and academic interchange between U.S. neurologists in Central and South America, Europe, and indeed the world. This has positioned him well to develop an outstanding cadre of worldwide authorities in sleep and its disorders as authors of his text.

My only word of warning is to Dr. Culebras. Neurosomnology is expanding at an increasing rate. He should be thinking about his next edition before this one sells out.

Robert C. Griggs, M.D.

Professor of Neurology, Medicine, Pediatrics, and Pathology
Chair of Neurology
University of Rochester School of Medicine & Dentistry

Editor-in-Chief
Neurology

Preface

The neurology of sleep, or neurosomnology, is the study of sleep from the neurological perspective. It focuses on the fabric of neurological mechanisms and manifestations that underlie sleep and its disorders, whether primary or secondary. Thus, in the neurology of sleep, the neuroanatomy and neurophysiology of sleep are studied with the intention of establishing a platform of basic neurological mechanisms upon which to build the discipline. It is not limited to the description of sleep manifestations in common neurological disorders, such as Parkinson's disease or multiple sclerosis, or of intrinsic sleep disorders such as narcolepsy and idiopathic CNS hypersomnia, but extends into dimensions of pathophysiology, treatment, and prevention. The neurology of sleep takes off from the premise that sleep is a function of the brain and that all sleep problems emanate from brain dysfunctions—whether structural as in brain tumors, degenerative as in fatal familial insomnia, neurochemical as in narcolepsy, neuromuscular as in sleep apnea, or behavioral as in insomnia. Some are primary and intrinsic, with the sleep dysfunction at the core of the condition as in narcolepsy, while others are secondary as in the sleep disorders associated with Parkinson's disease. In some instances, it is difficult to dissect primary from secondary since the sleep dysfunction is intimately embroidered into the substance of the neurological condition; thus, one cannot conceive the study of headaches without a basic understanding of the sleep alterations that follow or trigger them, or of epilepsy without knowledge of its relationship to sleep deprivation and sleep onset. No aspect of neurology is left untouched. Altertness, attention, concentration, memory, and mood states are so intimately connected with sleep that theories abound about the refreshment properties of sleep in brain circuits processing basic mechanisms.

Although sleep is a function of the brain, and thc neurology of sleep its corollary, sleep medicine remains a multidisciplinary body. So numerous are the ramifications and so extensive the reach of sleep and its dysfunctions that the specialist in neurology requires the collaboration of experts in other disciplines to attend to the vast field unfolded. Pulmonary specialists and cardiologists are carrying the study of sleep apnea and its treatment into areas where neurologists would have never gone. Psychiatrists and psychologists are developing a subdiscipline that studies the behaviors of patients with sleep alterations, applying treatment modalities distant from internal medicine or neurology. In the end, the neurology of sleep might prevail as the core discipline advancing the investigation of brain processes underlying sleep functions and dysfunctions, but, as in other areas of clinical medicine, transcendence of sleep beyond the traditional confines of neurology requires an interdisciplinary approach.

Although neuropsychiatrists, psychiatrists, psychologists, resident physicians, neuroscientists, and sleep specialists will also find this book useful, it is published with the neurologist in mind. It focuses on subjects of importance to the specialist in neurology, establishing a domain that is exclusive to the neurologist within sleep medicine while ratifying sleep as part of the scope of practice of the neurologist. The chapters have a clinical orientation, toward description of manifestations, diagnosis of nosologic entities, and treatment. Procedural aspects of sleep-laboratory function are not addressed except where important as an adjunct to the understanding of clinical manifestations.

The reader will find that some topics are addressed in more than one chapter. This does not represent duplication or scatter but, rather, diversity that enriches the book with different perspectives on the same subject. Where appropriate I have indicated the chapters in which complementary information on the same topic might also be found.

The authors are prestigious neurologists with an international name in the field of sleep disorders. They were invited to collaborate because of their expertise in the topic selected and their proven ability as communicators. Despite multiple other commitments and distracting obligations, they all complied diligently with the task given and should be commended for their superb effort.

Antonio Culebras

Contents

Contributors

Michael S. Aldrich, M.D. Professor, Department of Neurology, and Director, Sleep Disorders Center, University of Michigan Health System, Ann Arbor, Michigan

Gabriele M. Barthlen, M.D. Neurologist, Department of Pulmonary and Internal Medicine, Freiburg University Medical Center, Freiburg, Germany

Claudio Bassetti, M.D. Director, Sleep Disorders Center, Neurology Department, University Hospital (Inselpital), Bern, Switzerland

Ali G. Bassiri, M.D. Fellow, Center for Excellence in Sleep Disorders Medicine, Stanford University Medical School, Palo Alto, California

Donald L. Bliwise, Ph.D. Associate Professor, Department of Neurology, Emory University School of Medicine, and Director, Sleep Disorders Center, Wesley Woods Geriatric Hospital, Atlanta, Georgia

Sudhansu Chokroverty, M.D., F.R.C.P., F.A.C.P. Professor and Associate Chairman of Neurology; Chairman, Division of Neurophysiology; and Director, Center of Sleep Medicine, Department of Neurology, Saint Vincents Hospital and New York Medical College, New York, New York

Antonio Culebras, M.D. Senior Neurologist, Veterans Affairs Medical Center;

Professor of Neurology, Health Science Center, State University of New York; and Consultant, Sleep Center, Community General Hospital, Syracuse, New York

Christian Guilleminault, M.D. Professor, Center for Excellence in Sleep Disorders Medicine, Stanford University Medical School, Palo Alto, California

Elio Lugaresi, M.D. Professor of Neurology; Director, Institute of Clinical Neurology; and Director, Sleep Disorders Centre, University of Bologna, Bologna, Italy

Mark W. Mahowald, M.D. Director, Minnesota Regional Sleep Disorders Center, Hennepin County Medical Center, and Professor, Department of Neurology, University of Minnesota Medical School, Minneapolis, Minnesota

Pasquale Montagna, M.D. Associate Professor of Neurology, Institute of Clinical Neurology, University of Bologna, Bologna, Italy

Heikki Palomäki, M.D., Ph.D. Department of Clinical Neurosciences, University of Helsinki, Helsinki, Finland

Markku Partinen, M.D., Ph.D. Director, Haaga Neurological Research Center, and Department of Clinical Neurosciences, University of Helsinki, Helsinki, Finland

Giuseppe Plazzi, M.D. Assistant Professor, Institute of Clinical Neurology, University of Bologna, Bologna, Italy

Charles P. Pollak, M.D. Professor, Department of Neurology, The Ohio State University Medical Center, Columbus, Ohio

Federica Provini, M.D. Researcher, Institute of Clinical Neurology, University of Bologna, Bologna, Italy

Christine Quinto, M.D. Research Associate, Department of Neurology, Saint Vincents Hospital, New York, New York

Robert L. Rodnitzky, M.D. Professor and Vice Chairman, Department of Neurology, and Director, Movement Disorders Clinic, University of Iowa College of Medicine, Iowa City, Iowa

Carlos H. Schenck, M.D. Minnesota Regional Sleep Disorders Center and Department of Psychiatry, Hennepin County Medical Center, and Associate Professor, Department of Psychiatry, University of Minnesota Medical School, Minneapolis, Minnesota

Stephen H. Sheldon, D.O. Director, Sleep Medicine Center, Children's Memorial Hospital, and Assistant Professor, Department of Pediatrics, Northwestern University Medical School, Chicago, Illinois

Michael J. Thorpy, M.D. Director, Sleep-Wake Disorders Center, Montefiore Medical Center, and Associate Professor, Department of Neurology, Albert Einstein College of Medicine, Bronx, New York

Irina V. Zhdanova, M.D., Ph.D. Department of Brain and Cognitive Sciences, Massachusetts Institute of Technology, Cambridge, Massachusetts

1

Historical Perspective on Sleep and Man

Michael J. Thorpy
Montefiore Medical Center
and Albert Einstein College of Medicine
Bronx, New York

Sleep; King of all the gods and of all mortals,
harken now, prithee, to my word;
and if ever before thou didst listen, obey me now,
and I will ever be grateful to thee all my days.

—Homer, 14th Book of the *Iliad*

A rudimentary understanding of insomnia and sleepiness existed in ancient times, but specific sleep disorders, such as narcolepsy, began to be recognized only in the late 19th century. Differentiation between causes of sleepiness and insomnia has reached a peak within the last 50 years, especially since the development of sophisticated technology for the investigation of sleep.

Neurologists have made major contributions to the understanding of sleep, particularly since the end of the last century, when many different theories on the cause of sleep were rampant. Sleep is now recognized as a function of the brain, and the mechanism that underlies it has intrigued scientists since time began.

SLEEP IN PREHISTORIC AND ANCIENT TIMES

Sleep's the only medicine that gives ease.

—Sophocles, *Philoctetes*

The sleep patterns and sleep disorders of prehistoric man are unknown, and therefore we must speculate from the comparative physiology of animals and from evidence of other behaviors and illnesses. Theories on the phylogenetic development of sleep stages in mammals have been developed from information available on the mammal-like reptiles. The earliest form of life developed about 600 million years ago in the pre-Cambrian period, and mammal-like reptiles evolved approximately 250 million years ago. It was about 180 million years ago, when slow-wave sleep is believed to have appeared, that the monotremes (egg-laying mammals) evolved as a separate line from the therian (live-bearing) mammals; REM sleep (paradoxical sleep) appeared about 50 million years later (1).

The pattern of sleep and waking behavior in prehistoric man can be deduced from studies of nonhuman primates, such as apes and Old World monkeys, the animal groups phylogenetically closest to man. Sleep–wake patterns in nonprimates consist mainly of polyphasic episodes of rest and activity with frequent (up to 12) cycles of wakeful activity throughout the 24-hour day. Man has the most developed monophasic pattern, with one episode of consolidated sleep and one main episode of wakefulness. Some animals have a biphasic sleep–wake pattern, with a nap taken during the daytime, the pattern present, for instance, in the chimpanzee. The chimpanzee has a rather prolonged sleep episode from dusk to dawn of approximately 10 hours; however, during this time there are frequent, brief awakenings. The daytime is characterized by two long episodes of wakefulness and an approximately 5-hour midday nap, which also includes frequent brief wakefulness episodes.

An early polyphasic sleep pattern seems likely to have been characteristic of earliest man, particularly if man also attempted to sleep between dusk and dawn. There would have been frequent awakenings during the major sleep episode, as a single sleep episode of more than 10 hours appears unlikely. It is reasonable to predict that man first began to develop a monophasic sleep–wake pattern in the Neolithic period (since 10,000 B.C.). The chimpanzee's sleep pattern was probably similar to that present in man prior to the Neolithic period; Neanderthal Man (70,000 to 40,000 B.C.) may well have been in a transitional stage between a polyphasic sleep pattern and the monophasic pattern seen today.

There is evidence from studies of animal fossils that disease was present even before humans evolved. Medical evidence of such illnesses as pneumonia, arteriosclerosis, and parasitic disease has been found in the mummies of early Egypt, and it is reasonable to believe that disease in early man was associated with changes in sleep and wakefulness in a manner similar to that seen today. However, evidence also suggests that man's lifetime was much shorter during the Paleolithic and early Neolithic periods, averaging only about 30 to 40 years. The sleep disturbances of concern to the elderly today may not have been a problem in prehistoric man.

One can assume that prehistoric man would have attempted to treat sleep disturbances, but the nature of their efforts is unknown. Therapy probably resembled that utilized by sick animals, such as the removal of infective agents, eating various plants to induce emesis, and possibly even bloodletting. Certainly bloodletting became an increasingly frequent therapeutic means for treating disease, including sleep disorders, in more advanced ancient civilizations. Primitive societies, even today, consider many illnesses and diseases to be caused by gods, magic, and spirits, and therefore various forms of divination, such as the casting of bones, moving of beads, charms, fetishes, chanting, or the use of elaborate ceremonies, are invoked for therapeutic reasons. Such forms of treatment were probably applied by prehistoric man for disturbances of sleep and wakefulness.

Mesopotamians (ca. 3000 B.C.) thought illness was produced by irate gods, and so their gods were named for specific diseases, for example, Tiu, the god of headache, and Nergel, the god of fever. Treatment consisted largely of determining what misdeed had been committed by the sufferer, and then performing divination in an attempt to appease the gods. Plants, oils, minerals, and animal substances were ingested, inhaled, or given as suppositories or enemas. These agents were usually administered by a priest–physician, and strict codes were established for payment for medical services, as well as for punishment of the physician for inadequate treatment. It is likely that many punishments were administered for failure to relieve sleep disorders that would have been chronic and often difficult to cure, such as insomnia and narcolepsy.

The ancient medical papyruses of Egypt provide most of our current knowledge of ancient Egyptian medicine (2). The Chester Beatty papyrus, which was written around 1350 B.C., contains information on the interpretation of dreams. Dreams were regarded as being contrary predictions; for example, a dream of death meant a long life. However, the Georg Ebers papyrus (1600 B.C.), an extensive text on a variety of medical subjects, including treatment, has not been reported to contain any information on sleep disturbances. Ancient Egyptian medical practice consisted largely of praying to the gods and invoking the help of these divine healers. Thoth, who was a physician to the gods, and Imhotep were important gods of healing at that time. The ancient Egyptians were known for their attention to hygiene and cleanliness, and it is likely that such attention was also paid to sleeping habits.

Medical opinion at the time held that the body was made up of a system of channels (Metu), which conveyed air to all parts of the body. Because they believed that bodily fluids could enter this system of channels, the ancient Egyptians were particularly concerned about feces entering the Metu. Hence, the treatment of many illnesses was carried out by purging and enemas. Infective illnesses, including malaria, parasitic infections, smallpox, and leprosy, were common at that time. Wine and other mildly alcoholic drinks (as compared to distilled alcoholic products) were consumed in large amounts and were probably the earliest treatments for insomnia but may also have been important in its development. Medicinal plants were utilized, particularly the product of the opium poppy (*Papaver somniferum*), and hyoscyamine and scopolamine, derived from belladonna and nightshade (3). [The word *opium* is derived from the Greek word for "juice," as the drug is derived from the juice of the poppy. *Papaver somniferum* was coined at a much later date; *somniferum* was derived from the latin word *somnus* (the Roman god of sleep). In subsequent periods of history, opium (laudanum) was widely used as a treatment for insomnia, and it is likely that it was used as far back as the Sumerian age, which suggests that opium may have been the first hypnotic medication used.]

Bloodletting was commonly performed by the ancient Egyptians for the treatment of a variety of ailments and illnesses and perhaps for sleep disorders, particularly for disorders that produced excessive sleepiness or stupor. Medical treatment was widely available; the names of several hundred physicians have been documented in ancient Egypt. Herodotus (fifth century B.C.) wrote of the Egyptians: "Medicine with them is distributed in the following way: every physician is for one disease and not for several, and the whole country is full of physicians for the eyes; others of the head; others of the teeth; others of the belly, and others of obscure diseases."

It appears likely that some physicians specialized in insomnia, and possibly even in disorders that produced excessive sleepiness. There were certainly physicians who specialized in dream interpretation—for example, Artemidorus of Daldis, who wrote the major work on dreams, *Oneirocritica* (4).

Other civilizations that developed around the same time were those of ancient India and China. Early Indian medicine consisted mainly of magical and religious practices but also featured soundly based, rational treatments. Over 700 Indian vegetable medicines have been documented from ancient times and include the plant called *Rauwolfa serpentina* (reserpine). Rauwolfia was used for the treatment of anxiety, among other disorders, and was probably used to treat insomnia. In India, as in Egypt, infective illnesses were common, so physicians, who were largely from the Brahman or priestly caste, were viewed with great importance. Effective treatment of most illnesses is reported to have been dependent on four major factors: the physician, the patient, the medicine, and the nurse. Asoka (273–232 B.C.), a ruler of the Mauryan dynasty, reported that hospitals were established as early as in the third century B.C.

The ancient Chinese believed in the importance of the universe and environment in producing all things, including behavior and health. The basic principles of life were thought to derive from the interplay of two basic elements in nature: the active, light, dry, warm, positive, masculine Yang and the passive, dark, cold, moist, negative Yin. The proportions of Yin and Yang determined the Tao (the way), which determined right and wrong, good and bad, health and illness, etc. The basic Yin-Yang symbol is attributed to Fu Hsi (ca. 2900 B.C.), who originated the concept of eight interacting conditions, the "Pa kua." The Yin-Yang has since become the symbol for sleep and wakefulness. (This Yin-Yang symbol has been adopted by the American Sleep Disorders Association as its emblem.) The views of the Chinese on physiology were similar to those of the ancient Greeks; they too believed in a humoral system of physiology. The palpation of the pulse was important in the diagnosis of disease. To determine whether a patient had upset the Tao, not only were the patient's symptoms taken into consideration but also the social and economic status, the weather, and particularly the patient's dreams, as well as the dreams of other family members.

The most important medical compendium of the time was that produced by Yu Hsiung (ca. 2600 B.C.), the *Nei Ching* ("Canon of Medicine"). This manuscript mentioned five important methods of treatment: curing the spirit, nourishing the body, administering medications, treating the whole body, and the use of acupuncture and moxibustion (counterirritation by moxa, a combustible substance that is burned on the skin). It is most likely that these latter forms of therapy were applied to the sleep disorders. Massage and breathing exercises were also commonly employed, in a manner similar to that of Yoga. Herbal medicines were plentiful and consisted of extracts of virtually anything available, including minerals and metals, animal-derived products and waste products (3).

Two important Chinese remedies existed. One was ephedra (Ma Huang), a stimulant that contained ephedrine, derived from the "horsetail" plant and first described by the Red Emperor, Shen Nung (ca. 2800 B.C.). The second common medicinal herb was ginseng (a man-shaped root), which was used for stimulation as well as sedating purposes. Although commonly used by the Greeks at this time, opium does not appear to have been used in ancient China. Acupuncture was widespread and is believed to have been developed by the Yellow Emperor (Huang Ti) around 2600 B.C.(5). Acupuncture and moxibustion were used for treating virtually every illness and symptom and therefore may well have been administered for sleep disorders.

In ancient China, physicians were also highly regarded and were grouped into five categories: the chief physician, food physicians, physicians for simple diseases, ulcer physicians, and physicians for animals. They were rated according to their treatment results, and each doctor had to report his therapeutic successes and failures. Sleep was regarded by the Chinese as a state of unity with the universe and was therefore regarded as being very important for health. The Chinese philosopher Chuang-Tzu (300 B.C.) said, "Everything is one; during sleep the soul, undistracted, is absorbed into the unity; when awake, distracted, it sees the different beings."

Much of what we know about early Greek medicine is derived from the *Iliad* and *Odyssey* by Homer, a collection of traditions, legends, and epic poems. Homer (ca. 900 B.C.) based his epic works on the life of the ancient Greeks in the days of the Mycenaean Citadel of about 1200 B.C. The Mycenaeans, who came from mainland Greece in about 1600 B.C., conquered the Minoans, who had established a well-developed civilization in Crete at Knossus. This civilization was the setting for Homer's epics, which concerned an earlier period, but his writings included medical details that were probably derived from his own era. However, Homer's view of medicine in early Greece, called Homeric medicine, is the best representation of early Greek medical practices. The quotation from the *Iliad* that appears on page 1 reflects the importance that Homer ascribed to good, quality sleep. The god of sleep, Hypnos—from whose name come the terms *hypnotic* and *hypnotism*—was first mentioned in the 14th book of the *Iliad*, and was mentioned again in the *Theogony* of Hesiod (ca. 700 B.C.) about two centuries later (6).

Also mentioned in Homer was the chieftain Asclepios and his two sons: Machanon, who in subsequent centuries became known as the father of surgery, and Podalirios, the father of internal medicine. In subsequent years, Asclepios became known as the god of healing, and temples were erected in his honor, the first being established in about the sixth century B.C. in Thessaly or Ipidauros. The Asclepieian temples were a collection of several buildings, many of which were very elaborate and ornate. They consisted of a *tholos*, a round building that contained water for purification, and a main temple, which were separated by a building called the *abaton*. The abaton was a very important structure because it was where ill patients were placed for a cure. The cure consisted of an "incubation" ceremony in which the cure took place in each worshipper's dreams. The medical ceremony began at dusk, when the patient lay on a bed of skins to await a visit by Asclepios, the god of healing. During the night, the priest would visit each patient and administer a treatment, which often consisted of medicines derived from such animals as snakes and geese. On awakening the next morning after dreaming of Asclepios, the patient was expected to have been cured. This treatment was clearly the forerunner of sleep therapy, which has been practiced through the ages until the present day, particularly in Eastern countries. Although Asclepieian medicine was used to treat any type of illness, it was most effective for those of a psychological nature. Much of the healing was probably related to the impressive ceremony and the relaxation that occurred in conjunction with the setting. The priest–physicians instilled faith in the cures—not only in their patients but also in themselves. However, many attempted cures were in the realm of magic and fantasy.

A more rational style of medicine developed in around the fifth century B.C., due largely to the influence of the Greek scientist–philosophers, such as Thales and Pythagoras. Thales of Miletos (640–546 B.C.), who believed that water was an important basic element of all animal and plant life, made many contributions not only to medicine but also to geometry, astronomy, and mathematics. His direction in medicine was not inspired by mythological or religious beliefs but rather by observing natural processes of the environment. Around the same time, Pythagoras (ca. 530 B.C.) was born on an island off the coast of Asia Minor, and developed a school of medicine at Crotona in southern Italy. Pythagoras developed a philosophical approach to medicine that was based on the science of numbers and the spiritual universe, but the importance of diet, exercise, music, and meditation was emphasized. Alcmaeon (fifth century B.C.), of the Crotona school of medical thought, concentrated on man, and his basic belief was that health was harmony and disease was a disturbance of harmony (7). He considered the brain essential for memory and thought, a belief that Aristotle, who believed that the mind resided in the heart, would reject 100 years later. Alcmaeon proposed what was probably the first theory on the cause of sleep, when he postulated that sleep occurs when the blood vessels of the brain fill with blood; withdrawal of blood from the brain leads to waking. However, his major contribution to medicine was the detailed description of the optic pathways at the base of brain. His much more rational concepts of medicine have led some to consider him the first true medical scientist.

Around the time of Alcmaeon, a center of medicine was established in Sicily, and Empedocles (ca. 493–ca. 443 B.C.) was credited with the original concept that all things are composed of four basic elements: water, air, fire, and earth (the importance of these four elements had been established earlier) (7). Empedocles believed that sleep occurs when the fire in the blood cools, thus separating one of the four elements from the others. He believed that illnesses are due to either separation of the four elements or alterations in their balance. The principle of the balance of body humors, known as *humoralism*, became established medical doctrine around this time. In humoralism, health is believed to be based on the balance of four body fluids: blood, phlegm, and yellow and black bile. These fluids were usually seen during severe illnesses and disappeared when the crises were over.

Two other major schools of medicine were developed in the fifth century B.C., one at Cnidos and the other at Cos. At Cnidos, an elaborate classification system for diseases was devised in which each specific disease was ascribed to one symptom. In contrast, the school at Cos concentrated largely on the development of rational treatments and rational diagnostic principles.

> *In whatever disease sleep is laborious, it is a deadly symptom.*
>
> —Hippocrates, *Aphorisms*, II

Hippocrates (460–370 B.C.) was born on the island of Cos and was responsible for that school of medicine's direction. No individual in history has had more influence on medicine than Hippocrates, who produced many of the basic tenets that underlie the practice of modern medicine (8). He produced numerous works that are gathered in the *Corpus Hippocraticum*, which comprises not only his own writings but also those of others of the time. His approximately 72 books covered all aspects of medicine, including medical ethics, and are most widely known for the Hippocratic oath. In his writings, Hippocrates not only discussed his theory of the cause of sleep but also offered suggestions about the cause of dreams, which he considered to be of "medical" origin. He stated that "sleep is due to blood going from the limbs to the inner regions of the body.'' This statement was based on recognition of the importance of blood being warmed by the inner part of the body to produce sleep—a theory contrary to that proposed by Alcmaeon. Since Hippocrates believed that narcotics derived from the opium poppy could be useful in treatment, they were probably applied to treat insomnia at that time.

Following Hippocrates, the philosophers Plato and Aristotle had an important influence on medicine. Plato (ca. 429–347 B.C.), a teacher of Aristotle, developed many medical speculations. He influenced the practice of medicine to the extent that medical practice became more dogma than patient evaluation. For this reason, physicians who supported his doctrines were called ''dogmatists'' and their therapeutic endeavors relied largely on drastic purgings and bleedings. Aristotle (384–322 B.C.) believed that dreams are important predictors of the future but proposed a theory of sleep based on the effect of food ingestion (9,10). He suggested that food, once eaten, induces fumes that are taken into the blood vessels and then transferred into the brain, where they induce sleepiness. The fumes subsequently cool and return to the lower parts of the body, taking heat away from the brain, thereby triggering sleep. The sleep process continues as long as food is being digested. Following the Hippocratic era of medicine, Greek medicine began to develop in Rome, along with temples to Asclepios in 300 B.C.

Atomism, the concept that all physical objects are composed of atoms in an infinite number that undergo random motion, was first developed by Democritus of Abdera (ca. 420 B.C.) and Leucippus of Miletus (ca. 430 B.C.). Leucippus regarded sleep as a state caused by the partial or complete splitting-off of atoms. Democritus considered insomnia the result of an unhealthy diet and daytime sleeping as being a sign of ill health. Epicurus (ca. 300 B.C.) revived the theory of atomism and wrote extensively on sleep and dreams, although his own works have been lost. The Roman poet Titus Lucretius Carus (ca. 50 B.C.) wrote of the teachings of Epicurus on atomism, sleep, and dreams in a poem entitled ''De rerum natura.'' In this poem, the loss of central control that leads to loss of peripheral muscle control and to relaxation forms the foundation of a neural theory of sleep that took 2000 years to be expanded on: ''And so, when the motions are changed, sense withdraws deep within. And since there is nothing which can, as it were, support the limbs, the body grows feeble, and all the limbs are slackened; arms and eyelids droop, and the hams, even as you lie down, often give way, and relax their strength.''

Asclepiades of Bithynia (ca. 120–ca. 70 B.C.), another figure in Roman medicine, believed that the physician is more important than nature in curing disease. He used the term *phrenitis* for mental illness and invoked treatment that consisted of hygiene, opium, and wine. He was also the first to popularize the tracheostomy as a treatment for upper airway obstruction.

Cornelius Celsus (ca. 20 A.D.) and Caius Pliny the Elder (23–79 A.D.) substantially documented medical practice of their time. *De Medicina*, the work of Celsus, covered a wide range of topics, including history, preventive medicine, surgery, and anatomy. Pliny produced *Historia Naturalis*, a work that contained virtually every piece of medical information available. Although Pliny's writings were regarded as the mainstay of medicine right through the Middle Ages, the Greek Galen (129–ca. 200 A.D.) had a greater impact on the subsequent development of medicine (11,12). Galen's detailed writings contributed greatly to the knowledge of anatomy, and he outlined the important elements of diagnosis and treatment. He believed bloodletting was important in the treatment of many illnesses, but he also encouraged conservative treatments, such as diet, rest, and exercise. He utilized many herbal medicines, often in complicated combinations. The anatomical works of Galen reigned supreme in medicine until the works of Vesalius in the 16th century.

The Bible contains numerous references to sleep and dreams. Dreams were largely regarded as being predictors of the future (but less significant than in previous eras) (13). The Bible emphasized the importance of sleep and rest; the essential elements for good sleep were considered to be hard work, a clear conscience, freedom from anxiety, and trust in Jehovah (Ecclesiastes 5:12; Psalms 3:5, 4:8; Proverbs 3:24–26). Sleep disturbance was less likely to occur if one was content with life's lot, and sleeplessness would result from excessive worry about material possessions (Ecclesiastes 5:12).

SLEEP IN THE MIDDLE AGES AND THE RENAISSANCE

Long sleep at after-noones by stirring fumes
Breeds Slouth, and Agues
Aking heads and Rheumes.
—School at Salerno, *Regimen*: *Sanitatis Salernitanum* (1095–1224)

The time from the fall of Rome in 476 A.D. to the fall of Constantinople in 1453 A.D. is often referred to as the Middle Ages, the first 500 years of which were the Dark Ages. The Middle Ages comprise the medieval period, the Age of Faith, a time when medicine was greatly influenced by the rise of Christianity.

With the spread of the word of Christianity, man was convinced that the day of judgment was about to come, and disease was believed to be God's punishment. Prayer and good deeds were considered important for cures and to prevent illness. Concern for "thy neighbor" led to the establishment of facilities for the care of the ill, most of which were run with religious motives. Medicine involved strong religious mysticism, and there was a loss of the rational, clinical observation and management of disease that had begun to develop in earlier years. Monasteries that cared for the sick were established, but they scorned scientific, medical teaching. One of the first was Monte Cassino in Italy, founded by St. Benedict of Nursia (480–554 A.D.). It was in these times that the Temples of Asclepios were also popular for the treatment of illnesses by Incubatio. Although superstition and magic swept the Western world, some physicians with skill in observation and deduction—such as Alexander of Tralles (525–405 A.D.)—slowly advanced medical knowledge.

In the Moslem world, there was a similar religious approach to medicine. Although in Islam disease is regarded as a punishment by Allah, hospitals in Moslem countries were very much better than those in the West because of their improved sanitation and better and more spacious facilities. Physicians were largely of the Christian and Jewish faiths, but Moslem practitioners gradually helped spread medicine in the East. The Persian Razi (850–ca. 923) (also known as Rhazes in the West) wrote more than 200 books on many topics, including medicine (14). Avicenna (980–1037 A.D.), who also contributed to medical understanding, was regarded both in Islam and Christendom as being of equal importance to Galen (15,16). A little later, Moses ben Maimon (1135–1204 A.D.), also known as Maimonides, emerged as the most influential Jewish physician in Arabic medicine. He appeared to combine the views of Hippocrates, Galen, and Avicenna, but his primary focus was on philosophy. In the Misheneh Torah ("Hilchoth De'oth," Chapter 4, no. 4), Maimonides expressed his own opinion about how much and when a person should sleep: "The day and night consist of 24 hours. It is sufficient for a person to sleep one third thereof which is eight hours. These should [preferably] be at the end of the night so that from the beginning of sleep until the rising of the sun will be eight hours. Thus he will arise from his bed before the sun rises."

In the 10th century A.D., several medical schools came into prominence. Perhaps the first was that established at Salerno, not far from Monte Cassino. The school at Salerno developed a practical scientific approach to medicine, eschewing its neighbors' concentration on philosophy and religious mysticism. Several universities in France, including those at Montepellier and Paris, were also highly regarded. At Paris, the school had a medical rather than a surgical bias, being more influenced by the Church. At Montpellier, Greek practices were more in evidence.

By 1000 A.D., at the end of the Dark Ages, monastic medicine began to decline as the influence of the universities increased. Many hospitals were founded that are well known today, such as St. Thomas's and St. Bartholomew's in England and the Hôtel-Dieu in Paris. Here, diet was regarded as an important form of treatment, as were medications, particularly those derived from plant materials. One of the most commonly used medications at this time was theriac, which had been developed in the first century A.D.; it consisted of many substances derived from plants and animals, including snake flesh. Theriac would have been used for the treatment of a variety of sleep disorders, particularly those thought to be caused by poisons. Mysticism and astrology were important elements of medicine in the Middle Ages. Often the primary treatment considered was exorcism; however, purgatives and bloodletting were also still commonly employed.

In the 15th and 16th centuries, the works of Hippocrates were revived. Paracelsus (1493–1541), known as the "father of pharmacology," began using metals in treatment, often producing some outstanding cures (17). Although illnesses such as leprosy and the plague had largely disappeared, venereal diseases, including gonorrhea and syphilis, were rampant. Art and medicine became allied, as evidenced in the anatomical drawings of Michelangelo Buonarroti (1475–1564) and Albrecht Durer (1471–1528). Andreas Vesalius (1514–1564) produced one of the greatest medical books in history, *De Humani Corporis Fabrica* (18). Its detailed anatomical drawings surpassed those of Galen and Fabrica, and it became the anatomical cornerstone of scientific medicine in the centuries to come.

SLEEP IN THE 17th AND 18th CENTURIES

Methought I heard a voice cry, "Sleep no more!
Macbeth does murder sleep," the innocent sleep,
Sleep that knits up the ravell'd sleave of care,
The death of each day's life, sore labour's bath,
Balm of hurt minds, great nature's second course,
Chief nourisher in life's feast.

—*Shakespeare, Macbeth*, Act II (ca. 1605)

In the 17th century, medicine underwent a major change from the doctrines that had influenced it up to that time, such as Aristotelianism, Galenism, and Paracelsianism, to more scientifically directed theories, with the underlying teleological desire to accumulate knowledge on the way things work. This period, known as the Age of Scientific Revolution, included the major medical developments of Francis Bacon, William Harvey, and Marcello Malpighi.

The scientific revolution began with the theories of René Descartes (1596–1650), who rejected Aristotle's doctrines and developed theories based on mechanisms (19). In this regard he was similar to Francis Bacon (1561–1626), who espoused experimentation and utilitarianism. Descartes developed a hydraulic model of sleep, in which, when the pineal gland maintains fullness of the cerebral ventricles, there is alertness. The loss of "animal spirits" from the pineal causes the ventricles to collapse, inducing sleep.

Even Shakespeare made innumerable references to sleep in his writings, and it has been suggested that the playwright's clear descriptions of insomnia indicate that he himself suffered from this malady:

O sleep, O gentle sleep,
Nature's soft nurse, how have I frighted thee,
That thou no more wilt weight my eyelids down
and steep my senses in forgetfulness . . .

Medicine was now being viewed as an advancement in man's control over nature and was more soundly based on scientific principles. However, it was still a time to be speculative and philosophical about medicine: "He sleeps well who knows not that he sleeps ill" (Francis Bacon, *Ornatnentata Rationalia*, IV, quoted by Publilius Syrus, *Sententiae*).

The chemical principles of Paracelsus were advanced in the 17th century, and medicines, including the use of mercurials, began to take over from such treatments as purging and bloodletting. Illness was now considered something that attacks the body in a distinct manner, and the Galenic and earlier concepts that disease is a derangement of humors, the essential elements of the body, were starting to fade. Atomism, which had been proposed by Democritus, Leucippus, and Epicurus several centuries before the time of Christ, underwent a revival in the 17th century. It was supported by the findings of Jan Baptista Van Helmont (1577–1644), who coined the term *gas* and recognized that air is composed of a variety of gases. Robert Boyle (1627–1691) demonstrated the importance of air for life and the effect of gases under pressure, which led to the discovery that the reddening of venous blood occurred because of exposure of blood to gases contained in the air. However, the major discovery of the 17th century was that of William Harvey (1578–1657), who was the first to demonstrate that blood is pumped around the body by the heart.

It was against this background that the great neurologists Thomas Willis (1621–1675) and Thomas Sydenham (1624–1689) developed the principles and practice of clinical neurology. Willis made a number of contributions to the knowledge of various disorders in sleep, including restless-legs syndrome, nightmares, and insomnia. He recognized that a component of coffee could prevent sleep and that sleep is not a disease but primarily a symptom of underlying causes. His book *The Practice of Physick* (1692) devoted four chapters to disorders producing sleepiness and insomnia (20). Like Descartes, he believed that the animal spirits within the body undergo rest during sleep. However, he thought that animal spirits residing in the cerebellum become active during sleep to maintain a control over physiology, and that some of the "animal spirits" become intermittently unrestrained, leading to the development of dreams. He also described restless-legs syndrome, which he considered an escape of the animal humors into the nerves supplying the limbs, "when being a bed, they betake themselves to sleep, presently in the arms and legs, leapings and contractions of the tendons, and so great a restlessness and tossings of their members ensue, that the diseased are no more able to sleep, than if they were in a place of the greatest torture.'' Willis discovered that laudanum, a solution of powdered opium, was effective in treating restless-legs syndrome.

Due to the generally unhygienic living conditions, epidemics—mainly the plague, measles, smallpox, scarlet fever, and chicken pox—continued to rage through Europe at this time. Therapy was still based largely on practices of the past, such as purging, bloodletting, dietary restriction, exercise, and the use of such potions as theriac.

Although the 18th century is widely regarded as a period when the scientific foundation of medicine was extended from the principles laid down in the 17th century, this was not entirely the situation. Some medical theorists played an influential role in maintaining concepts of vitalism. George Stahl (1660–1734) was a strong proponent of the ''animal spirits'' concept of earlier years and decried Descartes' theory of a machinistic approach to medicine. Stahl also expounded his enthusiasm for such treatments as bloodletting to get rid of the unwanted spirits.

Despite some setbacks, a scientific approach to medicine continued with the works of Linnaeus and Von Haller. Karl Von Linne (1707–1778), called Linnaeus, made important contributions to the classifications of botany, zoology, and medicine (21). He emphasized the importance of cyclical changes in botany, which was nowhere more clearly presented than in his flower clock. The flower clock was developed on the principle that different species of flowers open their leaves at different times of the day. Therefore, a garden of appropriately selected flowers arranged in a circular pattern could provide an estimate of the time of day by the pattern of flower and leaf openings and closings.

Linnaeus' finding was an important early milestone in the development of the science of biological rhythms in plants and animals. As far back as in ancient Greece, there had been some recognition of variation in the behavior of plants and animals, not only on a seasonal basis but also on a daily basis. Even the Bible makes mention of seasonal change in the following passage from Ecclesiastes (3:1) ''To everything there is a season and a time to every purpose under the heavens.''

One of the first chronobiological experiments was carried out by Sanctorious (ca. 1657), who measured the cyclical pattern of change in a number of his own physiological variables. His experimental apparatus has been regarded as the first ''laboratory for chronobiology.'' Subsequently, the intrinsic pattern of circadian activity was demonstrated in the experiment performed by Jacques De Mairan in 1729, which was reported by M. Marchant (22). De Mairan placed a heliotrope plant in a darkened closet and observed that the leaves continued to open in darkness, at the same time of day that they had in sunlight. This experiment illustrated the presence of an intrinsic circadian rhythm independent of environmental lighting conditions. De Mairan also recognized the importance of this observation for understanding the behavior of patients: "This seems to be related to the sensitivity of a great number of bed-ridden sick people, who, in their confinement, are aware of the differences of day and night."

During the 17th and 18th centuries, medical schools rapidly expanded throughout Europe, with those north of the French-Italian Alps beginning to gain in prominence. The Swiss-born scientist Albrecht Von Haller (1708–1777), a pupil of Boerhaave of the University of Leiden, an important medical center in Europe, made major contributions to many scientific topics, including medicine. Von Haller performed numerous experiments on the nervous system and demonstrated the sensitivity of nerve and the irritability of muscle; in doing so he dispelled much of the mysticism of previous eras. Von Haller produced a major work, *Elementa Physiologiae*, in which he devoted 36 pages to the physiology of sleep and proposed a theory for its cause (23). In a vascular concept similar to that of Alcmaeon in the fifth century B.C., he believed that sleep is caused by the flow of blood to the head, which puts pressure on the brain, thereby inducing sleep. Von Haller's theory was expanded in the 19th century into the congestion theory of the causes of sleep, a theory that was still subscribed to into the early part of the 20th century. He also considered dreams a symptom of disease, "a stimulating cause, by which the perfect tranquility of the sensorium is interrupted."

The late 17th century was also the time of the discovery of oxygen by Karl Scheele (1742–1786) and Joseph Priestley (1733–1804), but it was Antione-Laurent Lavoisier (1743–1794) who coined the term *oxygen* and recognized its importance in the maintenance of living tissue. Despite the important advances in clinical medicine that occurred in the 17th century, there were very few therapeutic advances. Medications still consisted of potions developed from plant and animal tissues, and opium was still the main form of sedation, in a common formulation called "Hoffmann's Anodyne of Opium." However, the ancient practices of bleeding and purging continued to be widely prescribed throughout the 18th century. One particularly important medication was an herbal brew from the foxglove plant, *Digitalis purpurea*. This medication, discovered by William Withering in 1785, was most helpful in the treatment of dropsy (swelling of the limbs) caused by heart disease. This was also the time of the French Revolution, following which it was recognized that more humane care was necessary for people with psychiatric disease; Phillipe Pinel (1745–1826), who was a supporter of vitalism, has been considered the founder of modern psychiatry.

Despite the important advances in the science of medicine and in scientifically based principles of treatment, it was still a time of hoaxes and charlatanism. On the fringe of quackery was Franz Anton Mesmer (1734–1815), who utilized "animal magnetism" for a hypnotic treatment that led to the term *mesmerism*.

He enticed the gullible to undergo treatment in his darkened rooms, which were considered cradles of immorality. Mesmer was subsequently banished from Paris, despite producing some effective cures of hysteria by the use of hypnotic suggestion.

Perhaps the greatest advance made in the development of sleep medicine occurred in Bologna with Luigi Galvani's (1737–1798) demonstration of electrical activity of the nervous system. His findings led to the subsequent development of the field of electrophysiology and the gradual destruction of the humoralist theory of nervous activity.

With the development of the scientific approach to medicine, the discovery of atomism and animal electrophysiology, the advances in respiratory and cardiovascular physiology, and such treatment advances as quinine for malaria and digitalis for heart disease, medicine was about to enter its modern era, the 19th century.

SLEEP IN THE 19th CENTURY

What probing deep
Has ever solved the mystery of sleep?
—Thomas Aldrich (1836–1907), *Human Ignorance*

Medicine made rapid advances in the 19th century, due largely to the discovery of anesthesia, the practice of surgery, and the finding that microorganisms were a major cause of disease. This was the time of the Industrial Revolution; people came from the depressed countryside to the abhorrent working conditions and slums of the cities to be employed in factories. Although sanitation, as well as preventive medicine, was important, epidemics continued to rage in both Europe and the United States. Cholera and typhoid fever were just two of several infective illnesses that claimed many victims.

There were major advances in understanding the cause of sleep, and in the latter half of the century a number of specific sleep disorders were recognized. The anatomy of sleep and wakefulness was partially revealed through the animal experiments of two outstanding neuroanatomists of the time, P. Rolando (1773–1831) and Marie Jan Pierre Flourens (1794–1867). In 1809 Rolando demonstrated that a state of sleepiness occurred when the cerebral hemispheres of birds were removed (24). His experiments were replicated by Flourens in 1822 with the ablation of the cerebral hemispheres of pigeons (25): "Just imagine an animal which has been condemned to be permanently asleep, one that has been devoid even of the ability to dream during sleep; this is more or less the situation of the pigeon in which I had ablated the cerebral hemispheres."

The 19th century could be regarded as the "age of sleep theories" as some of the greatest physicians, psychologists, and physiologists turned their attention to explanations of the cause of sleep. Advances were made in the clinical recognition of sleep disorders, particularly the causes of daytime sleepiness, and several comprehensive books were written entirely on the physiological and clinical aspects of sleep. Much of what was known about insomnia and its causes, however, was only a slight expansion of earlier knowledge.

The theories of the cause of sleep can be placed into four main groups: *vascular* (mechanical, anemic, congestive), *chemical* (humoral), *neural* (histological), and a fourth group of theories that explain the reason for sleep rather than the physiological cause, *behavioral* (psychological, biological).

The vascular theories of sleep were the ones most widely disputed in the early part of the 19th century. They were based on the first rational theory for the cause of sleep, proposed by Alcmaeon in ancient Greece in the fifth century B.C. (7). Alcmaeon believed that sleep is caused by blood filling the brain and waking associated with the return of blood to the rest of the body, a concept consistent with the notions of ancient times, when it was recognized that brain disorders such as apoplexy were associated with stupor (*karos*). Hippocrates had an alternative theory; he believed that sleep is due to blood flowing in the opposite direction, from the limbs to the central part of the body (8). Von Haller, in the 18th century, agreed with Alcmaeon's concept and proposed that blood going to the head causes the brain to be pressed against the skull, thereby inducing sleep by cutting off the "animal spirits." Von Haller derived his beliefs from the views of his mentor, Hermann Boerhaave (1667–1738), who had presented a similar theory a few years earlier, in 1750. Johann Fredreich Blumenbach (1752–1840), a professor at Gottingen who is considered the founder of modern anthropology, was the first to observe the brain of a sleeping subject in 1795 (26). He noted that the surface of the brain was pale during sleep compared with wakefulness; contrary to earlier theories, he proposed that sleep was caused by the lack of blood in the brain. It was against this background of early sleep theories that the 19th-century researchers looked for the cause of sleep.

The theory that sleep is caused by congestion of the brain was the most accepted vascular theory in the first half of the 19th century. In 1830 Robert MacNish wrote a seminal volume on sleep and its disorders, *The Philosophy of Sleep* (27). MacNish supported the previous concept that sleep is due to the pressure of blood on the brain. In 1846 Johannes Evangelistica Purkinje (1787–1869), an outstanding neuroanatomist and professor of physiology and pathology at Breslau (Wroclaw, in modern Poland), proposed a slightly different theory on the cause of sleep that was consistent with the congestive concept (28,29). Purkinje proposed that the brain pathways (corona radiata) become compressed by blood congestion of the cell masses of the brain (basal ganglia), thereby severing neural transmission and inducing sleep. James Cappie wrote in detail in 1860 about the circulation of the brain, and was one of the last supporters of the congestion theory, which was finally contradicted by the findings of the outstanding clinical neurologist John Hughlings Jackson (1835–1911). In 1863 Jackson observed the optic fundi during sleep and reported that the retinal arteries became pale during sleep, which was consistent with Blumenbach's earlier findings (30). He therefore reasoned that brain congestion was not a cause of sleep.

The main alternative to the congestion theory was the idea that sleep is caused by insufficient blood in the brain (anemia). In 1854 William Alexander Hammond (1828–1900), the noted American physician, was the first in the 19th century to direct attention to the anemia theory, after observing the brain of a patient who had had a traumatic skull injury (31). The following year, Alexander Fleming supported the anemia theory after he performed an experiment in which he occluded the carotid arteries and induced a sleeplike state. One of the strongest advocates for the anemia theory was Frans Cornelius Donders (1818–1889), a professor at Utrecht in Holland, who carefully observed the cerebral circulation in animals through windows placed in the skull (32). Donders, and subsequently Angelo Mosso (1826–1910), who observed the cerebral circulation in humans with skull defects, believed that at sleep onset blood passes from the brain to the skin (33). Arthur Edward Durham (1833–1895), who wrote extensively on the topic in 1860, believed that the blood passed from the brain during sleep not only to supply the skin but also to supply the internal organs (34). The final advocates for the anemia theory of sleep were the physiologists William Henry Howell (1860–1945) and Sir Leonard Erskine Hill (1866–1952). Howell believed that the change in arterial blood pressure at the base of the brain is responsible for cerebral anemia (35). Hill extensively studied the cerebral circulation, and in 1896 reported the absence of a change in cerebral blood pressure during sleep (36). He believed that the brain does not become anemic or congested during sleep, and showed that intracranial pressure was normal during sleep compared with during wakefulness. By the end of the 19th century, the vascular sleep theories, based on congestion or anemia of the brain, were less enthusiastically supported. Subsequent research showed that changes during sleep do occur in both cerebral blood flow and intracranial pressure, but it was no longer believed that these changes are responsible for the cause of sleep.

The neural theories for the cause of sleep were based on mid-19th-century developments in the histological understanding of the central nervous system. Camillo Golgi (1843–1926) presented the first clear picture of the nerve cell and its processes. His studies were extended by Heinreich Waldeyer (1837–1921), who named the nerve cell—the neuron—and demonstrated an afferent axon and efferent dendrites. In 1890, Rabl-Ruckhardt developed a hypothesis, called "neurospongium," that during sleep there is a partial paralysis of the neuron prolongations, which prevents communication with adjacent nerve cells (37). Subsequently, Raphael Jacques Lepine (1840–1919), of Paris, in 1894 and Marie Mathias Duval (1844–1907) in 1895 proposed similar theories, agreeing that sleep is produced by retraction of ameboid processes of the nerve cell (38,39).

The outstanding histologist Santiago Ramon y Cajal (1852–1934) proposed that small cells called *neuroglia* interact between neurons and are able to promote or inhibit the transfer of information from one cell to another. Cajal, who in 1906 was awarded a Nobel prize along with Golgi for his work on neurohistology, suggested that the alteration in the transference of information by neuroglia could explain not only sleep but also the effect of hypnotic medications (40,41). In 1898 Ernesto Lugaro proposed an alternative histological theory, that sleep is due to expansion of the neuron processes (42). He believed that neural impulses inducing sleep pass through expanded processes (gemmules) to allow transmission between cells. (In the early 20th century, the theories relating movements to parts of the neuron were largely discredited and theories based on synaptic transmission of neurotransmitters became the prominent neural explanation for changes in sleep and wakefulness.)

The chemical theories of sleep originated with Aristotle, who believed that sleep results from "fumes" taken into the blood vessels following the ingestion of food—the fumes are transferred to the brain, where they cause sleepiness. Wilhelm Sommer, in 1868, proposed that sleep is due to lack of oxygen. Sommer's theory was developed from the work of Carl Voit and Max Pettenkofer, who had shown in 1867 that the body absorbs more oxygen during sleep than during the day (43). Edouard Fredreich Wilhelm Pfluger (1829–1910) became the main advocate for the oxygen hypothesis in 1875 (44). Thierry Wilhelm Preyer (1841–1897) suggested in 1877 that the accumulation of lactic acid during daytime fatigue leads to a deficiency of oxygen in the brain at night, causing hypoxemia and subsequent sleep (45). This theory led to several others on the accumulation of toxic substances, which included cholesterol and other toxic waste products. Perhaps the most widely disseminated theory was that of Leo Errera of Brussels, who believed that the accumulation of poisonous substances called "leucomaines" induces sleep by passing from the blood to the brain (46). The leucomaines were believed to be broken down gradually during sleep, leading ultimately to wakefulness. In 1895 Reymond Emil DuBois (1818–1896) proposed that sleep is a result of carbon dioxide toxicity, which in small amounts during wakefulness leads to sleep, but large accumulations during sleep induce wakefulness (47). Abel Bouchard (1833–1899), in 1886, presented the idea that sleep is due to toxic agents, excreted in the urine during sleep, that he called "urotoxins"; he also believed that diurnally produced urine contains toxic agents that produce wakefulness. The chemical theories continued to be popular at the end of the 19th century.

The behavioral theories of sleep developed from those of ancient times when general explanations were given for sleep. Although many behavioral theories were proposed over the years, the inhibition theory was the most popular; it was first alluded to in 1889 by Charles Edouard Brown-Sequard (1817–1894), an outstanding clinical neurologist and physiologist.

Brown-Sequard, who believed that most glands produce secretions that pass into the bloodstream, is also known as the father of endocrinology. Based on the previous work of Rolando (1809) and Flourens (1824), who had demonstrated that removal of the cerebral cortex was accompanied by a sleeplike state (25), Brown-Sequard proposed that sleep is due to an inhibitory reflex (48,49). The inhibitory theory of sleep was advanced with the experiment of Emil Heubel, of Kiev University in Russia, who suggested that sleep is triggered by the loss of peripheral sensory stimulation essential for the maintenance of alertness (50). Subsequently, the inhibitory theory of sleep was greatly expanded by the work of Ivan Pavlov in the early 20th century (51,52). Marie de Manaceine, in his 1897 book *Sleep: Physiology, Pathology, Hygiene and Psychology*, regarded sleep as the "resting state of consciousness," which was an appealing truism although it provided little information on the mechanism of sleep (53).

A few researchers believed that a specific site in the body is capable of inducing sleep. The thyroid had been considered a sleep-inducing gland, until it was recognized that its removal was not associated with insomnia. In 1849 Jonathon Osborne proposed that the choroid plexus was the "organ of sleep" (54). He reasoned that congestion of the choroid keeps the ventricles distended to produce sleep, and that contraction of the choroid is associated with wakefulness.

In the latter part of the 19th century, two neurologists, Maurice Edouard Marie Gayet and Ludwig Mauthner, reported clinical findings that eventually led to the discovery of the brainstem's role in sleep and wakefulness. In 1875 Gayet presented a patient with lethargy and associated eye-movement paralysis who had upper brainstem pathology at autopsy, which led Gayet to believe that the lethargy was due to a thalamic defect that produced impaired transmission from the brainstem to the cerebral hemispheres (55). Mauthner reported in 1890 a similar association between an eye-movement disorder and sleepiness but placed the site of the deficit at the brainstem level (56). These findings received little attention at the turn of the century because of the more popular vascular and chemical sleep theories.

The science of chronobiology made a few advances in the 19th century, largely through the studies of plant biologists such as Augustin Pyramus de Candolle (1778–1841), who demonstrated in 1832 that plants in constant conditions have a rhythm slightly different from a 24-hour cycle (57). In 1875 Wilhelm Friedrich Phillip Pfeffer (1845–1920) confirmed de Mairan's finding that plants have their own intrinsic rhythm in the absence of environmental influences. In 1845, James George Davy (1813–1895) reported circadian rhythms of his own core body temperature, and in 1866 William Ogle performed similar experiments:

> There is a rise in the early morning while we are still asleep, and a fall in the evening while we are still awake, which cannot be explained by reference to any of the hitherto mentioned influences. They are not due

to variations in light; they are probably produced by periodic variations in the activity of the organic functions.

The 19th century was a time of rapid clinical advances in medicine. The mesmerism of the early part of the 19th century gave way to hypnotism, a term coined in 1843 by James Braid (1791–1860). Subsequently, ether, nitrous oxide, and chloroform were used to induce anesthesia for surgery. Although at this time the main focus of academic medicine was in Europe, medical practice in the United States developed rapidly, and the major American university medical centers were established by the end of the 19th century. Medical practice became specialized with the development of ophthalmology, otolaryngology, and urology; neurology and psychiatry did not become separate specialties until the beginning of the 20th century. Bacteriology developed as a specialized area of medicine, and disease was no longer viewed as being due to supernatural causes but mainly as the result of infection. This was the time of Louis Pasteur (1822–1895), who firmly established the association between disease and microorganisms. Pharmacology was well established, although herbal treatments were still given because pharmacology was not able to keep up with the rapid development of clinical medicine. The first medication introduced specifically as a hypnotic was bromide in 1853, and other hypnotic medications introduced before 1900 included paraldehyde, urethan, and sulfonal.

Although the theories regarding the cause of sleep were the focus of attention in the second half of the 19th century, important contributions were made to sleep-disorder medicine. Hammond, who was well known for his contributions to medicine during the Civil War, wrote a book entitled *Sleep and Its Derangements* in 1869, based on his series of publications on the topic of insomnia (31). Silas Weir Mitchell (1829–1914), a well-known and influential neurologist in the United States, wrote a number of clinical articles on sleep, including the recognition of abnormal respiration during sleep, night terrors, nocturnal epilepsy, and the effect of stimulants on insomnia (58).

Perhaps the greatest clinical contribution in the field of sleep-disorder medicine was the first description in 1880 of narcolepsy by Jean Baptiste Edouard Gelineau (1828–1906), who derived "narcolepsy" from the Greek words *narkosis* (a benumbing) and *lepsis* (to overtake) (59). The term "cataplexy" for emotionally induced muscle weakness (a prominent symptom of narcolepsy) was subsequently coined in 1916 by Richard Henneberg (60). Although Gelineau was the first to clearly describe the clinical manifestations of narcolepsy, several patients had previously been described by Caffe in 1862 (61), Carl Friedrich Otto Westphal (1833–1890) in 1877 (62), and Franz Fischer in 1878.

The leading sleep disorder of the 20th century—obstructive sleep apnea syndrome—was described in 1836, not by a clinician but by the novelist Charles Dickens (1812–1870). In *The Posthumous Papers of the Pickwick Club*, he described Joe, the fat boy, who was always excessively sleepy (63). Joe, a loud snorer who was obese and somnolent, may have had right-sided heart failure that led to his being called "young dropsy."

More than 100 years later, obstructive sleep apnea syndrome became a well-recognized clinical entity. However, a number of writers in the 19th century did allude to some of the features of sleep apnea in their publications. In 1816 William Wadd, surgeon to the king of England, wrote about the relationship between obesity and sleepiness. George Catlin, a lawyer, described the breathing habits of the American Indian; in his 1861 book *Breath of Life*, he graphically portrayed the effects of obstructed breathing during sleep (64). William Henry Broadbent (1835–1907) in 1877 was the first physician to report the clinical features of the obstructive sleep apnea syndrome, and William Hill observed in 1889 that upper airway obstruction contributed to "stupidity" in children. The most notable description was provided by William Hughes Wells (1854–1919) in 1898; he cured several patients of sleepiness by treatment of upper airway obstruction (65).

THE 20th CENTURY

> *The interpretation of dreams is the royal road to a knowledge of the part the unconscious plays in the mental life.*
>
> —Sigmund Freud, *The Interpretation of Dreams* (1905)

Medicine in the 20th century is radically different from that of previous eras. The major advances have been the development of new diagnostic means, the recognition of infectious disease, the development of antibiotic medications, the elimination of most global epidemics, the development of surgery, and the treatment of cancer.

For the first time, objective diagnostic procedures complemented the physician's skill. X-rays were discovered in 1895 by Wilhelm Konrad Roentgen (1845–1923), and the first clinical application was reported in 1896. Widespread routine use of X-ray procedures began in the early 20th century; sophisticated brain-imaging techniques, such as computerized axial tomography (CAT) and nuclear magnetic resonance (NMR) scanning, began in the second half of the century.

The vascular theories of the cause of sleep were no longer popular. Although the chemical theories were briefly of interest because of the findings of Rene Legendre and Henri Pieron in 1907 (66,67), they were largely overshadowed by the behavioral theory of Ivan Petrovitch (1849–1936). Pavlov, who is regarded as one of the greatest physiologists of all time, published his initial lectures on conditional reflexes in 1927 (52). In them he expressed his belief that sleep is due to widespread cortical inhibition, describing it as "an inhibition which has spread over the great section of the cerebrum, over the entire hemispheres and even into the lower lying mid-brain."

Pavlov's studies on dogs showed that a continuous and monotonous stimulus would be followed by drowsiness and sleep. He reasoned that the continuous stimulus acts at a certain point of the central nervous system and leads to inhibition with resulting sleepiness. Although Pavlov's theories on conditioning were interesting, they held little information on physiological mechanisms. Vladimir Michailovitch Bekhterev (1857–1927) published his findings on human reflexology and sleep in 1894 (translated into English in 1932) (68). Bekhterev, who also believed that sleep was a general inhibition due to a loss of higher-level reflexes, defined it as "a reflex which has been biologically evolved for the purpose of protecting the brain from further poisoning by the products of metabolism, and which may be evoked, as an association reflex, by the conditions of fatigue."

Bekhterev's theory—similar to that of Edouard Claparede, who in 1905 characterized sleep as an "instinct" (69)—was subsequently influenced by the work of Legendre and Pieron; he believed that the biochemical process leading to the inhibition of the brain is the action of "hypnotoxins." Since then, electrophysiological studies have demonstrated that the passive, cortical inhibition proposed by Pavlov and Bekhterev does not occur; instead, the brain maintains its activity during sleep, particularly during rapid-eye-movement (REM) sleep.

Since the days of ancient Greece, it had been recognized that sleep consisted of two states: one associated with dreaming and the other with quiet sleep. Willis had noticed the difference in the 17th century, and believed that dream sleep was associated with release of the "animal spirits" from the cerebellum. However, the physiological changes of dreaming sleep were not reported until 1868, when Wilhelm Griesinger (1816–1868) noted the associated eye movements. Sigmund Freud, 5 years before the publication of his first book on dreams in 1900, recognized that paralysis of skeletal muscles during dream sleep prevents the dreamer from acting out dreams (70).

Sleep research, both basic and clinical, had its greatest period of growth during the second half of the 20th century. The advances in neurochemistry, electrophysiology, neurophysiology, chronobiology, pathology of sleep, sleep-disorder medicine, and the development of sleep societies are too many to list but a summary is presented below.

Neurochemistry

> *Our studies have established that the accumulation of the hypnotoxin produces an increasing need for sleep.*
>
> —Henri Pieron, *Le Probleme Physiologique du Sommeil* (67)

The most significant advance in the chemical theories came in 1907, when Legendre and Pieron provided evidence for an agent called "hypnotoxin," derived from the blood serum of sleep-deprived dogs. When introduced in dogs that were not sleep-deprived, hypnotoxin induced sleep. Although attempts to replicate Legendre's work were often unsuccessful, in 1967 John Pappenheimer and colleagues induced sleep with cerebrospinal fluid obtained from sleep-deprived goats. The transmissible chemical, called Factor S, was subsequently identified as a muramyl peptide in 1982 and is thought to act via the leukocyte monokine Interleukin-1. Finding alternative sleep factors has met with mixed success; the number of putative sleep factors has grown enormously in the last 20 years. However, in 1988 Osamu Hayaishi discovered that prostaglandin PGD2, found in the preoptic nuclei, was capable of inducing sleep in rats, leading to the speculation that the preoptic nucleus is the site of the perennial and elusive "sleep center."

Electrophysiology

> *Feeble currents of varying direction pass through the multiplier when electrodes are placed on two points of the external surface [of the brain].*
>
> —Richard Caton (71)

The most useful objective tools for diagnosing sleep disorders have proven to be electrophysiological techniques. Following Galvani's demonstration of the electrical activity of the nervous system in the late 18th century, Richard Caton (1842–1926) in 1875 demonstrated action potentials in the brains of animals, an important step in the development of the electroencephalograph (71). In 1929, Johannes (Hans) Berger (1873–1941), the first to record electrical activity in the human brain, demonstrated differences in activity between wakefulness and sleep (72). Berger's discovery led to the development of the electroencephalograph as a clinical tool for the diagnosis of brain disease. The electroencephalograph was applied to determine different sleep states in 1937, when Alfred L. Loomis, E. Newton Harvey (1887–1959), and Garret Hobart were able to classify sleep into five stages, from A to E (73).

Dreaming sleep was characterized in 1953 by Eugene Aserinsky and Nathaniel Kleitman. They demonstrated the occurrence of rapid eye movements during a stage of sleep that they called REM sleep (74). In 1957 William Dement and Nathaniel Kleitman discovered a recurring pattern of REM sleep and non-REM sleep during overnight electroencephalographic monitoring—a finding that made it clear that sleep no longer could be regarded as a homogeneous state (75). In 1968 Allan Rechtschaffen and Anthony Kales developed a scoring manual, *A Manual of Standardised Terminology: Techniques and Scoring System for Sleep Stages of Human Subjects*, which has become the standard in the field (76). The first report of an effective measure of daytime alertness was by Gary Richardson et al., in 1978 (77), whose study compared narcoleptics with normals by applying the Multiple Sleep Latency Test (MSLT) that had been conceived and developed by Mary Carskadon working with William Dement at Stanford University.

Neurophysiology

> Analysis of hypnogenic mechanisms has thus underlined the paramount importance of inhibition and disinhibition in the determination of sleep onset and maintenance—a striking illustration of Sherrington's visionary concepts.
>
> —Frederic Bremer (78)

In the early part of the 20th century, two schools of thought emerged regarding the neurophysiological basis of sleep and wakefulness. One characterized sleep as being due to disinhibition with release of an active "sleep center," and the other as due to a passive event, the result of inhibition of a "waking center." The theories proposed at the end of the 18th century by Mauthner and others assumed an interruption of peripheral sensory stimulation, allowing the cerebral cortex to produce sleep. This "deafferentation" theory had been suggested first by Purkinje in 1846 (28). The notion of a specific sleep center did not receive much support, as illustrated by the comment of the prominent clinical neurologist Jacques Jean Lhermitte (1877–1959) in 1910 (79): "We absolutely object to the thought of the existence of a nerve center attributed to the function of sleep. The conception of a center for sleep is erroneous, as it disavows the most simple principles of physiology."

Lhermitte was supported in 1914 by a pioneer of brain localization, Joseph Jules Dejerine, who said, "Sleep cannot be localized." However, in 1923, Constantin Von Economo (1876–1931) proposed a "center for regulation of sleep" based on anatomical and clinical studies of "encephalitis lethargica" at the Psychiatric Clinic of Wagner Von Jauregg in Vienna (80,81). Viral encephalitis reached epidemic proportions between 1916 and 1920, and Von Economo had the opportunity to correlate the clinical features of sleep disturbance with central nervous system pathology. His studies demonstrated inflammatory lesions in the posterior hypothalamus of patients with excessive sleepiness and lesions in the preoptic area and anterior hypothalamus of patients with insomnia (82). Von Economo, influenced by the studies by Pieron and Pavlov, suggested that the "sleep-regulating center" was controlled by substances circulating in the blood. These substances caused the sleep center to exert an inhibitory influence on the cerebral cortex, thereby leading to sleep. The same year in Zurich, Walter Rudolph Hess (1881–1973), who was awarded the Nobel prize with Egas Moriiz for his work in neuroanatomy, confirmed Von Economo's findings by demonstrating that stimulation of the central gray matter in the region of the thalamus induced sleep (83).

In 1929 Kleitman pointed to the cerebral cortex as the source of wakefulness, and proposed that sleep due to inactivity of the central nervous system is brought about by a reduction in peripheral stimulation because of fatigue. His hypothesis conformed to the "deafferentation" theory. Steven Walter Ranson (1880–1942) demonstrated in 1932 that lesions placed at the top of the brainstem produced sleepiness; experimentally, this was consistent with Von Economo's findings (84).

In 1935, Frederic Bremer, of the University of Brussels, experimentally gave support to the deafferentation theory (85). Bremer completely transected the midbrain, producing the *cerveau isolé* preparation in isolation of the cerebrum—and was able to show characteristic sleep patterns on the electroencephalogram. The studies up to this time were consistent with the concept that a lesion that prevents transmission of peripheral stimulation is important in the production of sleep. However, in 1939 Ranson showed that lesions of the lateral hypothalamus, in the absence of upper-brainstem lesions, were associated with sleep through a loss of the "waking center" (86). A few years later, Walle Jetz Harinx Nauta demonstrated that posterior hypothalamic lesions produced sleepiness whereas anterior hypothalamic lesions produced insomnia, thereby supporting the concept of a waking center in the posterior hypothalamus and a sleep center in the anterior hypothalamus (87). According to Nauta: "Whereas Ranson and his collaborators held that periods of sleep were caused by more or less intrinsic periodic decreases in activity of the waking center, we are inclined to attribute these decreases to the inhibitory influence of a sleep center."

Horace W. Magoun and Ruth Rhines, at the Northwestern University Medical School in Chicago, demonstrated in 1946 that the lower portion of the brainstem reticular formation was responsible for inhibiting skeletal muscle tone (88). This function of the lower brainstem had previously been alluded to in the clinical studies of Jackson in 1897. The fact that the lower reticular formation could have an inhibitory function through descending pathways led to the finding by Guiseppe Moruzzi and Magoun in 1949 that the brainstem reticular formation also had ascending pathways (89,90). This resulted in the discovery of the "ascending reticular activating system," which led to a new emphasis in the physiological investigation of sleep. Stimulation of the ascending reticular activating system produced electroencephalographic patterns of wakefulness. It was now recognized that the brainstem transection studies produced sleep not because of "deafferentation" of peripheral sensory input but because of the loss of the wakefulness stimulus from the ascending reticular activating system. As a result, sleep became regarded as a passive phenomenon.

At the beginning of the second half of the 20th century, research was concentrated on determining the neurophysiological basis for non-REM and REM sleep. Following the electrophysiological documentation of REM sleep, Michel Jouvet in 1959 demonstrated REM-sleep-related muscle atonia, and in 1965 that the brainstem, serotonin-containing neurons of the raphe nuclei were important in the maintenance of sleep (91). Subsequently, Jouvet demonstrated that the rostral raphe nucleus was important for non-REM sleep, whereas the caudal raphe nucleus was important in the maintenance of REM sleep. In 1975, Robert William McCarley and J. Allan Hobson proposed a reciprocal interaction model of REM and non-REM sleep, with rostral REM ''on'' cells and caudal REM ''off'' cells (92).

Chronobiology

> *Despite the multiplicity of its constituents, the circadian system often behaves like one unit which is characterized by the durability of its oscillations and its internal temporal order.*
>
> —Jürgen Aschoff (1981)

Auguste Henri Forel (1848–1931), a Swiss physician, is credited with stimulating the investigation of circadian rhythms as important time-measuring systems. His studies in 1910 on the accurate timing system of bees were consistent with those of Linnaeus in the 18th century on the opening of the flower petals at a given time of day. The circadian behavior of rodents was first reported by Curt P. Richter in his Ph.D. thesis in 1922 (93), and in 1935 Erwin Bunning was able to demonstrate the genetic origin of circadian rhythms in plants and subsequently developed a concept of ''biological clocks'' (94). In the early 1960s, Richter searched for the biological clock in extensive studies that culminated with the report in 1965 that lesions placed in the anterior-ventral hypothalamus produced disruption of circadian rhythms (90). Two groups acting independently in 1972, led by Robert Y. Moore and Victor B. Eichler, and F. K. Stephan and Irving Zucker, discovered the ''clock'' to be two small, bilateral nuclei in the anterior hypothalamus, which were subsequently called the suprachiasmatic nuclei (SCN) (96,97).

Jules Aschoff and Kurt Wever in 1962 investigated human circadian rhythms in the absence of environmental time cues, in an underground laboratory in Munich (98). They demonstrated a free-running pattern of sleep and wakefulness with a period longer than 24 hours. A similar free-running pattern was demonstrated in field experiments in 1974 by the speleologist Michel Siffre, who lived for three months without time cues on an ice glacier deep in the Franco-Italian mountains (99). Many human biological rhythms have recently been discovered, such as the 24-hour episodic secretory pattern of cortisol that was reported by Elliot David Weitzman (1929–1983) in 1966 (100). In 1978 Weitzman and Charles Czeisler demonstrated the internal organization of temperature, neuroendocrine rhythms, and the sleep–wake cycle in subjects monitored in an environment free of time cues for periods of up to six months. Sutherland Simpson (1863–1926) and J. J. Galbraith in 1906 had demonstrated that the light–dark cycle could influence mammal behavior (101), however, it was not until the 1980s that Czeisler and colleagues demonstrated the importance of the light–dark cycle in the entrainment of human circadian rhythms.

Pathology of Sleep

> *Five billion people go through the cycle of sleep and wakefulness every day, and relatively few of them know the joy of being fully rested and fully alert all day long.*
>
> —William Dement (1988)

Sleep disorders were poorly described at the turn of the century, and, other than narcolepsy and sleeping sickness, few specific sleep disorders were recognized. In addition to general medical illness, environmental effects and anxiety were viewed as the main causes of sleep disturbance. However, a gradual recognition of the multiplicity of sleep diagnoses began to parallel progress in psychiatry. Freud's book *The Interpretation of Dreams* led to the development of psychoanalysis, which was applied to the treatment of insomnia until the evolution of a more "organic" or "biological" psychiatric approach.

Psychoactive medications became widely used with the introduction of the phenothiazines in the 1950s, but hypnotic medications, particularly the barbiturates, had been in common usage since barbital was introduced in 1903. The 1960s saw the introduction of the benzodiazepine hypnotics, which largely replaced the barbiturates in the late 1970s. However, the 1980s saw a decline in the use of hypnotics with increased physician and public awareness of the disadvantages of chronic hypnotic use. Insomnia became recognized as a symptom rather than a diagnosis, and treatment was directed to the underlying physical or psychological causes. Several books on sleep had a major influence on the development of sleep-disorder medicine. Pieron's *Le Probleme Physiologique du Sommeil,* published in 1913, summarized the scientific sleep literature at that time (67). A similar approach was taken by Kleitman, who produced his monumental treatise *Sleep and Wakefulness* in 1939 (updated in 1963 to contain 4337 references) (102). The Association of Sleep Disorder Centers classification committee chaired by Howard Roffwarg produced the *Diagnostic Classification of Sleep and Arousal Disorders* in 1979 (103), which ushered in the modern era of sleep diagnosis and became the first classification to be widely used. The *Principles and Practice of Sleep Disorders Medicine*, edited by Meir Kryger, Thomas Roth, and William Dement in 1989, was the first comprehensive textbook on basis sleep research and clinical sleep medicine (104).

Increased knowledge about sleep and sleep disorders in general has resulted from the research of a few core sleep disorders, which include narcolepsy, obstructive sleep apnea syndrome, and the insomnias.

Following Gelineau's description in the late 19th century, narcolepsy was brought to general recognition in 1926 by the Australian-born neurologist William John Adie (1886–1935) (105), and stimulants were first used for treatment by Otakar Janota in 1931. In 1941 John Burton Dynes and Knox H. Finley applied the electroencephalograph to the diagnosis of narcolepsy (106), and the characteristic sleep-onset REM period of night sleep was discovered in 1960 by Gerald Vogel (107). Dement and colleagues at Stanford University developed a narcoleptic dog colony in the 1970s, which advanced the understanding of the biochemical and neuroanatomical bases of the disorder. The Multiple Sleep Latency Test was applied to the diagnosis by Richardson in 1978 (77), and the documentation of a strong association between the histocompatibility antigen HLA-DR2 and narcolepsy was made by Yutaka Honda and colleagues in 1984.

Following the reports of snoring, sleepiness, and obesity in the 19th century, Sir William Osler (1849–1919) referred in 1906 to Dickens' description of Joe (108): "An extraordinary phenomenon in excessively fat young persons is an uncontrollable tendency to sleep—like the fat boy in Pickwick."

Charles Sidney Burwell in 1956 brought general recognition to obstructive sleep apnea syndrome, which he called the "Pickwickian syndrome" (109), and the first objective documentation of polysomnographic features was simultaneously reported by Henri Gastaut and Jung in 1965 (110,111). Although the tracheotomy had been performed since the time of Asclepiades (first century B.C.), Wolfgang Kuhlo and Erich Doll reported in 1969 that it provided an effective treatment of the obstructive sleep apnea syndrome (112). Tanenosuke Ikematsu in 1964 popularized uvulopalatopharyngoplasty (UPP) surgery for the treatment of snoring (113), which was subsequently applied to the obstructive sleep apnea syndrome by Shiro Fujita in 1981 (114). In that same year, nasal continuous positive airway pressure (CPAP) treatment was described by Colin Sullivan, and it subsequently became the treatment of choice (115).

Another sleep-related breathing disorder called "Ondine's curse" was first reported by John W. Severinghaus and Robert A. Mitchell in 1962 (116). Named after the water nymph in Jean Giraudoux's play *Ondine* (117), this disorder was characterized by the failure of automatic ventilation that could lead to fatal apnea during sleep.

> Live! It's easy to say. If at least I could work up a little interest in living—but I'm too tired to make the effort. Since you left me, Ondine, all the things my body once did by itself, it now only does by special order . . . I have to supervise five senses, two hundred bones, a thousand muscles. A single moment of inattention, and I forget to breathe. He died, they will say, because it was a nuisance to breathe.
>
> —Jean Giraudoux, *Ondine*, Act III (117)

Insomnia received more interest in earlier centuries than in the first half of the 20th century, probably because of the availability of effective hypnotic medications. Frederick Snyder, in the 1960s, recognized and promoted the importance of psychiatric disorders in sleep medicine, especially depression: "Troubled minds have troubled sleep, and troubled sleep causes troubled minds."

The polysomnograph was applied to the investigation of patients with insomnia following the discovery of obstructive sleep apnea in 1965. Kales, in 1969, developed objective measures of hypnotic effectiveness. The concept of a conditioned insomnia (psychophysiological insomnia), first presented in *Diagnostic Classification of Sleep and Arousal Disorders* in 1979 (103), became recognized as a common form of insomnia. The "stimulus control" behavioral technique, developed by Richard Bootzin in 1978, was an effective treatment of insomnia (118), as was "sleep restriction therapy," developed by Arthur Spielman in 1987 (119).

Circadian-rhythm sleep disorders were recognized in the late 1970s, partly due to identification of the chronobiological features of "jet lag" and "shift work." Thomas Edison, whose development of the electric light bulb enabled shift work, had his own views on sleep: "In my opinion sleep is a habit, acquired by the environment. Like all habits it is generally carried to extremes. The man that sleeps four hours soundly is better off than a dreamy sleeper of eight hours."

The atypical, sleep-onset insomnia called the "delayed sleep phase syndrome," discovered by Weitzman and colleagues in 1981, led to a radically different form of treatment called "chronotherapy," based on chronobiological principles (120,121).

Many other sleep disorders have been discovered in the 20th century, including REM sleep behavior disorder by Carlos Schenck, in 1986 (122), paroxysmal nocturnal dystonia in 1981 (123) and fatal familial insomnia in 1986, by Elio Lugaresi (124), and food allergy insomnia by Andre Kahn in 1984 (125).

General and medical awareness of sleep disorders has dramatically increased since the 1970s through the contributions of sleep-disorder clinicians and the sleep societies. In addition to those mentioned, a few of the many who have contributed to this recognition are Roger Broughton, Michel Billiard, Christian Guilleminault, Peter Hauri, J. David Parkes, the late Pierre Passouant, and Bedrich Roth.

SLEEP-DISORDER MEDICINE

> *We have created a new clinical specialty, sleep disorders medicine, whose task is to watch over all of us while we are asleep.*
>
> —William Dement (1985)

Organized sleep-disorder medicine in the United States began with the founding of the Association for the Psychophysiological Study of Sleep (APSS) in 1961, an association composed of sleep researchers, many with clinical interests. Sleep research led to the investigation of sleep disorders, which resulted in the establishment in the early 1970s of clinical sleep-disorder centers for the diagnosis and treatment of patients. In 1976, the Association of Sleep Disorder Centers (ASDC) was founded.

The first sleep-disorder center to be engaged in active patient evaluation and treatment was established at Stanford University in California by William Dement. An accreditation process for sleep-disorder centers was established by the ASDC, and the first to be accredited in 1977 was the Sleep-Wake Disorders Unit, headed by Eliot Weitzman, at Montefiore Medical Center in New York.

In 1978, the medical journal *Sleep* was created to present research and clinical articles, and in 1979 a complete issue was devoted to the Diagnostic Classification of Sleep and Arousal Disorders. In 1978, the Association of Polysomnographic Technologists, founded by Peter Anderson McGregor, set standards of practice for polysomnographic technologists. In 1983 the Association for the Psychophysiology Study of Sleep was renamed the Sleep Research Society (SRS), and in 1984 the Clinical Sleep Society (CSS) was founded as the membership branch of the Association of Sleep Disorder Centers. In 1986, the Association of Sleep Disorder Centers, the Clinical Sleep Society, the Sleep Research Society, and the Association of Polysomnographic Technologists formed a federation called the Association of Professional Sleep Societies (APSS). The Association of Sleep Disorder Centers changed its name to the American Sleep Disorders Association (ASDA) in 1987.

With the increased recognition of the importance of sleep-disorder medicine, many international sleep societies have been founded, beginning with the European Sleep Research Society (ESRS) in 1971, the Japanese Society for Sleep Research (JSSR) in 1978, the Belgian Association for the Study of Sleep (BASS) in 1982, the Scandinavian Sleep Research Society (SSRS) in 1985, the Latin American Sleep Society (LASS) in 1986, the Sleep Society of Canada (SSC) in 1986, and the British Sleep Society (BSS) in 1989.

The 1990s saw major advances in sleep medicine and further worldwide recognition of sleep apnea and other sleep disorders. The dissemination of information on sleep moved to digital media with the release in 1994 of the first computerized textbook of sleep medicine, *SleepMultiMedia,* by Michael Thorpy, and in 1995 of the first Internet site devoted to providing an extensive list of links in sleep medicine, the Sleep Medicine Home Page. An online journal of sleep research, *Sleep Research Online* (SRO), was published by Michael Chase in 1998. Advances in information technology will play a major role in sleep medicine in the new millennium.

REFERENCES

1. Karmanova I. Evolution of Sleep. Basel: Karger, 1982.
2. Ebbell B. The Papyrus Ebers. London: Humphrey Milford, 1937.

3. Gunther RT. The Greek Herbal of Dioscorides. New York: Hafner, 1959.
4. White R. The Interpretation of Dreams: The *Oneircriticon* by Artemidorus. Park Ridge, NJ: Noyes Press, 1975.
5. Veith I. Huang Ti Nei—The Yellow Emperor's Classic of Internal Medicine. Baltimore: Williams and Wilkins, 1949.
6. Wittern R. Sleep theories in the antiquity and in the Renaissance. Horne J Sleep '88, 1989; 11–22.
7. Freeman, K. The pre-Socratic Philosophers. Cambridge, MA: Harvard University Press, 1966.
8. Chadwick J, Mann WN. Hippocratic Writings. London: Penguin Books, 1978.
9. Hett WS. Aristotle: *Parva Naturalia*. Cambridge, MA: Harvard University Press, 1964.
10. Wijsenbeek-Wijler H. Aristotle's Concept of Soul, Sleep and Dreams. Amsterdam: Adolf M Hakkert, 1978.
11. Siegel R. Galen on Psychology, Psychopathology, and Function and Diseases of the Nervous System. Basel: Karger, 1973.
12. Siegel R. Galen on the Affected Parts. Translation from the Greek text with explanatory notes. Basel: Karger, 1976.
13. MacKenzie N. Dreams and Dreaming. New York: Vanguard Press, 1965.
14. Ranking GS. The Life and Works of Rhazes. London: Frowde, 1914.
15. Gruner OCA. A Treatise on the Canon of Medicine of Avicenna. London: Luzac, 1930.
16. Gruner OCA. A Treatise on the Canon of Medicine of Avicenna. New York: M Kelly, 1970.
17. Pachter HM. Paracelsus, Magic into Science. New York: Schuman, 1951.
18. O'Malley CD. Andreas Vesalius. Los Angeles: University of California Press, 1965.
19. Descartes, René. Treatise of Man, 1632.
20. Willis, Thomas. The Practice of Physick, 1692.
21. Linnaeus C. Philosophia Botanica. Stockholme: Godofr Kiesewetter, 1751.
22. De Mairan, Jean. Observation Botanique: Histoire de l'Academie Royal des Sciences. Paris, 1729:35.
23. Von Haller A. Elementa Physiologiae Corporis Humani. 1769.
24. Rolando Luigi. Saggio sopra la vera strattura del cervello dell'uomo e degli animali e sopra la funzioni del sistema nervoso. Sassari, Stamperie di S.S.R.M. privilegiata, 1809.
25. Flourens, Pierre. Recherches Experimentales sur les Propriétés et les Fonctions du System Nerveux dans les animaux vertebres. Paris: Crévort, 1824.
26. Blumenbach, Johann. Anfangsgrunde de Physiologie, 1795.
27. MacNish, Robert. The Philosophy of Sleep. Glasgow: WR M'Phun, 1830.
28. Purkinje JE. Wachen, schlaf, traum und verwandte zustande. Handworterbuch der physiologie mit rucksicht auf physiologische pathologie. Wagner R III, ed. Bd Abth 1846; 2:412–480.
29. Kruta VJE. Purkyne's conception of the physiological basis of wakefulness and sleep. Scr Med Fac Med Brun 1967; 40:281–290.
30. Jackson, Hughlings. Ophthalmoscopic examination of sleep. Ophthalmic Hospital Reports 1863; 4:35–37.

31. Hammond, William. Sleep and Its Derangements. Lippincott: Philadelphia, 1873.
32. Donders, Frans. De bewegingen der hersenen en de veranderinger der vaatvulling van de pia mater. Nederlandsch Lancet 1849; 12:521–553.
33. Mosso, Angelo. Ueber die gegenseitigen benziehungen de bauch und brustathmung; Sulla circulazione del sangue nel cervello dell'uomo. Rome, 1880.
34. Durham, Arthur. The physiology of sleep. Guy's Hosp Reports, 3rd Series, 1860; VI: 149–173.
35. Howell, William. A contribution to the theory of sleep. J Exper Med 1897; 313–345.
36. Hill, Leonard. The physiology and pathology of the cerebral circulation. Brain, 1896.
37. Rabl-Ruckhardt. Sind die Ganglienzellen Amoboid? Neurologisches Centralblatt 1890; 9:199–200.
38. Lepine, Raphael. Revue de Medicine. Paris, 1894:727.
39. Duval, Matias. Hypothese sur la Physiologie des Centres Nerveux: Theorie Histologique du Sommeil. Soc de Biologie, 1895:85.
40. Cajal, Ramon y. Hipotesis Sobre el Mecanismo Histologico de la Association del Suevo y del Estado Vigil. Madrid, 1895.
41. Cajal, Ramon y. Histologie deu systeme nerveaux. Vol II. Translated and reprinted from first Spanish edition (Vol 1, 1899; Vol 2, 1904). Instituto Ramon y Cajal, Madrid, 1952.
42. Lugaro, Ernesto. Sulle modificazioni morfologiche funzionali dei dendriti delle cellule nervose. Rivista di Patologia Nervosa e Mentale, August 1898.
43. Sommer, Wilhelm. Neue theorie des schlafes. Zeitsch. f. Rationelle Medicine, Bd. XXXIII, 1868: 214ff.
44. Pfluger, Edouard. Theorie des Sclafes. Archiv F Physiol, Bonn, Bd X, 1875.
45. Preyer, Thierry. Ueber die urasache des schlafes, 1877.
46. Errera, Leo. Soc d'anthropologie de Bruxelles, t. 5, 1877.
47. Dubois, Reymond. Autonarcose carbon-acetonemique or sommeil hivernal de la marmotte. Revue de l'hypnotisme, 1895.
48. Brown-Sequard, Charles. On the Cause of the Torpidity of Tanrec. New York, 1854.
49. Brown-Sequard, Charles. Le sommeil normal, comme le sommeil hypnotique, est le resultat d'une inhibition de l'activite intellectuelle. Arch Physiol Norm Path 1889; 1:333–335.
50. Heubel, Emil. Abhangigkeit des wochen Gehirnzhstandes von seren Erregungen. Pfluger's Arch 1877; XIV.
51. Pavlov IP. On the identity of inhibition as a constant factor in the waking state with hypnosis and sleep. Q J Exp Physiol 1923; 13 bis:39–43.
52. Pavlov I. Lecture XV. Internal inhibition and sleep as one and the same process. Conditioned refexes: an investigation of the physiological activity of the cerebral cortex. Anrep GV, trans. Cambridge, England: Oxford University Press, 1927.
53. de Manaceine, Marie. Sleep: Its Physiology, Pathology, Hygiene and Psychology. London: Walter Scott, 1897.
54. Osborne J. Tending to prove that the choroid plexus is the organ of sleep. J Pract Med 1849; 977–982.

55. Gayet, Maurice. Affection encephalique. Arch Physiol Norm Pathol, 2nd ser, 1875; 7:341–351.
56. Mauthner, Ludwig. Pathologie und physiologie des schlafes. Wien Klin Wschr 1890; 3:445–446.
57. de Candolle, Augustin. Physiologie Vegetale. Vol 2. Paris: Brechet Jeune, 1832.
58. Weir Mitchell, Silas. Some disorders of sleep. Am J Med Sci 1890; 100:190–227.
59. Gelineau, Jean. De la narcolepsie. Gazette des Hopitaux 1880; 53:626–628, 635–637.
60. Henneberg R. Uber genuine narkolepsie. Neuro Centrabl 1916; 35:282–290.
61. Caffe. Journal des connaissances medical pratique, Aug 20, 1862.
62. Westphal, Carl. Eigenthumliche mit einschclafen verbundene anafalle. Arch Psych Nervenkr 1877; 7:631–635.
63. Dickens, Charles. The Posthumous Papers of the Pickwick Club. London: Chapman and Hall, 1836.
64. Catlin, George. The Breath of Life. New York: John Wiley & Sons, 1861.
65. Wells, William. Some nervous and mental manifestations occurring in connection with nasal disease. Am J Med Sci. 1898; 677–682.
66. Legendre R, Pieron H. Le rapports entre les conditions physiologiques et les modifications histologiques des cellules cerebrals dans l'insomnie experimentale. C Roy Soc Biol, 1907; 62:312.
67. Pieron H. Le Probleme Physiologique du Sommeil. Paris: Masson, 1913.
68. Bekhterev VM. General Principles of Human Reflexology. Murphy E, Murphy W, trans. New York: International Publishers, 1932.
69. Claparede E. Esquisse d'une theorie biologique du sommeil. Arch Psychol 1905; 4:246–349.
70. Freud S. The Interpretation of Dreams. Strachey J, trans and ed. London: Hogarth Press, 1958.
71. Caton, Richard. The electrical currents of the brain. Br Med J 1875; 2:278.
72. Berger H. Uber das eltrenkephalogram des menschen. Arch Psychiatry 1929; 87: 527–570.
73. Loomis AL, Harvey EN, Hobart G. Potential rhythms of the cerebral cortex during sleep. Science 1935; 71:597–598.
74. Aserinsky E, Kleitman N. Regularly occurring periods of eye motility, and concomitant phenomena during sleep. Science 1953; 118:273–274.
75. Dement W, Kleitman N. The relation of eye movements during sleep to dream activity: an objective method for the study of dreaming. J Exp psychol 1957; 53: 339–346.
76. Rechtschaffen A, Kales A. A Manual of Standardized Terminology and Scoring System for Sleep Stages of Human Subjects. Washington, DC: National Institutes of Health, 1968.
77. Richardson G, Carskadon M, Flagg W, et al. Excessive daytime sleepiness in man: multiple sleep latency measurements in narcoleptic and control subjects. Electroencephalogr Clin Neurophysiol 1978; 45:621–627.
78. Bremer F. Cerebral hypnogenic centers. Ann Neurol 1977; 2:1.
79. Lhermitte J. Les narcolepsies. Rev de Psychiat et de Psychol Exper 1910; 14: 265.

80. Von Economo C. Encephalitis Lethargica. Wien Med Wochenschr 1923; 73:777–782.
81. Von Economo C. Schlaftheorie. Ergebn Physiol 1929; 28:312–339.
82. Von Economo C. Die encephalitis lethargica, ibre nachrankheiten und ibre behandlung. Berlin: Urban and Schwarzenberg, 1929.
83. Hess W. Das schlafsyndrom als folge dienzephaler reizung. Helv Physiol Pharmkol Acta 1944; 2:305–344.
84. Ranson S, Ingram WR. Catalepsy caused by lesions between the mammillary bodies and third nerve in the cat. Amer J Physiol 1932; 101:690–696.
85. Bremer F. Cerveau isolé et physiologe du sommeil. C Roy Soc Biol 1935; 118: 1235–1241.
86. Ranson S. Somnolence caused by hypothalamic lesions in the monkey. Arch Neurol Psychiatry 1939; 41:1–23.
87. Nauta W. Hypothalamic regulation of sleep in rats: an experimental study. J Neurophysiol 1946; 9:285–316.
88. Magoun HW, Rhines R. An inhibitory mechanism in the bulbar reticular formation. J Neurophysiol 1946; 9:165–171.
89. Moruzzi G. The historical development of the deafferentation hypothesis of sleep. Proc Amer Philosophical Soc 1964; 108:19–28.
90. Moruzzi G, Magoun HW. Brain stem reticular formation and activation of the EEG. EEG Clin Neurophysiol 1949; 1:455–473.
91. Jouvet M, Delorme JF. Locus coeruleus et sommeil paradoxal. C Roy Soc Biol (Paris) 1965; 159:859–899.
92. McCarley R, Hobson J. Neuronal excitability modulation over the sleep cycle: a structural and mathematical model. Science 1975; 189:55–58.
93. Richter CP. A behavioristic study of the activity of the rat. Comp Psych Monographs 1922; 1:1–55.
94. Bunning E. Zur kenntis der erblichen tagesperiodiztat bei den primarblattern von Phaseolus Multiflorus. Jb Weiss Bot 1935; 81:411–418.
95. Rolando Luigi. Saggio sopra la vera strattura del cervelle dell'umo e degli animali e sopra la funzioni del sistema nervosa. Sassari, Stamperie di S.S.R.M. privilegiata, 1809.
96. Moore RY, Eichler VB. Loss of a circadian adrenal corticosterone rhythm following suprachiasmatic lesions in the rat. Brain Res 1972; 42:201–206.
97. Stephen FK, Zucker I. Circadian rhythms in drinking behavior and locomotor activity of rats are eliminated by hypothalamic lesions. Proc Natl Acad Sci USA 1972; 69:1583–1586.
98. Aschoff J, Wever R. Spontanperiodik des menschen bei ausschluss aller zeitgeber. Naturwissenschaften 1962; 49:337–342.
99. Siffre M. Beyond time. Briffault H, ed and trans. New York: McGraw-Hill, 1964.
100. Weitzman ED, Schaumburg H, Fishbein W. Plasma 17-hydoxy-corticosteroid levels during sleep in man. J Clin Endocrinol Metab 1966; 26:121–127.
101. Simpson S, Galbraith JJ. Observations on the normal temperature of the monkey and its diurnal variation, and on the effect of changes in the daily routine on this variation. Trans Roy Soc Edinburgh 1906; 45:65–106.

102. Kleitman N. Sleep and Wakefulness. Chicago: University of Chicago Press, 1939; revised, 1963.
103. Association of Sleep Disorder Centers. Diagnostic classification of sleep and arousal disorders. Sleep Disorders Classification Committee. Roffwarg H, chairman. Sleep 1979; 2:1–137.
104. Kryger M, Roth T, Dement W. Principles and Practice of Sleep Medicine. Philadelphia: WB Saunders, 1989.
105. Adie WJ. Idiopathic narcolepsy, a disease sui generis, with remarks on the mechanism of sleep. Brain 1926; 49:257–306.
106. Dynes JB, Finley KH. The electroencephalograph as an aid in the study of narcolepsy. Arch Neurol Psychiatry 1941; 46:598–612.
107. Vogel G. Studies in psychophysiology of dreams, III. The dream of narcolepsy. Arch Gen Psychiatry 1960; 3:421–428.
108. Osler W. The Principle and Practice of Medicine: Designed for the Use of Practicioners and Students of Medicine. 6th ed. New York: Apple, 1906.
109. Burwell CS, Robin ED, Whaley RJ, Bickelmann AG. Extreme obesity associated with alveolar hypoventilation—a Pickwickian syndrome. Amer J Med 1956; 21: 811–818.
110. Gastaut H, Tassinari CA, Duron B. Etude polygraphique des manifestations episodique (hypnique et respiratories), diurnes et nocturne, du syndrome de Pickwick. Rev Neurol 1965; 112:568–579.
111. Jung R, Kuhlo W. Neurophysiological studies of abnormal night sleep and the pickwickian syndrome. Prog Brain Res 1965; 18:140–159.
112. Kuhlo W, Doll E, Franck MD. Erfolgreiche behandlung eines Pickwick Syndroms durch eine dauertrachekanuele. Dtsch Med Wochenschr 1969; 94:1286–1290.
113. Ikematsu T. Study of snoring, 4th report. Therapy [in Japanese]. Jpn Otorhinolaryngol 1964; 64:434–435.
114. Fujita S, Conway W, Zorick F, Roth T. Surgical correction of anatomic abnormalities in obstructive sleep apnea syndrome: uvulopalatopharyngoplasty. Otolaryngol Head Neck Surg 1981; 89:923–934.
115. Sullivan CE, Issa FG, Berthon-Jones, Eves L. Reversal of obstructive sleep apnea by continuous positive airway pressure applied through the nares. Lancet 1981; i: 862–865.
116. Severinghaus JW, Mitchell RA. Ondine's curse—failure of respiratory automaticity while awake. Clin Res 1962; 10:122.
117. Giraudoux J. Ondine. Adapted by Valency M. New York: Random House, 1954.
118. Bootzin RR, Nicassio PM. Behavioral treatments for insomnia. In: Hersen M, Eissler R, Miller P, eds. Progress in Behavior Modification. Vol 6. New York: Academic Press, 1978:1–45.
119. Spielman AJ, Saskin P, Thorpy MJ. Treatment of chronic insomnia by restriction of time in bed. Sleep 1987; 10:45–56.
120. Weitzman ED, Czeisler CA, Coleman RM, Spielman AJ, Zimmerman JC, Dement W. Delayed sleep phase syndrome. Arch Gen Psychiatry 1981; 38:737–746.
121. Czeisler CA, Richardson GS, Coleman RM, et al. Chronotherapy: resetting the circadian clock of patients with delayed sleep phase insomnia. Sleep 1981; 4:1–21.

122. Schenck CH, Bundlie SR, Ettinger MG, Mahowald MW. Chronic behavioral disorders of human REM sleep: a new category of parasomnia. Sleep 1986; 9:293–308.
123. Lugaresi E, Cirignotta F. Hypnogenic paroxysmal dystonia: epileptic seizure or a new syndrome? Sleep 1981; 4:129–138.
124. Lugaresi E, Medori R, Montagna P, et al. Fatal familial insomnia and dysautonomia with selective degeneration of the thalamic nuclei. N Engl J Med 1986; 315:997–1003.
125. Kahn A, Mozin MJ,Casimir G, Montauk L, Blum D. Insomnia and cow's milk allergy in infants. Pediatrics 1985; 76:880–884.

2

Neurobiology and Segmental Neurology of Sleep

Antonio Culebras
Veterans Affairs Medical Center
State University of New York
and Community General Hospital
Syracuse, New York

INTRODUCTION

Sleep is a function of the brain. Like wakefulness, sleep originates in centers located in the brainstem, hypothalamus, thalamus and basal forebrain. The hemispheric cortex also intervenes in the development of sleep as a resonating organ, but appears to have no primary functions. Lesions of any nature affecting these segments of the nervous system will be reflected in an alteration of sleep and vigilance. Not all sleep disorders can be explained on a neuroanatomical basis suggesting neurochemical alteration of functions that remain to be uncovered.

While all sections of the brainstem intervene in maintaining wakefulness and in promoting sleep, there is a multisegmental core of nuclei important to all states and an aggregate of centers in the pons critical to the development of REM sleep. From brainstem areas, ascending and descending fibers carry the nervous impulses that execute all functions of sleep and maintain wakefulness.

NEUROBIOLOGY OF SLEEP

Reticular Formation

The reticular formation is the system central to sleep. It is a phylogenetically old part of the brain made up of diffuse aggregates of nerve cells traversed by fibers going in all directions (1). In general, large cells are restricted to the medial part while small cells occupy the lateral regions of the formation. The largest cells are found only at certain levels, such as the nucleus reticularis gigantocellularis of the medulla, and more rostrally in the nucleus reticularis pontis caudalis. Along the brainstem midline there are congregations of nerve cells collectively known as the raphe nuclei.

Nerve cells of the reticular formation project their axons rostrally and caudally with dendrites spreading out in a plane perpendicular to the long axis of the brainstem. The axons pass to the spinal cord from medullary and pontine nuclei in descending bundles known as the reticulospinal tract, and in ascending formations to the thalamus, while ascending and descending tracts reach other nuclei within the brainstem. Ascending fibers originate in the medulla, the lower pons–upper medulla, and the mesencephalon. Fibers originating in the mesencephalon reach targets that go beyond those of fibers coming from more caudal regions. Medullary and pontine fibers end in nonspecific thalamic nuclei, while projections from the mesencephalic formation reach the hypothalamus, the preoptic area, and the medial septal nucleus.

Afferent connections to the reticular formation come from the spinal cord via the spinoreticular tract and terminate mainly in the nucleus reticularis gigantocellularis of the medulla and in the nucleus reticularis pontis caudalis and oralis. The reticular formation also receives input from cranial nerve nuclei, the cerebellum, the lateral hypothalamus, the pallidum, the superior colliculus, and even the sensorimotor cortex.

In general, executive functions are mediated by nerve cells in the medial two-thirds of the reticular formation, while the lateral third works as an association area. There are also differences between levels, some acting preponderantly on the spinal cord and other levels on more rostral parts of the brain.

Wakefulness

To understand sleep generation, one must comprehend the origin of wakefulness. Neurons involved in promoting wakefulness are located in the reticular formation of the brainstem (ventral medullary, central pontine, and midbrain reticular formation), posterior hypothalamus, and basal forebrain (nucleus basalis of Meynert or substantia innominata, nucleus of diagonal band, and septal nucleus), subthalamus, and reticular nuclei of the thalamus (ventromedial, intralaminar, and midline thalamic nuclei). Wakefulness is maintained by tonic activity in the reticular activating system reinforced via collaterals by sensory input. The most powerful influences are acoustic and painful stimuli. Reticular system activation ascends via the brainstem reticular formation into the nonspecific thalamic system, from where it is transmitted to the cortex of the forebrain. An alternative extrathalamic route originates in the subthalamus, posterior hypothalamus, and basal forebrain projecting to the entire cortical mantle.

The electrophysiological expression of wakefulness is desynchronization of cortical electrical activity manifested in the electroencephalogram (EEG) by predominantly low-amplitude, fast, intermixed waveforms. Desynchronization of EEG rhythms is also observed in REM sleep. Both waking and REM sleep are activated states that show readiness of neuronal networks to receive afferent information. In wakefulness afferent stimuli come from the exterior, whereas in REM sleep afferent input is generated within the nervous system.

Tonically active catecholamine and acetylcholine containing neurons modulate the activity of subcortical and cortical neurons during wakefulness. Wakefulness is enhanced by histamine-containing neurons of the posterior hypothalamus and by glutamate-containing neurons located in brainstem, thalamus, and cortex.

Sleep

Non-REM Sleep

Sleep appears as the mechanisms maintaining wakefulness fade and sleep-promoting neurons become active. Transitional light sleep leading to synchronized sleep normally follows wakefulness. Synchronized sleep expresses the unified activity of many neuronal networks and is characterized by an EEG that shows high-voltage K-complexes, sleep spindles, and, as sleep deepens, high-voltage slow waves [slow-wave sleep (SWS)]. Neurons involved in the generation of synchronized sleep are found in the solitary tract nuclei of the medulla, raphe nuclei of the brainstem, reticular thalamic nuclei, anterior hypothalamus, preoptic area, basal forebrain, and orbitofrontal cortex.

Suppression of activity in the reticular arousal system releases the synchronous spindle oscillations of the thalamus. Sleep spindles are characterized by waxing and waning waveforms with a frequency of 12–14 cycles per second and a duration of 0.5–2 seconds. The presence of sleep spindles marks the onset of synaptic transmission blockade of afferent impulses through the thalamus as consciousness is lost. The reticular nucleus of the thalamus is the synchronizing pacemaker of EEG spindle oscillations (2). This nucleus forms a neuronal sheet that covers the rostral, lateral, and ventral surfaces of the thalamus. Bursts of activity in thalamocortical networks generate potentials and spike discharges within the spindle frequency in neocortical neurons that can be recorded with the surface EEG. This neuronal system is GABAergic, whereas cholinergic activation has an inhibitory effect, and thus sleep spindles disappear during activation of the cholinergic system that is associated with desynchronized REM sleep and wakefulness. The functional significance of sleep spindles is unknown. Clinical research has shown an increased density of sleep spindles in polysomnograms of patients with narcolepsy and idiopathic hypersomnia, suggesting a potential clinical usefulness as markers of excessive sleep (3).

Serotonin-containing neurons of the brainstem raphe inhibit sensory input and reduce motor activity, facilitating the emergence of slow-wave cortical activity. The thalamus also plays an important role in the genesis of EEG delta waves. The resonant thalamocortical loop transfers to the cortex action potentials and in turn drives thalamic cells by backward volleys. It should be noted, however, that slow waves persist in athalamic animals, perhaps because of in situ generation in cortical layers II, III, and IV (4).

Synaptic transmission through the thalamus is obliterated during drowsiness and blocked during synchronized sleep. This prevents the cortex from elaborating a response to afferent information. However, incoming stimuli that are powerful enough (loud noise, intense pain) bypass the thalamic blockade, causing cortical arousal. Synaptic transmission through the thalamus is enhanced during wakefulness and in REM sleep.

Serotonin-containing cells of the brainstem raphe nuclei (midline rostral and caudal midbrain, pontine and medullary tegmentum, and dorsolateral medulla) provide diffuse innervation to the brain and spinal cord. Alterations of this system produce insomnia, and serotonin antagonists such as parachlorphenylalanine (PCP)—which prevents the synthesis of serotonin by blocking the enzyme tryptophan hydroxylase—provoke severe insomnia that is reversed by the serotonin precursor 5-hydroxytryptamine, which bypasses tryptophan hydroxylase.

Other substances found in brain cells, such as adenosine, gamma-aminobutyric acid (GABA), opiates, somatostatin, and alpha-melanocyte-stimulating hormone, facilitate sleep. Adenosine neurons are located in the hypothalamus, and adenosine receptors are blocked by caffeine and xanthines in general. Benzodiazepines binding with receptors enhance the postsynaptic action of GABA and thus promote sleep. Neurons of the reticular nucleus of the thalamus and neurons of the anterior hypothalamus and basal forebrain are GABAergic.

REM Sleep

Rapid-eye-movement (REM) sleep—also known as desynchronized, paradoxical, active, and dream sleep—originates in brainstem centers. Unlike non-REM sleep, REM sleep is not organized in stages although "tonic" and "phasic" REM sleep are generally distinguished to recognize brief bursts of rapid eye-movement activity that characterize phasic REM sleep. In cats, phasic REM sleep is associated with bursts of ponto-geniculo-occipital (PGO) waves believed to be the pacemaker of myoclonic activity, causing twitching of facial muscles, limbs, and tail; variations in blood pressure, heart rate, and respirations; and dream events.

REM sleep is characterized by an apparently unrelated constellation of phenomena that are generated in different areas of the pons and caudal midbrain. The usage of various nomenclatures for nuclei in the brainstem of the cat, the most studied experimental animal, has created confusion (5). No center has been shown to function as the unique generator, although most authors would accept that the lateral portion of the nucleus reticularis pontis oralis [using Brodal's (1) terminology], ventral to the nucleus locus coeruleus, is the brain region most critical for the production of REM sleep. Others refer to the pedunculopontine (PPN) and the laterodorsal (LTD) nuclei in the dorsolateral region of the midbrain–pontine junction as the centers containing the most important aggregates of cholinergic neurons intervening in REM sleep (6). The PPN is a parabrachial nucleus found just lateral to the superior cerebellar peduncle in the midbrain and rostral pons. Cholinergic output from the PPN–LDT complex reaches specific and nonspecific thalamic nuclei as well as the substantia innominata and the posterior lateral hypothalamus (7). All these centers project diffusely to the cortex providing the PPN–LDT cells with a neuromodulatory role of cortical activity. A principal afferent system to the PPN–LDT complex comes from the internal segment of the globus pallidus and the pars reticulata of the substantia nigra (6).

Localized lesions in the tegmentum of the pons abolish REM sleep; pharmacological agents stimulating cholinergic transmission facilitate, whereas monoaminergic agents suppress, REM sleep. Many reticular neurons in the dorsolateral part of the pons display a high discharging rate in REM sleep, a low discharging rate in non-REM sleep, and absence of activity in wakefulness. These "REM sleep-on" neurons were considered the generators of REM sleep by Sakai et al. (8). Noradrenergic neurons localized in the locus coeruleus and serotonergic neurons in the brainstem raphe exhibit tonic and regular discharge rates in the waking state, decreased discharge rates in non-REM sleep, and cessation of firing in REM sleep. These monoaminergic cells are termed "REM sleep-off" neurons and may have a gating or inhibiting effect on the generators of REM sleep. Based on this counterbalance system, Steriade and McCarley (9) proposed that "REM sleep-on" neurons have an executive role in REM sleep whereas "REM sleep-off" neurons are inhibitors. Their interaction would determine the periodicity and duration of REM sleep. The arousal threshold in REM sleep is variable in humans in contrast with evidence in animals of a high arousal threshold in the context of a desynchronized EEG resembling the waking state. The purpose of REM sleep remains unknown; however, a correlation has been observed between active brain growth, brain development, and complexity of REM sleep.

The events comprising REM sleep include the following.

1. Desynchronization of cortical EEG rhythms characterized by low-voltage fast waves that arise as a result of activation of large nerve cells in the central midbrain reticular formation.
2. Hippocampal theta rhythms are highly synchronized theta waves in the range of 4–8 Hz, present continuously through REM sleep in the cat. Studies with deep electrodes have shown that theta rhythms are generated in the pyramidal cells of CA1 in the dentate gyrus and in the

medial entorhinal cortex of the hippocampus. Input comes from the medial septal nucleus and from the nucleus pontis oralis in the brainstem. They represent a stark contrast to desynchronized neocortical EEG activity.

3. Sawtooth waves are highly stereotypical trains of frontocentral, bilaterally synchronous, and symmetric surface positive waves with a frequency of 2–5 Hz, an amplitude of 20–100 μV, and a mean duration of 252 ms. These peculiar waveforms appear in trains of three or more consecutive waves with an angle greater than 80° to the baseline. Sawtooth waves precede the onset of the first episode of REM. In fact, Sato et al. (10) have described a sequence of events characterized by a generalized body movement followed by muscle-tone reduction, a train of sawtooth waves, and, finally, the first episode of REM activity heralding the onset of REM sleep. These authors have reported mean onset times for each event that are predictable and potentially usable for clinical research of reticular system conductivity. The origin of sawtooth waves is unknown.
4. Muscle atonia is a pronounced reduction in postural tone, sparing the oculomotor muscles and the diaphragm, that persists during REM sleep. Cells in the peri–locus coeruleus area, ventral to the nucleus locus coeruleus, become active and stimulate via the tegmentoreticular tract inhibitory nerve cells of the magnocellular reticular nucleus in the medial medulla (Figure 1), probably the same inhibitory area described by Magoun and Rhines (11). This region is a well-known inhibitory center of spinal motoneurons mediated via the reticulospinal tract. Postsynaptic inhibition is the principal mechanism responsible for atonia of the somatic musculature during REM sleep. Suppression of muscle tone in REM sleep is mediated by acetylcholine and glutamate in brainstem nuclei and by glycine in the spinal cord (12).

   Abolition of muscle atonia during REM sleep has been studied experimentally in the cat (8) and recognized clinically in humans. REM sleep without atonia can be induced by lesions placed in dorsolateral portions of the nucleus reticularis pontis oralis, just ventral to the locus coeruleus, or with bilateral interruption of the tegmentoreticular tract in the pons. The condition facilitates dream enactment and the release of stereotypical behaviors both in the experimental animal (oneiric behavior) and in humans (REM sleep behavior disorder—see Chapter 9). Similar episodes have been observed in cats with localized lesions in ventromedial portions of the medulla (13). The reverse condition—atonia without REM sleep—has been provoked experimentally by injecting carbachol, a potent cholinergic substance, in the dorsal pons in the same region that when injured causes REM sleep without atonia.

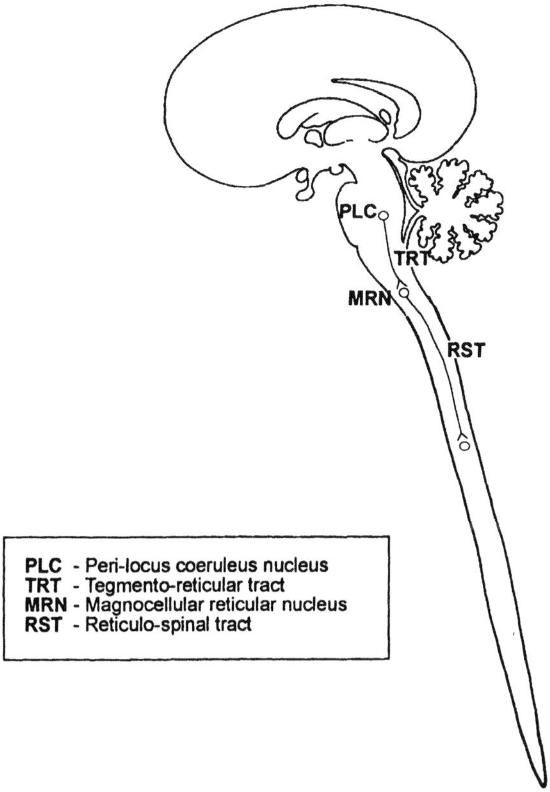

Figure 1 Muscle atonia generation. Cells in the peri–locus coeruleus area, ventral to the nucleus locus coeruleus, become active in REM sleep and stimulate via the tegmento-reticular tract the inhibitory nerve cells of the magnocellular reticular nucleus in the medial medulla. This region is an inhibitory center of spinal motoneurons, an action mediated via the reticulospinal tract. (From Ref. 63.)

More extensive injections can cause REM sleep. Activation of atonia without REM sleep may underlie the clinical phenomenon of cataplexy. Induction of cataplexy with laughter and other emotions in narcolepsy, as well as occurrence of symptomatic cataplexy in individuals with midbrain lesions (14), suggests that the REM sleep–muscle atonia system is modulated by supratentorial centers.

5. Ponto-geniculo-occipital (PGO) spike generation accompanies rapid eye movements and other phasic motor events of REM sleep (9) such as twitching of facial and acral muscles in the cat and variations in

blood pressure, heart rate, and respiration. PGO spikes originate in the dorsolateral pontine tegmentum bordering the brachium conjunctivum and reach the lateral geniculate nucleus. Each half of the pons functions as an independent generator of PGO spikes, and the pathway for propagation can be interrupted unilaterally by lesions in the rostral pons. PGO spikes can be triggered by cholinergic stimulation. Serotonin inhibits PGO waves, and serotonin depletion, such as produced by PCP, may trigger continuous PGO activity. Upon reaching neocortical areas, PGO waves trigger fragmentary imagery that we recognize as dreams.

6. Rapid eye movements are the rapid, saccadic, conjugate eye movements in the horizontal, vertical, and sometimes oblique planes that give name to this state of sleep. Horizontal eye movements originate in the periabducens area of the dorsomedial pons, and vertical eye movements are generated in the midbrain reticular formation. Horizontal and vertical eye movements appear in bursts throughout REM sleep, at times in conjunction with other phasic events related to PGO waves.
7. Myoclonia, or muscle twitches, are brief clonic contractions of facial and acral limb muscles (and of the tail in animals) that appear throughout REM sleep. Although muscle atonia is the predominant input reaching motoneurons during REM sleep, for reasons as yet unknown, overpowering breakthrough excitatory potentials reach motoneurons at irregular intervals, causing group unit discharges that trigger myoclonic jerks and rapid eye movements (12). The stimulus for phasic muscle twitches originates in cells located in the reticular nucleus pontis caudalis and nucleus gigantocellularis (15), an area that projects monosynaptically via the reticulospinal tracts to forelimb and hindlimb motoneurons and the facial nucleus.
8. Dream generation: subjects awakened from REM sleep report a dream experience 85% of the time. It is thought that PGO waves traveling to lateral geniculate nuclei and forebrain systems provide excitation of the forebrain and the substrate for dream visual experiences. Sensory system activation during dream experiences always includes the visual system (16). Auditory experiences appear in 65% of dreams. Spatial experiences such as flying, floating, or sinking, presumably associated with vestibular excitation, are considerably less common, while experiences involving tactile, taste, and smell perceptions are rare. Pain is almost never a component of dreams.

    Organized lower-extremity activity appears in most dreams. Experimental evidence indicates that cortical and subcortical motor structures mediating complex organized movements are activated during dream generation (17). According to the activation-synthesis hypothesis of Hobson and McCarley (18), nonrandom, ineffectual motor excitation of brainstem generators of complex motor activity, such as walking or running, incorporates as a corollary subjective experiences elaborated in the forebrain.

9. Other phenomena: during REM sleep in animals, there is abolition of thermoregulatory responses and the animal enters a poikilothermic state (19). Humans do not display physiological patterns indicative of complete cessation of thermoregulation similar to those observed in mammals. Nonetheless, there is evidence in humans of two separate processes of temperature regulation linked to REM and non-REM sleep. The preoptic-anterior hypothalamic nuclei intervene in thermoregulatory responses to the local hypothalamic temperature that represents the dominant feedback signal.

   Cardiorespiratory fluctuations, including variations in blood pressure, heart rate, and respiration, appear as a result of phasic activation of centers in the medial and lateral parabrachial nuclei of the pons, which in turn exert a modulatory influence over bulbar neurons. Respiratory fluctuations of REM sleep are controlled directly by neural mechanisms originating in the pneumotaxic centers of the brainstem and do not depend on peripheral changes (oxygen saturation, CO_2 content, or pH of blood).

   Even though most dreams are not sexually oriented, males have penile erections during REM sleep, from infancy (2 to 4 months) to senescence. In adolescence, tumescence time equals or surpasses REM sleep duration and occupies more sleep time than at any other age. Electrical stimulation of ventral tegmental points in the midbrain and of ventrolateral sites in the pons have elicited erections in the squirrel monkey (20).

   During REM sleep, cerebral blood flow, flow velocities (21), and metabolism increase as waves of increased intracranial pressure appear. Cardiac output declines while urine volume decreases. Phasic changes in parasympathetic output occur and sympathetic tone is lost. Sweating decreases or disappears.

CHRONOBIOLOGY

Many physiological cycles are coupled to the unending geocosmic rotation of day and night, recurring every 24 hours in periods that are called circadian (near 24 hours) (see Chapter 7). Subsidiary cycles, like entrained cogwheels, occur in compliance with the primary sleep–wake rhythm, and these in turn trigger other subservient cycles in a chain of events that touches virtually every aspect of the biological economy. Zucker reported in the early 1970s (22) that lesions of the interbrain or hypothalamus of the rat eliminate the activity–rest cycle of the animal. The area of the hypothalamus critical for this behavior was localized to a small cluster of cells situated above the optic chiasm called the suprachiasmatic nucleus (SCN). When the SCN was obliterated bilaterally, the rats continued to move and drink but the periodicity of the functions organized in accordance to the light–dark cycles disappeared entirely. Non-REM and REM sleep were still generated, but their occurrence failed to show periodicity or coupling with external cues.

The SCN of the anterior hypothalamus is the principal pacemaker of the circadian system. SCN rhythmicity is intrinsically generated. The earliest presence of SCN in humans occurs during the 18th week of gestation (23). It is not clear whether the SCN plays an executive autonomous role before birth, since there is evidence that circadian rhythms present in the fetus may be driven by the mother. It appears that melatonin that crosses the placental barrier mediates the entrainment of the fetal SCN to the circadian rhythm of the mother. After birth, entrainment to external factors—mainly light—occurs gradually over the first weeks and months of postnatal development. This is expressed by the eventual consolidation of sleep to the nocturnal period (24). The daily sleep–wake cycle is one of the most prominent manifestations of circadian rhythmicity, and its correct development in compliance with expected parameters over the first few months of life suggests a healthy integrated biological system.

Photoendocrine Reflex

Afferent projections to the SCN come primarily from retinal photoreceptors, and also from brainstem serotonergic raphe nuclei, cholinergic forebrain neurons, and pedunculopontine tegmental nuclei. Efferent projections reach the area ventral to the paraventricular nucleus in the hypothalamus by way of a dorsal pathway that appears to be the major efferent tract. From the paraventricular nucleus, efferents secondarily reach many other areas of influence of the SCN, including the pineal gland (Figure 2).

Using autoradiographic techniques, Moore and Lenn (25) demonstrated neural projections linking the retina to the SCN that were capable of conveying direct photic information to the suprachiasmatic pacemaker. This system is unique to mammals; birds and lizards have encephalic photoreceptors that permit direct photic entrainment. Transection of the retinohypothalamic tract or elimination of the retinal photoreceptors by enucleation abolishes circadian rhythms, showing the critical role of this projection in synchronizing the circadian pacemaker with the light–dark cycle.

Melatonin

Melatonin synthesized in the pineal gland from tryptophan and serotonin (see Chapter 6) is the hormone that exerts the most potent regulatory effect on the SCN

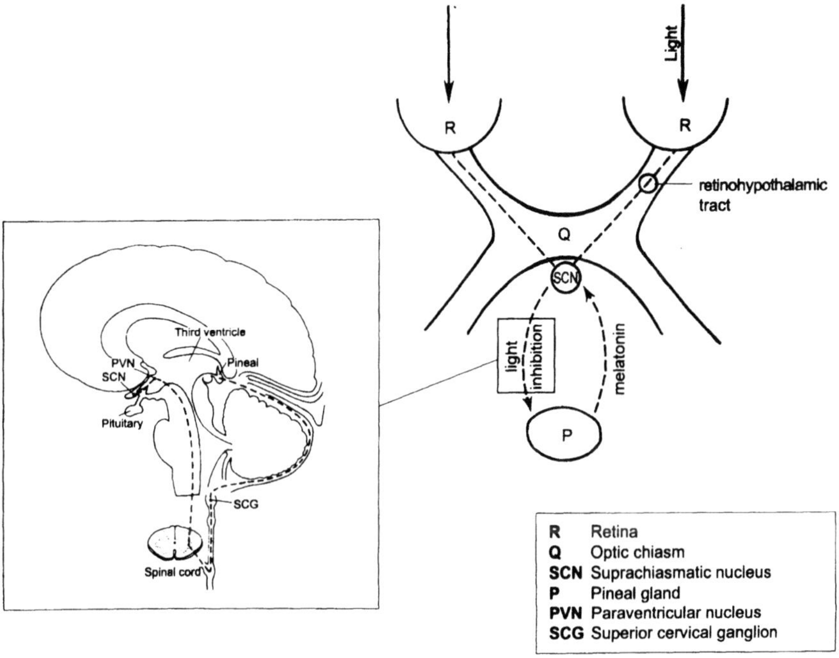

Figure 2 Retinohypothalamic tract and photoendocrine reflex. Light striking on the retina generates stimuli that are transmitted via the retinohypothalamic pathway to the SCN and then to the paraventricular nuclei. From here they travel with fibers of the medial forebrain bundle and reticular formation to reach the intermediolateral nucleus of the spinal cord. They pass to preganglionic adrenergic prolongations of the sympathetic nervous system that transmit them to the superior cervical ganglion. Postganglionic prolongations travel with the internal carotid sympathetic nervous plexus to reach their final destination in the pineal gland. Light inhibits and darkness stimulates melatonin secretion.

rhythm independently of the sleep–wake rhythm. It may act by synchronizing uncoupled rhythms. Light inhibits melatonin secretion whereas darkness releases its secretion, indicating that light stimuli relayed via the retinohypothalamic tract and the SCN play a critical role in the photoendocrine reflex (26) (Figure 2). In this reflex, impulses triggered by light travel via the retinohypothalamic pathway to the SCN and then to the paraventricular nuclei. From here they are transmitted via fibers of the medial forebrain bundle and reticular formation to the prolongations of the sympathetic nervous system that relay them to the superior cervical ganglion (27) and then to postganglionic prolongations that travel with the internal carotid sympathetic nervous plexus to their final destination in the pineal gland. Individuals with degenerative dysautonomia of any origin may have alteration or abolition of the melatonin rhythm, a phenomenon that has been observed in ganglionectomized animals (28). This includes patients with diabetes and spinal-cord section. It is unknown whether a similar alteration occurs in patients with Parkinson's disease and multisystem atrophy.

Melatonin reduces sleep latency and promotes sleep; its deficiency may have an important role in the development of insomnia among elderly people in whom controlled-release melatonin-replacement therapy improves sleep quality (29).

There are segments of the 24-hour cycle when the circadian system is highly responsive to light and other times when it appears to be resistant. Exposure to light in the evening phase-delays, or lengthens, the cycle, whereas exposure in the early morning causes a phase-advance, or shortening. On the other hand, during the middle of the day there is no circadian response to light cues. A reduction in SCN volume has been observed with progressive age, and in humans a shrinkage of the SCN has been identified in dementia, perhaps in connection with the major circadian dysrhythmia observed in this condition (30).

Cortisol

Cortisol secretion, a marker of ACTH release, occurs during the night, peaking in the early morning. It declines during daytime hours, reaching a nadir shortly before an individual retires to bed. Cortisol secretion is very resistant to change and persists even if sleep is eliminated, as in coma, or is delayed, as in the jet-lag syndrome.

Growth Hormone

The largest bursts of growth hormone (GH) secretion occur at night in association with the first cycle of slow-wave sleep (SWS), approximately 60 minutes after falling asleep. The sleep-related rise of GH is resistant to peripheral metabolic variations and fails to respond to pharmacological interventions that modify the waking-state response. SWS-related GH secretion is greater in children than in adults and tends to disappear in old age. The evidence suggests that SWS-related GH secretion is regulated by neural pathways that are different from those intervening in the wake-state release and independent of metabolic influences. Sleep deprivation in children may cause disruption of sleep-related GH release, with ominous consequences for normal growth. In fact, emotionally deprived children who sleep poorly tend to be of short stature (31). Sleep-laboratory investigation of patients with myotonic dystrophy and others with vascular or surgical lesions involving the dorsomedial nucleus of the thalamus and/or thalamocortical connections has revealed loss of plasma GH rises that are normally associated with the slow-wave phase of sleep (32), suggesting a role for this nucleus in the neural regulation of GH.

NEUROANATOMICAL CORRELATES

Sleep is a function of the brain and thus defined structural lesions may cause predictable alterations of sleep (33). The correlation is much less precise than that observed with motor or sensory functions, since sleep is a state of being of the brain. However, as increasingly detailed vicarious functions are studied, the correlation with neuroanatomical lesions becomes more and more sharply defined. Clinically observed correlations are studied in the next section following a rostrocaudal plan.

Telencephalon

Cerebral Hemispheres

The cerebral hemispheres are not primordial in the generation or maintenance of sleep, although considerable modulation of brainstem functions occurs as a result of the activity of subcortical nuclei. Anencephalic infants without thalami have survived for up to 85 days exhibiting periods of sleep and crude behaviors (34). Patients with extensive cortical injury eventually show cyclical changes in electroencephalographic activity suggestive of sleep–wake alternation (35). Survivors of large hemispheric stroke have increased slow-wave sleep while retaining normal percentages of REM sleep (36).

There is very little clinical information on the effects of human lesions involving the basal forebrain area, a region that has been heavily implicated in sleep mechanisms in the cat. In humans there are temporary increases in wakefulness following frontal leukotomy (37), but 10 years or more after the operation there is an increase in slow-wave sleep (38).

Although cortical structures do not appear to play an executive role in sleep, it is likely that cortical influences reach lower diencephalic and midbrain centers. Early studies by Nauta showed that stimulation of the "limbic forebrain–midbrain circuit" promotes sleep whereas damage causes insomnia along with neurovegetative disturbances (39). Recent evidence showing that the major output nuclei of the basal ganglia (internal segment of the globus pallidus and pars reticulata of the substantia nigra) reach the PPN–LDT region of the brainstem where REM sleep is generated suggests a rich pathophysiology that remains to be uncovered. Indeed, behavioral sleep alterations in disorders typically associated with dysfunction of the basal ganglia, such as Parkinson's disease, obsessive-compulsive disorder, and Tourette's syndrome, suggest that circuits intrinsic to the basal ganglia intervene heavily in sleep mechanisms (6).

Thalamus

Ablation of the thalamus in the cat leads to persistent and severe insomnia (4). Diffuse lesions of the thalamus in humans cause ipsilateral decrease or abolition of sleep spindles (40). Loss of stage 2 and of sleep spindles after hemispheric stroke is a poor prognostic sign for recovery (41). The dorsomedial nucleus has been implicated in sleep phenomena. In patients with myotonic dystrophy, nerve cells of the dorsomedial nuclei exhibit cytoplasmic inclusion bodies that manifest neuronal damage probably responsible for hypersomnia, apathy, mental decline, and "slow alpha" rhythms (42). Several clinical observations have linked lesions of the dorsomedial nuclei of the thalamus with loss of growth-hormone secretion during slow-wave sleep in patients with myotonic dystrophy (43) and in patients with stroke (36). Lugaresi and co-workers (44) (see Chapter 8) have described familial fatal insomnia with dysautonomia and a dreamlike state with dream enactments in patients with degenerative lesions of the dorsomedial and anterior nuclei of the thalamus, an observation suggesting that the thalamus plays an important role in integrating and expressing sleep (45).

Other Basal Ganglia

Descending output from the internal segment of the globus pallidus and the pars reticulata of the substantia nigra reaches the PPN–LDT region, providing opportunity for supratentorial modulation of sleep rapid eye movements, muscle atonia, and other REM-sleep-related phenomena. Furthermore, these pathways serve as an anatomical substrate linking the pathophysiology of REM sleep with conditions such as Parkinson's disease, schizophrenia, obsessive-compulsive disorder, attention-deficit disorder, and Tourette's syndrome (6) that manifest sleep behavioral alterations.

Diencephalon: Hypothalamus

Lesions of the posterior hypothalamus decrease wakefulness. Similar effects are obtained in cell destructions of the basal forebrain nuclei (substantia innominata or nucleus basalis of Meynert, nuclei of the diagonal band and septum), suggesting the existence of a waking center in the posterior hypothalamus and basal forebrain that projects to the cortical mantle.

Von Economo (46), in his classic studies in brains of patients dying with encephalitis, showed that lesions of the anterior hypothalamus were associated with insomnia, whereas lesions of the posterior hypothalamus and mesencephalic tegmentum correlated with lethargy and hypersomnia. Von Economo's observations were made in brains with lesions of encephalitis that were too diffuse to draw conclusive results. They had the virtue, however, of drawing attention to the hypothalamus as a brain area important to sleep and waking mechanisms.

Neuroendocrine rhythms related to sleep are modulated by structures as diverse as the amygdaloid nuclei, thalamus, midbrain, and the limbic system, but integrated at the hypothalamic level. There is clinical evidence indicating that hypothalamic damage causes various neuroendocrine dysfunctions that are usually manifested by loss of the ACTH-cortisol rhythm, hyperprolactinemia, and absence of slow-wave-sleep-associated growth-hormone secretion (47). The SCN, connected with the external environment through the retinohypothalamic tract, plays a leading role in the organization of circadian rhythmicity. Damage to this region may be responsible for circadian dysrhythmia, as observed in Alzheimer's disease and other degenerative disorders that affect the hypothalamus.

Hypothalamic tumors are associated with hypersomnia. Symptomatic narcolepsy may occur in lesions of the floor of the third ventricle involving the hypothalamus. Patients with diencephalic lesions have genuine sleep attacks (and not prolonged subalertness), abnormal presence of REM-sleep episodes in daytime sleep-latency tests, and cataplexy. There is some evidence that the dopaminergic tone of the hypothalamus is reduced during the symptomatic phase of the Kleine-Levin syndrome (48), a periodic hypersomnia associated with hyperphagia and hypersexuality in young men.

Brainstem

Transection of the midbrain in the cat immediately caudal to the third nerve nuclei (cerveau isolé) (49) initially produces slow-wave synchronized sleep without alternation along with loss of response to painful stimuli, and continuous spindles in the EEG; REM sleep is absent (5). If the transection is made lower in the brainstem, in the junction between the spinal cord and medulla (encephale isolé), wakefulness gradually returns and after a few days spontaneous periods of EEG desynchronization can be identified. REM sleep without atonia may be observed in this preparation (5). These experiments led to the development of the concept of the reticular activating system, synchronized and desynchronized states, and the discovery of REM-sleep centers.

Mesencephalon

Rostral segments of the reticular activating system are in close proximity with the third nerve nuclei in the medial midbrain. Lesions in this region almost invariably cause a reduction in the level of alertness, paresis of vertical gaze, and pupillary abnormalities. In infarction of the paramedian midbrain territory in "top of the basilar" occlusion, there is persistent sleepiness associated with pupillary dilatation, paresis of vertical gaze, and loss of convergence (50). Peduncular hallucinosis occasionally observed in this syndrome is characterized by development of colorful, intense, visual hallucinations, probably related to the dream phenomena of REM sleep. Lesions of the pars reticulata of the substantia nigra have also been associated with hallucinations (51). Peduncular hallucinosis always occurs in patients with sleep alterations, verifying its genesis in lesions of the midbrain adjacent to structures of the reticular system that intervene in sleep–wake mechanisms.

Cataplexy—the sudden loss of muscle tone, predominantly in antigravity muscles (see Chapter 16)—may progress from cranial nerves to upper and lower limbs or affect only one side of the body. Symptomatic cataplexy associated with sleep paralysis and sleep attacks appears in patients with rostral brainstem lesions invading the floor of the third ventricle (52). Recent reports indicate that a lesion of the midbrain without hypothalamic involvement would be sufficient to trigger cataplexy and sleep paralysis (53). Such lesions may disengage from rostral brainstem inhibition the atonia-generating system of the peri–locus coeruleus area.

Lesions of the lower mesencephalon–upper pons tegmentum involving the peri–locus coeruleus area are responsible for the syndrome of REM sleep without atonia. Motor behavior driven by a dream is called phantasmagoria. Full expression of the syndrome occurs with bilateral pontine lesions involving the peri–locus coeruleus area or the tegmentoreticular tract. In REM-sleep behavior disorder, muscle atonia fails to develop during REM stage as a result of the destruction of the atonia generator in the peri–locus coeruleus area or its disconnection from the muscle-tone inhibitory center of Magoun and Rhines (nucleus reticularis magnocellularis) in the medulla. This nucleus transmits impulses to the spinal motoneurons via the ventrolateral reticulospinal tract, resulting in muscle atonia (Table 1).

Pons

Profound alterations or abolition of non-REM and REM sleep in humans (54), along with reduction in total sleep time, occur with extensive lesions of the pontine tegmentum. Not uncommonly, sleep alterations are associated with paresis of lateral conjugate gaze (55). Patients with locked-in-syndrome of vascular origin, with lesion extending into the pontine tegmentum, experience loss of REM and non-REM stages.

Loss of non-REM sleep may occur with lesions of the median raphe in the pons and midbrain, a phenomenon consistent with experiments in the cat showing

Table 1 Brainstem Level and Effect of Damage on Sleep Mechanisms

Lesion location	Effect
Rostrocentral midbrain tegmentum	Intense sleepiness, vertical-gaze palsies, hallucinations
Dorsal pontine tegmentum	Profound insomnia, horizontal-gaze palsies
Pontomedullary junction	Cardiorespiratory alterations, loss of muscle atonia in REM
Medulla	Prominent cardiorespiratory alterations, loss of muscle atonia in REM

that damage to serotonergic nuclei of the median raphe causes persistent insomnia.

Medulla

Medullary lesions may affect the ability to breathe during sleep. Bilateral medullary damage can cause complete failure of automatic respiration that is undistinguishable from Ondine's curse. In acute bulbar poliomyelitis, there is widespread damage to brainstem reticular formation and involvement of respiratory centers that determine alteration of the respiratory function (56). It is conceivable that in bulbar poliomyelitis damage occurs to pneumotaxic centers of the pons and respiratory centers of the medulla as well as to reticular nerve cells maintaining tonic wakefulness in the midbrain region. Patients with the postpolio syndrome and a history of bulbar manifestations such as drowsiness are more likely to develop sleep apnea syndrome in parallel with other manifestations typical of the disorder (57). Central apneas in patients with the postpolio syndrome and a history of bulbar symptoms appear more commonly in non-REM sleep, suggesting reduction in forebrain control of compromised bulbar respiratory centers during non-REM sleep (58). In the Arnold-Chiari malformation, compression of medullary centers involved in respiration may cause nonobstructive sleep apnea, or obstructive sleep apnea if pharyngeal motor centers are also involved (59).

Spinal Cord

Patients with high spinal-cord lesions commonly complain of disordered sleep (60), and obstructive sleep apnea has been reported in patients with cervical cord damage. It has been suggested that the respiratory alteration is the consequence of excessive workload imposed on the diaphragm, which is the only source of ventilation, as shown by paradoxical retraction of the ribcage (61). Alveolar hypoventilation, obesity, and medications such as baclofen are contributing factors.

Peripheral Nerves and Muscle

Dysfunctions of the peripheral nervous system and muscles may affect sleep (see Chapter 20). Included in this pathophysiological group are alterations of the lower motor neuron, the neuromuscular junction, and muscle. Diaphragmatic and chest-wall muscle weakness, excessive respiratory muscle fatigability, restrictive lung disease, weakness of the pharyngeal wall, and obesity are causes of sleep-related respiratory insufficiency in patients with a neuromuscular disorder.

The physiological reduction of muscle tone in non-REM sleep and the virtual loss of activity of intercostal muscles with preservation or enhancement of diaphragmatic drive in REM sleep create a unique series of circumstances. Focal deficit of diaphragmatic function is characterized by REM-sleep-related nocturnal breathlessness and respiratory failure. As a result, sleep-related hypoxemia, nocturnal fragmentation of sleep, and decreased daytime function occur.

Diaphragmatic weakness is the major determinant of ventilatory compromise in patients with neuromuscular disease (62). The diaphragm may be weak in isolation or as part of a generalized muscle involvement. Diaphragmatic muscle weakness becomes specifically manifest during REM sleep, when the diaphragm is physiologically the only effective muscle pump. Patients with neuromuscular disease may also have restrictive lung disorder as a consequence of chest-wall muscle weakness. Inspiratory upper-airway resistance and obstructive sleep apnea may develop if there is weakness of pharyngeal muscle dilators causing increased upper-airway resistance or a tendency to pharyngeal-wall collapse.

Phrenic nerve damage causing diaphragmatic paralysis may occur in diffuse neuropathies and in motor neuron disease. The phrenic nerve originates in the phrenic nucleus situated in the ventral medial cell column of the cervical ventral gray horn, extending from C3 to the caudal part of C5. Unilateral paralysis may be asymptomatic, but bilateral paralysis is invariably symptomatic and may be life-threatening because of ventilatory insufficiency, which becomes more severe when the patient is supine and particularly profound during REM sleep. Undiagnosed bilateral diaphragmatic paralysis may lead to acute cardiopulmonary failure and death. Phrenic nerve paralysis has been reported in patients with Charcot-Marie-Tooth disease (hereditary motor and sensory neuropathy) complicated with diabetes mellitus, spinal cord injury, poliomyelitis, Guillain-Barré syndrome, diabetes, diphtheric neuropathy, beriberi, alcoholic neuropathy, brachial plexus neuropathy, lead neuropathy, trauma, ALS, myotonic dystrophy, Duchenne muscular dystrophy, and paraneoplastic syndrome.

REFERENCES

1. Brodal A. Neurological Anatomy in Relation to Clinical Medicine. 3rd ed. New York: Oxford University Press, 1981:394–447.
2. Steriade M. Basic mechanisms of sleep generation. Neurology 1992; 42(suppl 6): 9–18.
3. Bové A, Culebras A, Moore JT, Westlake RE. Relationship between sleep spindles and hypersomnia. Sleep 1994; 17:449–455.
4. Villablanca J. Role of the thalamus in sleep control: sleep-wakefulness studies in chronic diencephalic and athalamic cats. In: Petre-Quadens O, Schlag J, eds. Basic Sleep Mechanisms. New York: Academic Press, 1974:51–81.
5. Siegel JM. Brainstem mechanisms generating REM sleep. In: Kryger MH, Roth T, Dement WC, eds. Principles and Practice of Sleep Medicine. 2nd ed. Philadelphia: WB Saunders, 1994:125–144.
6. Rye DB. Contributions of the pedunculopontine region to normal and altered REM sleep. Sleep 1997; 20(9):757–788.
7. Szymusiak R. State of the art review. Magnocellular nuclei of the basal forebrain: substrates of sleep and arousal regulation. Sleep 1995; 18(6)478–500.
8. Sakai K, Sastre JP, Salvert D, et al. Tegmento-reticular projections with special

reference to the muscular atonia during paradoxical sleep in the cat: an HRP study. Brain Res 1979; 176:233–254.
9. Steriade M, McCarley RW. Brainstem control of wakefulness and sleep. New York: Plenum Press, 1990.
10. Sato S, McCutchen C, Graham B, Freeman A, Albertini-Carletti I, Alling DW. Relationship between muscle tone changes, sawtooth waves and rapid eye movement during sleep. Electroencephalog Clinical Neurophysiol 1997; 103:627–632.
11. Magoun HW, Rhines AR. An inhibitory mechanism in the bulbar reticular formation. J Neurophysiol 1946; 9:165–171.
12. Chase MH, Morales FR. The atonia and myoclonia of active (REM) sleep. Annu Rev Psychol 1990; 41:557–584.
13. Schenkel E, Siegel JM. REM sleep without atonia after lesions of the medial medulla. Neurosci Lett 1989; 98:159–165.
14. Fernández JM, Sadaba F, Villaverde FJ, Alvaro LC, Cortina C. Cataplexy associated with midbrain lesion. Neurology 1995; 45:393–394.
15. Vertes RP. Brainstem control of the events of REM sleep. Prog Neurobiol 1984; 22:241–288.
16. McCarley RW, Hoffman EA. REM sleep dreams and the activation-synthesis hypothesis. Am J Psychiatry 1981; 138:904–912.
17. Hess CW, Mills KR, Murray NMF, Schriefer TN. Excitability of the human motor cortex is enhanced during REM sleep. Neurosci Lett 1987; 82:47–52.
18. Hobson JA, McCarley RW. The brain as a dream state generator: an activation-synthesis hypothesis of the dream process. Am J Psychiatry 1977; 134:1335–1348.
19. Heller HC, Glotzbach S, Grahn D, Radeke C. Sleep-dependent changes in the thermoregulatory system. In: Lydic R, Biebuyck JF, eds. Clinical Physiology of Sleep. Clinical Physiology Series, American Physiological Society. New York: Oxford University Press, 1988:145–158.
20. MacLean PD, Denniston RH, Dua S. Further studies on cerebral representation of penile erection: caudal thalamus, midbrain and pons. J Neurophysiol 1963; 26:273–293.
21. Hajak G, Klingelhofer J, Schulz-Varszegi, et al. Relationship between cerebral blood flow velocities and cerebral electrical activity in sleep. Sleep 1994; 17(1):11–19.
22. Stephan F, Zucker I. Circadian rhythms in drinking behavior and locomotor activity of rats are eliminated by hypothalamic lesions. Proc Nat Acad Sci 1972; 69:1583–1586.
23. Reppert SM, Weaver DR, Rivkees SA, Stopa EG. Putative melatonin receptors in a human biological clock. Science 1988; 242:78–81.
24. Kleitman N, Engelmann TG. Sleep characteristics of infants. J Appl Physiol 1953; 6:269–282.
25. Moore RY, Lenn NJ. A retino-hypothalamic projection in the rat. J Comp Neurol 1972; 146:1–14.
26. Meijer JH, Rietveld WJ. Neurophysiology of the SCN circadian pacemaker in rodents. Physiol Rev 1989; 69:671–707.
27. Tamarkin L, Baird CJ, Almeida OFX. Melatonin: a coordinating signal for mammalian reproduction? Science 1985; 227:714–720.
28. Grubaugh W, et al. Effects of pinealectomy in pony mares. J Reprod Fertil 1982; 32(suppl):293–295.

29. Garfinkel D, Laudon M, Nof D, Zisapel N. Improvement of sleep quality in elderly people by controlled-release melatonin. Lancet 1995; 346:541–544.
30. Swaab DF, Fliers E, Partiman TS. The suprachiasmatic nucleus of the human brain in relation to sex, age, and senile dementia. Brain Res 1985; 342:37–44.
31. Powell GF, Hopwood NJ, Barrett ES. Growth hormone studies before and during catch-up growth in a child with emotional deprivation and short stature. J Clin Endocrinol Metab 1973; 37:674–679.
32. Culebras A. Thalamic lesions and the endocrine system. In: Guilleminault C, et al., eds. Fatal Familial Insomnia: Inherited Prion Diseases, Sleep and the Thalamus. New York: Raven Press, 1994:87–100.
33. Culebras A. Neuroanatomic and neurologic correlates of sleep disturbance. Neurology 1992; 42(suppl 6):19–27.
34. Nielsen JM, Sedgwick RP. Instincts and emotions in an anencephalic monster. J Nerv Ment Dis 1949; 110:387–394.
35. Autret A, Carrier H, Thommasi M, Jouvet M, Schott B. Etude physiopathologique et neuro-pathologique d'un syndrome de décortication cérébrale. Rev Neurol 1975; 131:491–504.
36. Culebras A, Miller M. Dissociated patterns of nocturnal prolactin, cortisol and growth hormone secretion after stroke. Neurology 1984; 34:631–636.
37. Hauri P, Hawkins DR. Human sleep after leucotomy. Arch Gen Psychiatry 1972; 26:469–473.
38. Culebras A. Update on disorders of sleep and the sleep-wake cycle. Psychiatr Clin North Am 1992; 15:467–489.
39. Nauta WJ, Haymaker W. Hypothalamic nuclei and fiber connections. In: Haymaker W, Anderson E, Nauta WJH, eds. The Hypothalamus. Springfield, IL: Charles C Thomas, 1969:136.
40. Jurko MF, Andy OJ, Webster CL. Disordered sleep patterns following thalamotomy. Clin Electroencephalogr 1971; 2:213–217.
41. Hachinski V, Mamelak M, Norris JW. Sleep morphology and prognosis in acute cerebrovascular lesions. In: Meyer JS, Lechner H, Reivich M, eds. Cerebral Vascular Disease. Amsterdam: Excerpta Medica, 1977.
42. Culebras A, Feldman RG, Merk FB. Cytoplasmic inclusion bodies within neurons of the thalamus in myotonic dystrophy. J Neurol Sci 1973; 19:319–329.
43. Culebras A, Podolsky S, Leopold NA. Absence of sleep-related growth hormone elevations in myotonic dystrophy. Neurology 1977; 27:165–167.
44. Lugaresi E, Medori R, Montagna P, et al. Fatal familial insomnia and dysautonomia with selective degeneration of thalamic nuclei. N Engl J Med 1986; 315:997–1003.
45. Lugaresi E. The thalamus and insomnia. Neurology 1992; 42(suppl 6):28–33.
46. von Economo C. Sleep as a problem of localization. J Nerv Ment Dis 1930; 71:249–259.
47. Culebras A, Magaña R. Neurologic disorders and sleep disturbances. Sem Neurol 1987; 7(3):277–285.
48. Chesson AL, Levine SN, Kong LS, Lee SC. Neuroendocrine evaluation in Kleine-Levin syndrome: evidence of reduced dopaminergic tone during periods of hypersomnolence. Sleep 1991; 14:226–232.

49. Bremer F. Cerveau isolé et physiologie du sommeil. C Roy Soc Biol (Paris) 1935; 118:1235–1242.
50. Caplan LR. Top of the basilar syndrome. Neurology 1980; 30:72–79.
51. McKee AC, Levine DN, Kowall NW, Richardson EP. Peduncular hallucinosis associated with isolated infarction of the substantia nigra pars reticulata. Ann Neurol 1990; 27:500–504.
52. Aldrich MS, Naylor MW. Narcolepsy associated with lesions of the diencephalon. Neurology 1989; 39:1505–1508.
53. Fernández JM, Sadaba F, Villaverde FJ, Alvaro LC, Cortina C. Cataplexy associated with midbrain lesion. Neurology 1995; 45:393–394.
54. Forcadas MJ, Zarranz JJ. Insomnio y alucinaciones tras lesiones vasculares del tegmento protuberancial en et hombre. Neurologia 1994; 9:211–223.
55. Autret A, Laffont F, Toffol B, Cathala HP. A syndrome of REM and nonREM sleep reduction and lateral gaze paresis after medial tegmental pontine stroke. Arch Neurol 1988; 45:1236–1242.
56. Plum F, Swanson A. Abnormalities in central regulation of respiration in acute and convalescent poliomyelitis. Arch Neurol Psychiatry 1958; 80:267–285.
57. Steljes DG, Kryger MH, Kirk BW, Millar TW. Sleep in postpolio syndrome. Chest 1990; 98:133–140.
58. Dean AC, Graham BA, Dalakas M. Sleep apnea in patients with postpolio syndrome. Ann Neurol 1998; 43:661–664.
59. Balk RA, Hiller FC, Lucas EA, Scrima L, Wilson FJ, Wooten V. Sleep apnea and the Arnold-Chiari malformation. Am Rev Respir Dis 1985; 132:929–930.
60. Bonekat HW, Andersen G, Squires J. Obstructive disordered breathing during sleep in patients with spinal cord injury. Paraplegia 1990; 28:292–398.
61. Braun SR, Giovannoni R, Levin AB, Harvey RF. Oxygen saturation during sleep in patients with spinal cord injury. Am J Phys Med 1982; 61:302–309.
62. Culebras A. Sleep and neuromuscular disorders. Neurologic Clinics 1996; 14:791–805.
63. Culebras A. Clinical Handbook of Sleep Disorders. Boston: Butterworth-Heinemann, 1996.

3

Disorders of Development and Maturation of Sleep, and Sleep Disorders in Infancy, Childhood, and Cerebral Palsy

Stephen H. Sheldon
Children's Memorial Hospital
and Northwestern University Medical School
Chicago, Illinois

INTRODUCTION

Disorders of the brain are often associated with severe sleep disturbances. Frequently, children with neurological disabilities experience chronic sleep–wake problems related to circadian timing of sleep, sleep-related seizure disorders, sleep-related movement disorders and sleep-related breathing disorders. Many respond poorly to traditional therapeutic intervention. Established treatments include behavioral management, chronotherapy, phototherapy, faded response cost programs, sedatives, hypnotics, and antidepressants. These are often unsuccessful in the youngster with a chronic disabling condition of the central nervous system (CNS). Some therapeutic approaches may even exacerbate symptoms or result in respite for only a few days.

Presenting symptoms can range from profound sleep-onset difficulties at desired bedtimes, inability to consolidate sleep, inability to maintain sleep, irregular sleep–wake schedules, rapidly changing sleep–wake schedules, obstructive sleep apnea syndrome, problems with central control of breathing, seizures, movement disorders, and arousal disorders. Presence of multiple symptoms is the rule, rather than exception. Sleep deprivation and fragmentation of sleep continuity occurs and considerable performance problems, as well as delay in the response to rehabilitative efforts, can result. Interestingly, not only do these disorders of sleep and the sleep–wake cycle deeply affect the patient and his or her quality of life, but they often result in sleep disturbances and decreased quality of life for the entire family.

This chapter addresses normal development and CNS, anatomical correlates, and the effect that specific CNS abnormalities might have on sleep and the sleep–wake cycle. Finally, suggestions regarding management are considered.

NORMAL AND ABNORMAL DEVELOPMENTAL AND ANATOMICAL CORRELATES OF THE CNS AND SLEEP

The CNS is the predominate organ system governing sleep, its components, and the sleep–wake cycle. Major CNS alterations occur throughout fetal life, neonatal life, infancy, and childhood. Understanding these changes is essential in assessing the patient with CNS dysfunction during wakefulness and during sleep. Indeed, a comprehensive awareness of maturational changes during sleep may provide insight into management.

Genetic and environmental factors are important in determining morphological and electrophysiological development of the CNS. Differentiation begins very early in the evolution of the embryo as a thickening of the dorsal ectoderm into the neural plate. This single layer of cells rapidly enlarges in number, stratifies, and develops two folds and a neural groove. This central groove fuses to become the neural tube giving rise to the substance of all neural elements whose cell bodies and supporting elements lie within the brain and spinal cord (1).

Early in the fourth postconceptional (PC) week, the prosencephalon subdivides the forebrain into the telencephalon and diencephalon. Telencephalon represents primordial development of the cerebral hemispheres, and diencephalon is destined to become the area containing the optic vesicles. Rhombencephalon develops later into the cerebellum and pons. Myelencephalon is the primitive medulla oblongata and matures somewhat later in embryogenesis.

During regional differentiation, structural flexure begins. Three regions can be identified: cephalic flexure (region of the midbrain), cervical flexure (junction of the brain and spinal cord), and pontine flexure (junction of the metencephalon and myelencephalon). In addition, the lumen of the neural tube undergoes dramatic changes during this time which correspond to regional specialization. The lumen in the area of the telencephalon extends into the paired future cerebral hemispheres and will ultimately become the lateral ventricles. The lumen within the telencephalon and diencephalon will become the third ventricle. Cerebral aqueduct develops from the lumen in the mesencephalon. The lumen of the metencephalon and myelencephalon becomes the fourth ventricle.

Neuronal activity appears to be important in migration of neurons to appropriate positions within the CNS, degree of dendritic branching, and strength of synaptic interconnections (2). Mitosis and migration continue throughout development, and completion of location of individual neurons occurs about one year after PC term. Two internal processes result in a high degree of neuronal activity: the waking state and active—rapid-eye-movement (REM)—sleep. It is possible that these two states are important during prenatal and early postnatal life for appropriate ultrastructural development of the CNS.

Centers responsible for control of sleep and the sleep–wake cycles are contained in areas that will develop from the diencephalon. Appropriate diencephalic maturation is essential for normal sleep to occur. All neuronal activity that eventually reaches the cortex passes through the diencephalon, with the sole exception of that originating from olfaction. The third ventricle is contained within the diencephalon. During the seventh week of development, a small evagination appears from the caudal wall of the third ventricle. This eventually becomes glandular and forms the pineal body, which is responsible for secretion of melatonin.

Melatonin plays an important role in regulating the sleep–wake cycle, presumably through entrainment to light–dark cycling. Secretion is highly responsive to afferent neural activity via the retinohypothalamic tract. It increases in a dark environment and decreases when the retina is exposed to light. Although data regarding the function of melatonin are conflicting, evidence exists that it affects the timing of sleep through its effect on circadian organization (3). Exogenous melatonin has been noted to be useful in regulating sleep in some sleep disorders (4) and in improving sleep in some neurologically handicapped children (5). It seems likely, therefore, that disorders of development of the diencephalon as well as acquired disorders that affect development or function of cells in the caudal wall of the third ventricle can result in significant sleep–wake disorders.

After the seventh PC week, thalamic regions undergo differentiation and neuronal fibers separate the massive gray matter of the walls of the thalamus into numerous thalamic nuclei. Similarly, the walls of the hypothalamus contain hypothalamic nuclei, the optic chiasm, suprachiasmatic nucleus, and the neural lobe of the stalk of the body of the pituitary gland. The hypothalamus eventually becomes the executive region for regulation of all autonomic activity including core body temperature, temperature regulation, and sleep. Since the suprachiasmatic nucleus becomes the governing region for circadian timing of many major physiological functions (the biological clock), it seems clear that dysfunctional development of, or injury to, the ventral region of the diencephalon can result in profound symptoms related to the sleep–wake cycle.

Cerebral hemispheres become prominent during the sixth PC week. They expand rapidly until they cover the diencephalon and mesencephalon. Telencephalon becomes the most specialized and complex portion of the brain. Telencephalon can be quite sensitive to changes in intrauterine environment. In the presence of decreased neuronal electrical activity secondary to hypoxemia from any cause, abnormal concentrations of cellular elements, decreased dendritic branching, and lack of synaptic strength to develop essential and mature neural networks may result.

DISORDERS IN DEVELOPMENTAL MATURATION: NEUROANATOMICAL CORRELATES

Culebras (6) has comprehensively described neuroanatomical and neurological correlates of a wide variety of sleep abnormalities. Lesions of the medial mesencephalon almost invariably cause a reduction in the level of alertness. Symptomatic cataplexy, characterized by active inhibition of skeletal muscle tone, has been described in patients with rostral brainstem tumors that invade the floor of the third ventricle (7). Disorders of the lower mesencephalon and upper pons tegmentum involving the peri–locus coeruleus region are responsible for symptoms of REM sleep without atonia (8) whereas extensive pontine tegmental lesions cause a reduction in total sleep time, alterations in or abolition of non-REM sleep states and REM sleep, and paralysis of lateral gaze (9).

Disorders involving the medullary regions of the CNS commonly affect respiratory centers. A wide variety of sleep-related breathing problems are seen in youngsters with Arnold-Chiari malformation (10,11). Central apnea, increased periodic breathing during REM and non-REM sleep, central hypoventilation syndrome, and prolonged expiratory apneas can occur. If motor centers controlling pharyngeal musculature are involved, obstructive sleep apnea may also be present.

Many other correlations can be identified. Hypothalamic lesions have been associated with hypersomnia; diffuse lesions of the thalamus lead to either ipsilateral decrease or complete abolition of sleep spindles and represent a useful electrographic sign of thalamic abnormalities (12). The cerebral hemispheres, although not primordial in the generation or maintenance of non-REM and REM sleep, do have a modulating influence. Patients with extensive cortical laminar necrosis fail to exhibit slow waves or spindles during non-REM sleep, but can express cortical desynchronization during REM sleep (13). Finally, space-occupying lesions of the CNS may cause sleep–wake disturbances or specific sleep disorders by virtue of their location. They may also cause symptoms indirectly through the development of increased intracranial pressure, hydrocephalus, or both.

DISORDERS IN DEVELOPMENTAL MATURATION: POLYSOMNOGRAPHIC CORRELATES

Although still in its infancy, the clinical discipline of pediatric sleep medicine and the study of sleep disorders in infants and children are becoming increasingly focused on dysfunctions of the brain. Concentration on the study of the sleeping brain has been termed by Culebras as "neurosomnology" (14). Physiological function of most other organ systems differs significantly from that in the waking state and there are clear ontogenetic changes that occur in sleep and its structure. Studying longitudinal changes of multiple physiological variables during sleep in the laboratory might be termed "developmental polysomnography" (15). Evaluation of maturation of sleep within the context of normal and abnormal human development might provide a sensitive method of analysis.

It has been shown that the EEG is an excellent method for measuring brain maturation (16). Each conceptional age reveals a characteristic pattern. The important features of normal EEG ontogeny, therefore, tend to reflect normal development. An apparent delay of the appearance of these EEG patterns might reflect an arrest or delay in maturation of the CNS. It has been proposed that close attention to stages of brain maturation in normal and abnormal EEGs, as well as the normal progression of state development during sleep, might allow more accurate timing of brain insult in infants with neurological sequelae.

Comprehensive polysomnography utilizing an EEG array that provides greater detail than the standard montage recommended for adult polysomnography is recommended for the neonatal and pediatric patient. However, diagnosing ontogenetic EEG variations must be performed with caution, since abnormalities in the EEG reflect general pathophysiological processes but show little specificity for particular disease (17).

Other polysomnographic variables can be important in assessment of developmental maturation. Recording of eye movements and EMG along with EEG might improve specificity. Recording of eye movements during sleep provides important information regarding identification of state. Eye-movement density and bursts of saccades may hold special significance in prediction of mental development and morbidity secondary to neonatal illness. Becker and Thoman (18) evaluated the occurrence of "REM storms" in newborn infants and again at 3, 6, and 12 months of chronological age. The amount of rapid eye movements within each 10-second interval of active sleep was rated on a scale based on frequency and intensity of eye movements. The Bayley scale of mental development was administered to the cohort of infants at 12 months of age. Interestingly, a significant negative correlation was found between the frequency of REM storms and Bayley scores. By 6 months of age, REM storms seemed to express dysfunction or delay in the development of central inhibitory feedback control for sleep organization and phasic sleep-related activities.

The degree of phasic EMG activity during sleep may also reflect maturity of the developing brainstem. Gross movements, localized body movements, and phasic muscle activity are controlled by the CNS at different organizational levels. Phasic motor activity is ontogenetically more simple and decreases early during development. Gross movements are quite complex and require a greater degree of central integration. The type and frequency of muscle activity during sleep might, therefore, add to information regarding integrity of the CNS. Hakamada and coworkers (19) studied various motor activity in term newborns with significant illnesses. Generalized body movements, localized tonic movements, and generalized phasic movements were evaluated. Patients with minimally depressed EEG background activity showed an increase in generalized movements and localized tonic movements during quiet sleep. In contrast, patients with markedly severe EEG abnormalities showed an increase in phasic movements. It was concluded that a significant decrease in generalized body movements or an increase in generalized phasic muscle activity might indicate a poor prognosis for particular infants. However, the presence of even small amounts of localized tonic movements suggested preservation of cortical function. Nonetheless, diagnostic use of polysomnography and its components becomes most cost-effective when applied to specific problems.

SPECIFIC SLEEP DISORDERS IN INFANTS AND CHILDREN

Sleep disorders that occur in adults also occur in children. Disorders of sleep and the sleep–wake cycle differ from adult disorders in etiology, pathophysiology, morbidity, and treatment. Indeed, symptomatology can be dramatically different, and childhood sleep disorders are frequently overlooked or overshadowed by clinical problems that appear and are evaluated during the day. It must be remembered that disordered sleep can underlie meaningful daytime symptoms, and can exacerbate other medical disorders.

There is often considerable delay in diagnosis of disordered sleep in the neonate, infant, and child. Brouillette and colleagues (20) have described significant delays in the diagnosis of sleep-disordered breathing, and have demonstrated profound morbidity. In 22 patients with documented obstructive sleep apnea, mean delay in referral for 20 patients first evaluated after the neonatal period was 23 ± 15 months. Almost three-quarters of patients studied developed serious sequelae, including cor pulmonale, failure to thrive, permanent neurological deficits, behavioral disturbances, hypersomnolence, and developmental abnormalities.

In this section, common primary sleep-related disorders in children are discussed, including sleep-related breathing disorders, sleep-related seizures, partial arousal disorders, movement disorders associated with sleep, and sleep–wake schedule disorders. Focus is placed on clinical presentation, laboratory diagnosis, and management considerations.

Sleep-Related Paroxysmal Disorders

Sleep-related paroxysmal disorders may be differentiated into epileptiform and nonepileptiform abnormalities. Interictal EEG evaluations may or may not be helpful in diagnosis. Often, spells do not occur in the laboratory and comprehensive assessments and management must be based on clinical grounds. Continuous monitoring of EEG activity and other physiological functions during polysomnography in the sleep laboratory may be quite helpful in differentiating seizure disorders from nonepileptic paroxysmal disturbances.

Sleep-Related Paroxysmal Disorders Associated with Seizures

A wide variety of paroxysmal motor disorders may occur during sleep. These recurring spells must be differentiated from sleep-related nonepileptic motor activity. The sleep of patients with true seizures is typically fragmented (21). Abnormal sleep patterns may, however, indicate a toxic effect of medication or CNS injury.

Interictal epileptiform activity tends to increase during light stages of non-REM sleep and to be suppressed during REM sleep. This is particularly true in patients suffering from partial complex seizures (22). Sleep deprivation increases the rate of focal interictal epileptiform discharges, most markedly in stage 2 non-REM sleep. Some epileptic seizures appear almost exclusively during sleep—for example, the Landau-Kleffner syndrome, manifested by continuous spike-and-wave activity during sleep in young children and associated with hyperkinesia, neuropsychological disturbances, and progressive aphasia (23).

There is much literature confirming the observation that epileptic seizures occur in specific relation to the sleep–wake cycle (24). Sleep deprivation is a common mechanism to promote seizures in the laboratory, especially in patients with temporal-lobe seizure disorders (25). Although absence seizures are recognized clinically only during the day, fluttering of the eyelids can be observed during sleep in conjunction with paroxysmal bursts of three-cycles-per-second spike-and-wave activity (26). Partial complex seizures originating in the frontal lobe occur most characteristically during non-REM sleep. Of the sleep-related complex seizures in patients studied by Cadilhac (27), almost two-thirds occurred during non-REM sleep. Approximately 16% of seizures studied were isolated to REM sleep, and 20% occurred in both non-REM and REM sleep states. There is also a strong correlation between seizures and sleep in patients with benign partial epilepsy with centrotemporal spikes (Rolandic epilepsy) (24).

In addition to the facilitatory effect of sleep on seizure activity, seizure frequency may be affected by the presence of other sleep-related disorders. For example, six of seven patients with obstructive sleep apnea syndrome and partial epilepsy studied by Divinsky and colleagues (28) experienced a significant reduction in the frequency of seizure activity and severity after successful treatment of the sleep-related breathing abnormality.

Clinical differentiation of epileptic and nonepileptic spells that occur during sleep can often be difficult. Reviewing this issue, Stores (29) was able to divide these diagnostic dilemmas into three categories. The first group consists of nonepileptic primary sleep disorders often associated with motor phenomena and with similar presentations. These include some nightmares and sleep terrors, non-REM-sleep partial-arousal disorders, and REM-sleep motor disorders. The second group comprises primary sleep disorders with motor components that can be incorrectly diagnosed as epilepsy and includes the partial-arousal disorders, REM-sleep motor disorder, sleep-related rhythmic-movement disorders (such as jactatio capitis nocturnes), some symptoms associated with obstructive sleep apnea, automatic behaviors, idiopathic CNS hypersomnia, and sleep-related enuresis. Finally, in the third group are some epileptic disorders that occur during sleep and may be mistaken for sleep disorders. These consists of nocturnal complex partial seizures of the temporal lobe and, particularly of frontal-lobe origin, nocturnal hypnogenic dystonia, episodic nocturnal wanderings, and nonconvulsive status epilepticus.

Hypnogenic Paroxysmal Dystonia

Hypnogenic paroxysmal dystonia, first described by Lugaresi in 1981 (30), is a rare disorder characterized by stereotypical, choreoathetotic movements and dystonic posturing during non-REM sleep. Symptoms may begin in childhood and be mistaken for normal (or abnormal) behavior patterns or other stereotypical movement disorders. Episodes may be brief, lasting less than a minute, or prolonged, persisting for hours. The eyes are often open and vocalizations may occur. If episodes occur frequently or are recurrent during a single sleep period, significant sleep disruption may occur. There are rhythmic, sometimes violent, stereotypical movements (e.g., kicking, thrashing) of the limbs and/or trunk associated with dystonic posturing of the hands, feet, arms, legs, and/or face. At the termination of an episode, patients may be coherent, but rapidly return to sleep.

Polysomnography usually reveals episodes arising out of stage 2 non-REM sleep (although it has been reported to occur in slow-wave sleep as well). An EEG pattern of arousal may occur a few seconds preceding an episode. Significant movement artifact is seen in the EEG. Clear epileptiform activity during a spell is somewhat controversial. Radiographic studies and magnetic resonance imaging are notably normal. It is unknown whether hypnogenic paroxysmal dystonia is associated with central nervous system (or other) pathology.

Symptoms generally run a chronic course and may persist for many years. Carbamazepine, in small doses, has ameliorated symptoms in some patients.

Sleep-Related Nonepileptic Paroxysmal Disorders: The Parasomnias

Parasomnias are classified as dysfunctions associated with sleep, sleep stages, or partial arousals from sleep (31). The disorders in this group have strikingly dissimilar presentations but can share many clinical and physiological characteristics. Often parasomnias present clear symptomatology (e.g., sleepwalking, headbanging, bruxism). Manifestations arise early in childhood and may appear to parents and health care practitioners as normal, benign, or behavioral in origin. As the child ages, benign characteristics can become exaggerated and dramatic. However, few pathophysiological abnormalities can be identified, despite occasionally severe paroxysmal features (32). As with all other disorders of sleep and wakefulness, evaluation begins with a comprehensive history and physical examination. Special attention must be paid to a detailed description of the events.

Neurodevelopmental landmarks must be carefully assessed. Sleep–wake schedules, habits, and patterns require delineation. Morning wake time, evening bedtime, bedtime rituals, and naptime rituals should be described. The presence of excessive daytime sleepiness, snoring, or restlessness during sleep should be ascertained. Information about the presence (or absence) of concurrent medical illnesses and whether the patient is taking any medications or drugs should be obtained in the clinical interview.

A complete physical examination must be performed, and emphasis placed on a comprehensive neurological and developmental assessment. The existence of developmental delays or symptoms suggestive of neurological disorders might indicate an organic basis for the patient's presenting symptoms. Evidence of other medical disorders should be assessed as signs of possible contributing or coexisting factors.

Laboratory evaluations should be guided by the presenting signs and symptoms. A urine drug screen may be helpful if it is suspected that the symptoms are side effects of medication. Polysomnography is often indicated. An expanded EEG electrode array is recommended. A more extensive EEG montage than typically recorded during polysomnography is often helpful in differentiating a non-epileptic parasomnia from sleep-related seizures. Concomitant video recording of the patient while sleeping is indispensable and can clearly demonstrate motor manifestations and chronicle stereotypical movements. Attempts should be made to obtain at least 400 minutes of natural *nocturnal* sleep. It is often helpful to have the patient drink fluids and avoid urination prior to settling since bladder distention may precipitate some parasomnias. The need for all-night as well as routine EEG recordings and radiographic studies depends on the presenting situation, nighttime manifestations, and clinical symptomatology.

Sleep–Wake Transition Disorders

These parasomnias occur mainly during transitions from wakefulness to sleep, from sleep to wakefulness, or from one sleep stage to another. All can occur in otherwise healthy children and may be regarded as manifestations of altered normal physiology. Symptomatology can vary from mild movements during sleep to violent, alarming behavior. All have the potential to result in discomfort, pain, injury, anxiety, embarrassment, and disturbance of sleep.

Rhythmic movement disorders: non-epileptic stereotypical parasomnias Although the phenomenon of stereotypical movements during sleep has been recognized for many years, little is known of the etiology. Stereotypical nonepileptic parasomnias are characterized by repetitive, meaningless movements or behaviors. Large muscle groups are involved, and manifestations include rhythmic, repetitive movements such as body-rocking, head-banging, head-rolling, and body-shuttling. They are typically associated with transition from wakefulness to sleep, may be sustained into light sleep, and/or occur after arousal from sleep. Children are usually normal—developmentally, behaviorally, and medically. Movements may be alarming, and parents often become concerned for the child's physical and mental well-being. Injury sometimes occurs.

Stereotypical movements occur in normal infants and children. Lack of rhythmic activity during infancy has occasionally been associated with developmental delays. When stereotypical movements during wakefulness persist into older childhood and adolescence, a coexisting psychogenic component may be present. Stereotypical movements may be a form of attention-getting behavior or a mechanism of self-stimulation or self-soothing, in developmentally disabled children.

Rhythmic movements can be observed in two-thirds of normal children by 9 months of age. The incidence of head-banging ranges from 3 to 6.5%, body-rocking from 19.1 to 21%, and head-rolling in 6.3% of the normal population. By 18 months of age, the prevalence decreases to less than 50%, and to approximately 8% by 4 years of age. This consistent decrease and spontaneous resolution of symptoms as the child grows and develops would be consistent with a maturational origin of the disorder.

At times, motor activity and head-banging are violent and physical injury can occur, although it is uncommon. Cutaneous ecchymosis and callus formation can result. However, more serious injuries, including subdural hematoma and retinal petechiae, have been reported. Rhythmic movements usually decrease in intensity and often resolve spontaneously between 2 and 4 years of age. Rarely, symptoms persist into adolescence and adulthood.

Diagnosis is based on identification of characteristic symptoms in the absence of other medical and/or psychiatric disorders. Polysomnography demonstrates typical rhythmic movements during the immediate presleep period and may persist into stage 1 non-REM sleep. Occasionally, activity is noted after spontaneous arousal. It can occur during slow-wave sleep, but it is rare during REM sleep. Focal, paroxysmal, and/or epileptiform EEG activity associated with the stereotypical activity are absent; however, a full-montage EEG may be necessary to rule out epilepsy. Sleep architecture, stage progression, and stage volumes are typically normal.

Parasomnias Associated with Slow-Wave Sleep: Arousal Disorders

Arousal disorders are thought to be due to impaired or "partial" arousal from slow-wave sleep. A hierarchical model may exist, since a continuum of manifestations of each of these disorders of sleep seems to be present. Symptoms most often begin in childhood and resolve spontaneously, although occasionally they persist into adolescence and adulthood. Manifestations are quite alarming, and injury often occurs.

Arousal disorders present with bizarre, dramatic symptoms and share a number of features. All seem to occur during stage 3–4 sleep; confusion, disorientation, and amnesia for the events are present; and episodes can be precipitated by external stimuli. In contrast, forced arousal from REM sleep is more often followed by rapid awakening, clear thought processes, and vivid dream recall.

Partial-arousal disorders occur more frequently during periods of stress, in the presence of fever, after sleep deprivation, and in patients with hypersomnolence syndromes. Partial arousals normally occur at the end of slow-wave sleep periods, during ascent to lighter sleep stages. Because of the depth of slow-wave sleep and the high arousal threshold in children, these arousal disorders may represent conflicting interaction between the mechanisms generating slow-wave sleep and arousal. Chronobiological triggers that control sleep-stage cycling may be more likely to result in a partial arousal if the sleep schedule is chaotic. There may be internal desynchronization and the internal arousal stimulus may come at the "wrong time," resulting in incomplete arousal and manifest characteristics of both states. As the child develops, these CNS mechanisms mature, synchronization occurs, and symptoms resolve spontaneously.

Confusional arousals: sleep drunkenness Confusional arousals, or sleep drunkenness, consists of partial arousals from slow-wave sleep during the first half of the sleep period. Episodes are sudden and startling, and may be precipitated by forced awakenings. Children may appear to be awake during the episode, but do not respond appropriately to commands and resist being consoled. Confusion and disorientation are prominent. Attempts to abort the "attack" may in fact make the symptoms more severe and violent.

Factors that result in increased slow-wave sleep or impair arousal may precipitate or exacerbate confusional arousals. Hypersomnia secondary to rebound from sleep deprivation, narcolepsy syndrome, idiopathic hypersomnia, or obstructive sleep apnea may exacerbate symptoms. Confusional arousals are frequently seen in patients with narcolepsy syndrome after prolonged daytime naps (those longer than 60 minutes that contain slow-wave sleep). Stress, anxiety, fever, and excessive exercise may precipitate attacks. Organic pathology is rarely noted, although CNS lesions of the periventricular gray matter, reticular activating system, or posterior hypothalamus have been reported in some patients. Injuries during confusional arousals are common if there is displacement of the patient from the bed.

The onset of symptoms is usually prior to 5 years of age. Children gradually arouse from slow wave sleep, and may moan or mumble unintelligibly. Symptoms then escalate significantly. Patients may thrash about in bed or fall from the bed to the floor. During the episode, the child appears profoundly confused and disoriented. Combativeness and aggressiveness may occur and consolation or restraint may result in exacerbation of symptoms. Episodes may be brief, lasting for only a few minutes, or prolonged, lasting for several hours. There is usually retrograde and/or anterograde amnesia of the event. There may be associated night terrors or somnambulism. Enuresis may occur during or following the episode, resulting in difficulties in differentiating these spells from partial complex seizures.

Diagnosis is based on identification of confusion, disorientation, agitation, and/or combativeness upon arousal, most often during the first one-third to one-half of the night. Associated amnesia of the event is present. Clearly identifiable medical and/or psychiatric disorders are rarely present on clinical evaluation. Partial complex seizure disorders with confusional automatisms need to be ruled out. Polysomnography reveals sudden arousal from slow-wave sleep, brief periods of delta activity, stage 1 theta patterns, recurrent microsleeps, and/or poorly reactive alpha activity. Focal, paroxysmal, and/or epileptiform activity are absent from the EEG. Symptoms may peak during middle childhood, and then undergo spontaneous remission. The clinical course is usually benign (although frightening). Physical injury can occur and the child must be protected from trauma during the episode.

Somnambulism: sleepwalking Somnambulism may vary in presentation from simple sitting up in bed to agitated running and aggressive, violent behavior during sleep. A complex series of automatic behaviors are manifested that on the surface may appear to be purposeful. As with other partial-arousal disorders, somnambulistic episodes occur out of slow-wave sleep, during the first third of the sleep period. Episodes may be quite alarming. Patients are uncoordinated and clumsy during the walking episode. Injuries are common. Because of the high incidence of trauma during such events, agitated somnambulism should be considered a potentially fatal disorder and the major goal of management is to protect the child from harm.

Somnambulism has been reported to occur in 1 to 15% of the population. It occurs with greatest frequency during childhood, decreasing significantly during adolescence, and is uncommon in adults. Because episodes vary in frequency, intensity, and length, parental reports are unreliable; the true incidence is therefore unknown. There appears to be an equal sex distribution. There also appears to be a significant familial pattern, but clear genetic transmission has not been identified.

Although somnambulism usually begins in middle childhood—between 4 and 8 years of age—onset may occur at any time after the child develops the ability to walk. Symptoms range from simple sitting up in bed to extremely agitated, semipurposeful automatisms and frantic running. Most often, the child will wander around the house and can perform complex tasks, such as unlocking doors, taking food from the refrigerator, and eating—he or she may even leave the house. Often the behaviors are meaningless and unusual. Verbalizations may occur, but are usually garbled, confused, and meaningless. Eyes are often open and the child may appear awake, but behaviors are only semipurposeful. There may be choreiform movements of the arms and head. Often, enuretic episodes occur and the child may urinate (or attempt to urinate) in unusual places around the house. During a somnambulistic spell the child is extremely difficult to wake, although complete arousal is possible, in which case confusion and disorientation are usually present. Motor activity can cease spontaneously, and the child may lie down and return to sleep in unusual places around the home or return to bed without ever becoming alert.

A number of factors may precipitate somnambulistic events, notably fever and sleep deprivation. Any disorder that can produce significant disruption of slow-wave sleep, such as obstructive sleep apnea, may trigger sleepwalking, as can urinary bladder distention in the susceptible patient or external noise. A number of medications can exacerbate the disorder, including thioridazine, prolixin, perphenazine, desipramine, and chloral hydrate.

Polysomnography typically reveals an arousal from stage 3 or 4 sleep during the first half of the sleep period. Most of the background EEG activity is obscured by muscle artifact. Seizure activity is notably absent.

Although clinically, difficult, somnambulism should be differentiated from other disorders of arousal, such as confusional arousals and night terrors. Displacement from the bed and calm nocturnal wanderings are less common with confusional arousals. Night terrors are more typically associated with the appearance of intense fear and panic and are less likely to be associated with displacement from bed (although displacement from bed is more common with night terrors than nightmares). Intense autonomic discharges and an initial scream herald a sleep terror and are not present in somnambulism. Nocturnal seizure disorders typically reveal epileptiform discharges during the events; however, the interictal EEG may be normal. REM-sleep behavior disorder, as described in children, is associated with clear verbalizations and seemingly purposeful movements.

Sleep terrors: pavor nocturnus Sleep terrors are third in a continuum of partial arousals from slow-wave sleep. The onset of a sleep terror (in contrast to the gradual onset of confusional arousals) is sudden, abrupt, striking, and frightening. These arousals are associated with profound autonomic discharges and behavioral manifestations of intense fear. As with other partial arousals, the exact prevalence of sleep terrors is unknown.

Onset of symptoms is usually between 2 and 4 years of age. Although most frequent during childhood, sleep terrors can occur at any age. As with other nonepileptic parasomnias, precipitating factors include fever, bladder distention, sleep deprivation, and CNS-depressant medication. Symptoms tend to significantly decrease during puberty and rarely persist into adolescence and adulthood. Psychopathology is rare in children.

A sleep terror begins suddenly. The child typically sits upright in bed and emits a piercing scream. Severe autonomic discharge occurs. Eyes are usually widely open and pupils may appear dilated. Tachycardia, tachypnea, diaphoresis, and increased muscle tone are present. During the episode the child is unresponsive to efforts to console, and parental efforts often exacerbate autonomic and motor activity. During a spell, the youngster may run hysterically around the house, sometimes running wildly into walls, furniture, or windows. Episodes of extreme agitation are commonly associated with injury. Unintelligible vocalizations and enuresis can occur. As in other partial-arousal disorders, if the child is awakened from a spell, he or she may be confused and disoriented and may not remember the event. In contrast to confusional arousals, episodes of sleep terrors are usually brief, lasting only a few minutes, and subside spontaneously.

Diagnosis is based on identification of the above symptoms and exclusion of organic pathology. Polysomnography reveals sudden arousal from slow-wave sleep during the first third of the major sleep period. Sleep terrors, however, can occur out of slow-wave sleep at any time during the night. Partial arousals without motor manifestation occur more frequently in children with sleep terrors than in normal children. Autonomic discharges during these partial arousals are identified by the presence of tachycardia without full-blown symptoms.

Sleep terrors require differentiation from sleep-related epilepsy with automatisms. In these patients, EEG may show abnormal discharges from the temporal lobe, although nasopharyngeal leads may be required to identify the focus of abnormal activity. Epileptic events may also be distinguished from disorders of partial arousal by the presence of a combination of clinical features and stereotypical behaviors, and the fact that they may occur during any part of the sleep period as well as during wakefulness. Identification of epileptiform activity, however, does not completely rule out the presence of a partial arousal, since they may occur concomitantly in the same patient.

Therapeutic Considerations

There is no clear consensus regarding when a partial-arousal parasomnia requires treatment. Symptoms are usually mild, occur less than once per month, and result in injury to neither the child nor the parents. In mild cases, explanation of partial-arousal disorders and reassurance of the parents may be all that is necessary. Sleep hygiene should also be discussed. Parents should be encouraged to let the event run its course and to intervene minimally. Interventions should focus on preventing injury and simply guiding the child back to bed. Too vigorous intervention may prolong the episode.

Parents can be alerted of a quiet somnambulistic episode by an alarm system (for example, a bell on the doorknob of the child's room). Appropriate sleep hygiene is essential. Sleep deprivation should be avoided and regular sleep–wake schedules maintained. Brief daytime naps might be attempted, and a period of quiet activity or relaxation techniques instituted prior to bedtime. Fluids after the evening meal should be limited and the child encouraged to empty his or her bladder immediately prior to bedtime. Fevers, if present, should be appropriately treated.

Severity of partial arousals are considered moderate when symptoms occur less than once per week and do not result in harm to the patient or to others. In these cases, reassurance and a behavioral approach (including behavior training, enforcement of good sleep hygiene, psychotherapy, and/or hypnosis) have been successful.

In severe cases—when episodes occur almost nightly or are associated with injury—nondrug approaches are considered first. Drug treatment, when used, should be prescribed for a short period of time and be used in conjunction with sleep-hygiene and behavioral management. Medication should be discontinued when symptoms have been under good control for approximately 3–6 months.

The most commonly prescribed medication is diazepam. However, lorazepam or clonazepam in small doses is also quite effective. Dosage should be adjusted to the needs of the child. Prolonged use of medication increases the potential for side effects and complications. The young child generally responds well to both behavioral and medicinal approaches.

Parasomnias Usually Associated with REM Sleep

The parasomnias previously discussed have been related to dysfunctions associated with sleep-state transitions and partial arousal from non-REM stage 3 and 4 sleep. Parasomnias have also been reported to occur out of REM sleep. In many cases, manifestations are dissimilar and can be differentiated on clinical grounds alone. Certain REM-sleep parasomnias, however, may share symptoms with partial-arousal disorders. Some frequently occur in children (e.g., nightmares), while others are extremely rare and have only recently been described in children (e.g., REM-sleep behavior disorder). Discussion of disorders rarely encountered in children is included below because their importance to the practitioner may become clear when they are more completely understood and dysfunction associated with the sleeping state is further delineated in children.

Nightmares: anxiety dreams A nightmare is a frightening dream that may awaken the youngster from REM sleep. There is usually vivid recall of disturbing dream content, anxiety, and mild autonomic manifestations. Often an anxiety dream contains elements of danger to the individual. After sudden arousal from REM sleep, the youngster is oriented to the environment with clear sensorium. Dream content usually involves an experience of immediate and credible threat to survival, security, or self-esteem.

Dream anxiety attacks occur in REM sleep, and are often associated with the longest, most intense REM period, during the last third of the night. Because of REM hypotonia, major body movements are rare; however, REM-sleep fragmentation, increased phasic activity, and frequent movement arousals and awakening with clear mentation are typical. Manifestations are generally mild and vocalizations are rare. Although autonomic activity increases during nightmares, it is generally mild, differentiating it from a sleep terror. There is good recall of the disturbing dream and the child functions well upon waking. Sleep terrors are brief and return to sleep is rapid after cessation of the spell. With nightmares, however, a prolonged waking episode with difficulty returning to sleep is common. In addition, nightmares are generally not associated with violent outbursts, there is no displacement from the bed (until the child awakens), and injuries are quite rare. Return to sleep is generally delayed, but the child often responds well to parental intervention.

Diagnosis of anxiety dreams is based on the identification of the mild manifestations of disturbing dreams occurring during the early morning hours, absence of intense autonomic activation, clear recall of the dream, appropriate functioning and alertness upon awakening, and a good response to parental interventions. Polysomnography may reveal an abrupt arousal from REM sleep. The REM period from which the child awakens is usually the longest and most intense period of the night. It occurs later in the sleep period, during early morning hours, and is associated with mild tachycardia and tachypnea. Increased eye-movement frequency may be noted. Focal, paroxysmal, and epileptiform EEG activity are absent.

Nightmares must be differentiated from sleep terrors, REM-sleep behavior disorder, and epilepsy. Sleep terrors usually are more vivid, are frightening to the observer, occur during the first third of the sleep period, and are associated with severe autonomic discharges. There is fragmented recall, the child is confused upon waking, somnambulism and agitated sleepwalking is common, and many suffer injuries. REM-sleep behavior disorder has recently been described in children. Symptoms are similar to those seen in the adult patient. In the adult, there is sudden arousal from REM sleep associated with significant purposeful motor activity. Similar symptoms may be seen in patients with posttraumatic stress disorder in which there is state dissociation including, but not limited to, increases in chin muscle tone, phasic activity, major body movements during REM sleep, and periodic limb movements. Partial complex seizures may occur in any stage of sleep or wakefulness, and automatisms and stereotypy are common. Seizure episodes are associated with abnormal EEG activity.

Sleep paralysis Sleep paralysis is characterized by absence of voluntary motor activity at the beginning of a sleep period (hypnogogic) or immediately after awakening (hypnopompic). The patient is conscious and aware of his or her environment, but feels paralyzed. All muscle groups are involved; however, the diaphragm and extraocular muscles are spared. Active inhibition of alpha and gamma motor neurons is present and similar to that seen during REM sleep and cataplexy. Sleep paralysis typically lasts only several minutes and subsides spontaneously. Occasionally, attacks can be aborted by rapid movements of the eyes or by being touched. Hypnogogic or hypnopompic hallucinations are unusual, but can occur and add to anxiety.

Isolated episodes of sleep paralysis can occur in normal individuals. Frequent spells are reported in patients with narcolepsy and in "familial sleep paralysis." Onset is usually during adolescence, but symptoms may begin during childhood. Children have difficulty describing the events and may appear asleep during the episode. Parents are unaware of the child's sleep paralysis since the atonia can be aborted by touching or shaking.

The clinical course varies significantly. Most cases are isolated and may be exacerbated by sleep deprivation, excessive sleepiness, stress, or irregular sleep–wake schedules, or after acute changes in sleep phase. Sleep paralysis runs a more chronic course in patients with narcolepsy and in the familial form of the disorder.

Diagnosis of sleep paralysis is based on identification of presenting symptoms. These may be quite difficult to interpret in children. A youngster complaining to the parent of an inability to "get up" or "wake up" is far more common than a child's reporting inability to move after awakening. Sleep paralysis associated with narcolepsy can be differentiated from the isolated form by the absence of chronic excessive daytime sleepiness, sleep attacks, hypnogogic hallucinations, and cataplexy. Atonic generalized seizures occur during wakefulness and may or may not be associated with changes in levels of consciousness. Syncope occurs during wakefulness as well, and is most commonly associated with altered levels of consciousness.

Polysomnography usually reveals significant decrease in skeletal muscle tone in the presence of a normal waking EEG pattern and conjugate eye movements. Occasionally, patients may enter sleep during an episode of sleep paralysis and reveal an EEG pattern consistent with stage 1 sleep. True sleep-onset REM periods may occur.

REM sleep behavior disorder REM-sleep behavior disorder (RBD), or REM-sleep motor anomaly (RMA), has been described in adults (33). There is evidence that a similar syndrome also occurs during childhood (34). Nonetheless, RBD is an unusual disorder, characterized by the appearance of elaborate, sometimes purposeful movements during REM sleep. There is a paradoxical increase in muscle tone and patients seem to be acting out their dreams. Violent behavior such as punching, kicking, leaping out of bed, and running are reported and often correspond with dream mentation. Injuries to the patient and to bed partners are common.

Cases of RBD have been reported in pediatric patients (34), and further understanding of this disorder may reveal the incidence and prevalence to be higher than current descriptions suggest. The majority of cases are idiopathic; however, neurological disorders have been identified in approximately 40% of affected adults.

Polysomnography reveals increased muscle tone, which persists throughout sleep. There is often a paradoxical increase in muscle tone during REM sleep, increased phasic activity, and excessive limb- or body-jerking. Complex behaviors occur out of REM sleep, but no epileptiform activity is noted on EEG during the complex movements. Interestingly, RBD in adults responds well to benzodiazepines, especially clonazepam.

Management Considerations

Imperative in management of youngsters with nonepileptic partial-arousal disorders is a stepwise approach. Education of parents and reassurance may be the only requirements. It is essential that the child be protected from injury, especially if spells are frequent, there is displacement from the bed, or the child is significantly agitated and violent. Behavioral management includes close attention to sleep hygiene, adequate total sleep time, and limited intake of nocturnal fluids. Fever should be evaluated and treated appropriately. Sleep deprivation should be avoided, and sources of stress and anxiety identified and appropriately addressed. If motor manifestations are present, an alarm system should be established to alert parents or caretakers to episodes—a bell on a doorknob may be all that is needed. If medications are indicated, benzodiazepines are typically the drugs of first choice. Clonazepam in small doses (e.g., 0.25 mg orally at bedtime) is quite effective for both non-REM and REM disorders. Unfortunately, because of the long half-life of clonazepam, a "hangover effect" can occur and the youngster may do poorly and exhibit excessive sleepiness the following day. Lorazepam in similarly small doses has been quite successful. Small doses of diazepam at bedtime may be most appropriate for partial-arousal parasomnias that occur only during the first third of the sleep period. If RBD is suspected, appropriate psychological, neurological, and/or psychiatric evaluations should be considered. As previously stated, RBD has been associated with posttraumatic stress disorder in adults, and preliminary data may support a similar phenomenon in children.

CEREBRAL PALSY

Sleep problems commonly occur in patients with cerebral palsy (CP). Alterations of the sleep–wake cycle and specific primary sleep disorders may increase morbidity. Often, quality of life of the youngster and family is profoundly affected.

Physiological changes occurring during sleep affects specific reflexes in children with CP. Alterations in the H reflex during sleep were studied in 13 children with cerebral palsy (eight with spastic tetraplegia, two with a mixed form of cerebral palsy without spasticity, and three with hypotonic diplegia or tetraplegia) (35). In normal children, the maximum H reflex progressively decreases in amplitude from wakefulness to REM sleep. In hypertonic patients, there is only a slight decrease in the H reflex in non-REM sleep and no significant change in REM sleep; the amplitude of the H reflex is always greater than that in the control group. In the dystonic and hypotonic patients, the results obtained are similar to those of the control group. In spastic patients—as opposed to the control, dystonic, and hypotonic groups—normal balance between the function of supraspinal systems regulating the amplitude of the spinal reflexes during wake and sleep is altered, probably through the scarce functionality of the supraspinal inhibitory structures.

Youngsters with CP are often less physically active than their healthy peers. Children with spastic diplegia were compared to normal controls in an analysis of their physical activity during the day and during sleep (36). It was determined that children with spastic diplegia are considerably less active than their healthy peers. This is often significant in stabilization of the sleep–wake cycle, in which there is a correlation of regularly scheduled physical activity during the day and improvement of sleep at night. Regular exercise as part of a comprehensive sleep-hygiene program is important in stabilization of the sleep–wake cycle and can improve sleep in some youngsters.

Disturbances in the sleep–wake cycle have also been evaluated electroencephalographically in children with CP. Classification of the background EEG was well correlated with the disturbances of sleep cycle, which was also related to the interval after the hypoxic insult (37). The relationship between sleep states and EEG patterns also had a close correlation with the classification and became progressively disturbed with increasing severity of the background EEG. Each grade of the background EEG abnormality had a different prognostic significance according to the time of the recording. The one in the first week offered the best prognostic value. A disturbance of sleep—if it exists—always runs parallel with the course of the disease (38).

Sleep EEG patterns were studied in 23 mentally retarded children with CP (from 4 months to 5 years) and 39 reference mentally retarded children of no abnormality with the exception of psychomotor retardation (39). In the CP cases, there was an absence of EEG patterns characteristic of wakefulness, inability to differentiate non-REM sleep states, absence of non-REM characteristics and non-REM sleep without spindles, and absence of REM sleep. In addition, short sleep times and long waking times during the night were often noted.

Melatonin concentration in blood, urine, or saliva may become a useful marker of the circadian rhythm in disorders of biological rhythms (40). Of particular interest to the pediatric population will be the potential application of melatonin treatment in establishing or re-establishing circadian rhythms in infants and children maintained for long periods under artificial light conditions, as encountered in intensive care units, and in the treatment of sleep and other rhythm disorders associated with developmental delay or blindness. Care must be taken in utilization of melatonin in youngsters with neurological deficits, especially those with intractable seizure disorders. There may be a proconvulsant effect of exogenous melatonin in some children with CP and seizure disorder (41). Until a clear understanding of efficacy and side effects of melatonin is obtained, it should be reserved for youngsters with chronic neurological disabilities not associated with epilepsy and sightless youngsters who are unresponsive to light–dark cycling.

Infants and children with myelomeningocele, hydrocephalus, and Arnold-Chiari malformation often exhibit symptomatic apnea or hypoventilation. In a study of 18 asymptomatic infants, Ward and colleagues (42) have shown that asymptomatic infants with myelomeningocele had longer total sleep time, more episodes of apnea 6 seconds or longer as a percentage of total sleep time, and lower mean heart rate than did control infants. This suggested that asymptomatic infants with myelomeningocele have a high incidence of ventilatory-pattern abnormalities during sleep. This is currently being studied in a multicenter retrospective analysis of respiratory patterns in children with this CNS abnormality.

To assess hypoxic and hypercapneic arousal response in children with myelomeningocele and apnea, Ward and colleagues (43) evaluated 11 infants in the presence of controlled hypoxemia and six infants with controlled hypercarbia challenges. During hypoxemia, only two infants with myelomeningocele aroused in comparison to eight of nine control infants. Similarly, during hypercarbia, arousal occurred in only three infants with myelomeningocele compared to all seven control infants. Three infants with myelomeningocele subsequently died. It was concluded that infants with myelomeningocele, Arnold-Chiari malformation, and apnea or hypoventilation have arousal deficits to normal respiratory stimuli.

SLEEP–WAKE DISORDERS ASSOCIATED WITH BIOLOGICAL RHYTHMS

Children suffering from chronic debilitating neurological disabilities frequently experience disorders of the sleep–wake cycle related to intrinsic biological (circadian) rhythms. In addition to disordered sleep architecture and composition, many youngsters (and their families) will endure significant disorganization of the timing of sleep. Such disturbances may cause significant lifestyle disarray, affect daytime functioning and performance, and contribute to resistance to therapeutic interventions during daytime hours.

Delayed Sleep-Phase Syndrome

Sleep-phase delay is common during childhood and is seen in many youngsters with and without neurological abnormalities. Bedtime struggles are common, and sleep-onset difficulties can be profound. Once the child is asleep, continuity and architecture may be normal, unless early morning waking is required or sleep-maintenance difficulties also are present. If the child has early morning responsibilities, he or she may experience extreme difficulty arousing. Excessive daytime sleepiness will most likely occur, especially during early morning hours. This may be manifested by actual sleep attacks (unintentional sleep episodes), attentional problems, behavioral abnormalities, and/or hyperactivity. Youngsters with delayed sleep-phase syndrome function best in the afternoon or early evening. Spontaneous sleep offset when no responsibilities are present tends to be quite late in the morning, often extending into the afternoon. On weekends, recovery may occur due to the ability to sleep later in the day, only to have the problem recur during weekdays.

Treatment focuses principally on sleep hygiene. A firm, stable time of morning sleep offset is essential. Advancing bedtime will follow. Faded bedtimes with response cost is an appropriate behavioral intervention. If the youngster is not asleep within a reasonable period of time (e.g., 20–30 minutes after lights out), he or she may be removed from bed to perform quiet tasks until drowsiness is identified, and then placed back into bed. Slowly advancing bedtime after sleep onset occurs relatively rapidly will assist in changing and ultimately fixing timing of the major sleep period. Although there is typically a rapid response to this type of intervention, it may take somewhat longer in the youngster with developmental or neurological disability. It is sometimes necessary to give children with significant neurological abnormalities medication that delays sleep onset. Chloral hydrate and benzodiazepines are most commonly prescribed. If chloral hydrate is used, dosage should be adequate to assist in sleep onset.

REFERENCES

1. Martin JH, Jessell TM. Development as a guide to the regional anatomy of the brain. In: Kandel ER, Schwartz JH, Jessell TM, eds. Principles of Neural Science. 3rd ed. New York: Elsevier, 1991:296–308.
2. Oksenberg A, Marks G, Farber J, et al. Effect of REM sleep deprivation during the critical period of neuroanatomical development of the cat visual system. Sleep Res 1986; 15:53.
3. Armstrong SM, Cassone VN, Chesworth MJ, Redman JR, Short RV. Synchronization of mammalian circadian rhythms by melatonin. J Neural Trans S 1986; 21:375–394.
4. Dahlitz M, Alvarez B, Vignau J, English J, Arendt J, Parkes JD. Delayed sleep phase syndrome response to melatonin. Lancet 1991; 333:1121–1124.
5. Jan JE, Espezel H, Appleton RE. The treatment of sleep disorders with melatonin. Dev Med Child Neurol 1994; 36:97–107.
6. Culebras A. Neuroanatomic and neurologic correlates of sleep disturbances. Neurology 1992; 42(suppl 6):19–27.
7. Stahl SM, Layzer RB, Aminoff MJ, et al. Continuous cataplexy in a patient with a midbrain tumor: the limp-man syndrome. Neurology 1980; 30:1115–118.
8. Hendricks JC, Morrison AR, Mann GL. Different behaviors during paradoxical sleep without atonia depend on pontine lesion site. Brain Res 1982; 239:81–105.
9. Autret A, Laffont F, de Toffol B, et al. A syndrome of REM and non-REM sleep reduction and lateral gaze paresis after medial tegmental pontine stroke: CT scans and anatomical correlation in four patients. Arch Neurol 1988; 45:1236–1242.
10. Balk RA, Hiller FC, Lucas EA, et al. Sleep apnea and the Arnold-Chiari malformation. Am Rev Respir Dis 1985; 132:929–930.
11. Ward SL, Jacobs RA, Gates EP, Hart LD, Keens TG. Abnormal ventilatory patterns during sleep in infants with meningomyelocele. J Pediatr 1986; 109:631–634.
12. Jurko MF, Andy OJ, Webster CL. Disordered sleep patterns following thalamotomy. Clin Electroencephalogr 1971; 2:213–217.
13. Autret A, Carrier H, Thommasi M, et al. Etude physiopathologique et neuro-pathologique d'un syndrome decortication cerebrale. Rev Neurol (Paris) 1975; 131:491–504.
14. Culebras A. The neurology of sleep. Neurology 1992; 42(suppl 6):6–8.
15. Sheldon SH. Evaluating sleep in infants and children. New York: Lippincott-Raven, 1996:276.
16. Tharp BR. Electrophysiological brain maturation in premature infants: an historical perspective. J Clin Neurophysiol 1990; 7:302–314.
17. Binnie CD, Prior PF. Electroencephalography. J Neurol Neurosurg Psychiatry 1994; 57:1308–1319.
18. Becker PT, Thoman EB. Rapid eye movement storms in infants: rate of occurrence at 6 months predicts mental development at 1 year. Science 1981; 212:1415–1416.

19. Hakamada S, Watanabe K, Hara K, Miyazaki S, Kumagai T. Body movements during sleep in full-term newborn infants. Brain Dev 1982; 4:51–55.
20. Brouillette RT, Fernbach SK, Hunt CE. Obstructive sleep apnea in infants and children. J Pediatr 1982; 100:31–40.
21. Baldy-Moulinier M, Touchon J, Besset A, et al. Sleep architecture and epileptic seizures. In: Degen R, Neidermeyer E, eds. Epilepsy, Sleep and Sleep Deprivation. Amsterdam: Elsevier, 1984:109–118.
22. Rossi GF, Colicchio G, Pola P. Interictal epileptic activity during sleep: a stereo-EEG study in patients with partial epilepsy. Electroencephalogr Clin Neurophysiol 1984; 58:97–106.
23. Hirsch E, Marescaux C, Maquet P, et al. Landau-Kleffner syndrome: a clinical and EEG study of five cases. Epilepsia 1990; 31:756–767.
24. Bourgeois B. The relationship between sleep and epilepsy in children. Sem Pediatr Neurol 1996; 3:29–35.
25. Rajna P, Veres J. Correlation between night sleep duration and seizure frequency in temporal lobe epilepsy. Epilepsia 1993; 34:574–579.
26. Niedermeyer E. Sleep electroencephalogram in petit mal. Arch Neurol 1965; 12: 625–630.
27. Cadilhac J. Complex partial seizures and REM sleep. In: Sterman MB, Shouse MN, Passouant P, eds. Sleep and Epilepsy. New York: Academic Press, 1982:315–324.
28. Divensky O, Ehrenberg B, Harthlen GM, et al. Epilepsy and sleep apnea syndrome. Neurology 1994; 44:2062–2064.
29. Stores G. Confusions concerning sleep disorders and epilepsys in children and adolescents. Br J Psychiatry 1991; 158:1–7.
30. Lugaresi E, Cirignotta F. Hypnogenic paroxysmal dystonia: epileptic seizure or a new syndrome? Sleep 1981; 4:129–138.
31. American Sleep Disorders Association. International Classification of Sleep Disorders, Revised: Diagnostic and Coding Manual. Rochester, Minnesota: American Sleep Disorders Association, 1997:141–181.
32. Sheldon SH. Pediatric Sleep Medicine. Philadelphia: WB Saunders, 1992:119–135.
33. Schenck CH, Hurwitz TD Mahowald MW. REM sleep behavior disorder. Am J Psychiatry 1988; 145:652.
34. Sheldon SH, Jacobsen JJ. REM sleep motor disorder in children. Child Neurology 1998; 13:257–260.
35. Cherubini E, Frascarelli M, Riccardi B, Valenti C, Ricci G. Changes in the monosynaptic reflex during wakefulness and sleep of children with cerebral paralysis. Rivista di Neurologia 1978; 48:228–241.
36. van den Berg-Emons HJ, Saris WH, de Barbanson DC, Westerterp KR, Huson A, van Baak MA. Daily physical activity of school children with spastic diplegia and of healthy control subjects. J Pediatr 1995; 127:578–584.
37. Watanabe K, Miyazaki S, Hara K, Hakamada S. Behavioral state cycles, background EEGs and prognosis of newborns with perinatal hypoxia. Electroenceph Clin Neurophysiol 1980; 49:618–625.
38. Laffont F, Autret A, Minz M, Beillevaire T, Gilbert A, Cathala HP. Polygraphic study of nocturnal sleep in three degenerative diseases: ALS, oligo-ponto-cerebellar atrophy, and progressive supranuclear palsy. Waking Sleeping 1979; 3:17–30.

39. Shibagaki M, Kiyono S, Takeuchi T. Nocturnal sleep in mentally retarded infants with cerebral palsy. Electroenceph Clin Neurophysiol 1985; 61:465–471.
40. Cavallo A. The pineal gland in human beings: relevance to pediatrics. J Pediatr 1993; 123:843–851.
41. Sheldon SH. Proconvulsant effects of oral melatonin in neurologically disabled children. Lancet 1998; 351:1254.
42. Ward SL, Jacobs RA, Gates EP, Hart LD, Keens TG. Abnormal ventilatory patterns during sleep in infants with myelomeningocele. J Pediatr 1986; 109:631–634.
43. Ward SL, Nickerson BG, van der Hal A, Rodriguez AM, Jacobs RA, Keens TG. Absent hypoxic and hypercapneic arousal responses in children with myelomeningocele and apnea Pediatrics 1986; 78:44–50.

4

Sleep-Related Respiratory Physiology in Infancy, Sleep Apnea Syndromes in Infancy and Childhood, and Polysomnography

Gabriele M. Barthlen
Freiburg University Sleep Center
Robert Koch Hospital
Freiburg im Breisgau, Germany

Stephen H. Sheldon
Children's Memorial Hospital
and Northwestern University Medical School
Chicago, Illinois

SLEEP-RELATED RESPIRATORY PHYSIOLOGY IN INFANCY

The Newborn

Sleep Characteristics

By 30 weeks gestational age, sleep can be differentiated into active (REM) sleep and quiet (non-REM) sleep. Active sleep is characterized by general muscular atonia, rapid eye movements, and irreguar respiration (1).

In the newborn, sleep onset begins with REM sleep. After a few months of age, this changes to an adult pattern, in which REM usually begins 90 minutes after sleep onset. An infant spends approximately 70% of a 24-hour period asleep, compared to about 30% for an adult. Also different from adults is the total time spent in REM sleep: over 50%, compared to approximately 20% in an adult (2).

Respiratory Characteristics

Respiratory adaptation to sleep is the most tenuous from birth to 3 months of age because of the following physiological factors: total sleep time is high and the predominating sleep stage is REM sleep, with its marked respiratory variability.

Mechanical factors also play a role: the diaphragm is flat and thus less efficient than the dome-shaped diaphragm of older children. In addition, the compliant chest wall moves inward with inspiration when the stabilizing effect of the intercostal musculature is lost during active (REM) sleep, leading to less efficient ''paradoxical breathing'' and decreased lung volumes (3). To avoid hypoventilation, there must be increased diaphragmatic activity, which can lead to diaphragmatic fatigue (4). Breathing in newborns with neuromuscular disorders involving the diaphragm and intercostal muscles is further compromised, and may lead to noctumal hypoxemia and hypercarbia.

Newborns are nosebreathers because of a narrow upper airway, a relatively large epiglottis, and a horizontally located tongue (5). Newborns with nasal obstruction may suffer respiratory impairment. Also, ventilatory response to hypoxia is different in the newborn, who initially reacts to hypoxemia with increased ventilation, as does the older child or adult, but then with a reduction in ventilation (6).

3 Months to 1 Year of Age

Sleep Characteristics

After 3 months of age, sleep characteristics change toward a more mature pattern, with emergence of vertex sharp waves (stage 1) and sleep spindles (stage 2).

Respiratory Characteristics

During non-REM sleep, respiratory rate falls, upper-airway muscle tone diminishes, airflow resistance increases, and minute ventilation decreases (7). During REM sleep, varying tidal volumes with an irregular respiratory rate are normal, and occasional apneas and hypopneas can be seen.

Summary

In summary, infants have mainly active (REM) sleep, and begin their sleep period with REM sleep. Starting at age 3 months, they develop a sleep pattem similar to that of older children and adults. Normal respiratory patterns during REM sleep—which, as noted, represents most of the newborn's state—are rare apneas and hypopneas, short periods of hypoventilation, minor oxygen desaturations, minimal hypercarbia, irregular respiration, varying tidal volumes and respiratory rates, paradoxical respiratory effort, and nosebreathing.

SLEEP-APNEA SYNDROMES IN INFANCY AND CHILDHOOD

Apnea of Prematurity

Apnea of prematurity (AOP) is defined as excessive periodic breathing with pathological apnea in a premature infant. Almost half of all premature infants manifest periodic breathing during the neonatal period. Periodic breathing occurs with greater frequency as gestational age decreases, and is present in almost all newborns less than 28 weeks gestation (8). AOP occurs in about half of all infants with periodic breathing. It is thought to be related to immaturity of the brainstem respiratory centers, central and peripheral chemoreceptors, and pulmonary reflexes.

Even though many respiratory pauses in the premature infant are central, there is evidence suggesting that half of all apneas in premature infants may be obstructive or mixed in origin (9). In these immature—and often ill—newborns, complex neuromuscular events required to maintain pharyngeal patency during respiration are easily overwhelmed (10).

AOP is often responsive to medical treatment. Treatment of recurrent, clinically significant apnea in a premature infant should ensure adequate oxygenation and ventilation. Physical stimulation may be all that is necessary. Continuous positive airway pressure, supplemental oxygen, and/or mechanical ventilation may also be required.

Methylxanthines are currently the most widely used medications in the treatment of AOP (11). Although theophylline has been shown to reduce the number of apneic episodes and lessen development of respiratory failure (12), it does not shorten the clinical course of AOP. Caffeine has also been shown to produce a significant increase in ventilation (mainly, it appears, by increasing central inspiratory drive), tidal volume, and mean inspiratory flow. Both caffeine and theophylline have similar effects on episodes of apnea; however, caffeine seems to have an earlier effect on respiratory rate. Side effects of tachycardia, arousal, and gastrointestinal intolerance are more frequently observed with theophylline than with caffeine (13). Aminophylline has been shown to be associated with a decrease in cerebral blood flow (14). Caffeine provides stable plasma levels and has a significantly longer plasma half-life, allowing the prescription of only one daily maintenance dose.

Nasal continuous positive airway pressure (CPAP) is quite effective in resolving obstructive apneas in premature and very young infants. Central apneas, on the other hand, are unaffected by nasal CPAP, although oxygenation has been shown to increase whether or not apnea is present (15). For central apneas in premature infants, methylxanthine treatment appears to be significantly superior to CPAP (16).

Doxapram, a potent respiratory stimulant, has been used experimentally to treat AOP. It appears to affect both peripheral chemoreceptors and central respiratory centers (17). Doxapram infusions have been used in preterm infants when therapeutic concentrations of theophylline had failed to control episodes of central apnea (18).

Characteristics of Pathological Apnea

Sleep apnea can be pathological depending on the event's length, frequency, and associated symptoms (Table 1). Occasional respiratory pauses of less than 10 seconds, without significant hypoxemia or hypercarbia, are normal.

Still under debate are the number of apneas and hypopneas per hour of sleep—the apnea/hypopnea index (AHI)—and the degree of oxygen saturation and hypercapnia that is considered normal or abnormal. Drops in O_2 saturation of >1 to 2% and rises in CO_2 values of >5 to 10 mm Hg are generally considered abnormal.

There is often considerable delay in diagnosis of sleep-disordered breathing in the neonate, infant, and child. Brouillette and colleagues (19) have described significant delays in the diagnosis of sleep-disordered breathing, and have demonstrated profound morbidity. In 22 patients with documented obstructive sleep apnea, mean delay in referral for 20 patients first evaluated after the neonatal period was 23 $\pm$ 15 months. Almost three-quarters of patients studied developed serious sequelae, including cor pulmonale, failure to thrive, permanent neurological deficits, behavioral disturbances, hypersomnolence, and developmental abnormalities.

Table 1 Characteristics of Pathological Apnea

Duration longer than 20 seconds
Associated with
Significant O_2 desaturation
Significant hypercarbia
Cyanosis
Pallor
Hypotonia
Bradycardia

Sleep-Apnea Syndromes in Infancy

In infancy up to 6 months of age, the following special definitions apply.

Obstructive apnea is a respiratory pause equal to two breaths with less than 20% baseline airflow (see Figure 1). Up to one such pause per hour of sleep is considered normal. Obstructive apnea can be prolonged and associated with cardiac deceleration (generally occurring during the last third of the apnea), oxygen desaturation, and elevation of end-tidal CO_2 (E_tCO_2) after airflow resumes.

Hypopnea is a respiratory pause equal to two breaths with less than 80% baseline airflow. Up to two of such pauses per hour of sleep is considered normal.

Partial obtruction is a period of paradoxical respiratory effort (chest and abdominal respiratory movements in opposite directions) associated with O_2 desaturations of >2% and/or CO_2 rises above 50.

Central apnea: airflow <80% of baseline for over 20 seconds with absent respiratory effort (see Figure 2). This period can be shorter than 20 seconds if the event is associated with O_2 desaturations >4%, a drop in O_2 saturation below 92%, a rise in CO_2 >50 mm Hg, bradycardia of <70 bpm, or cyanosis or pallor. Prolonged central apnea, related to absence of both inspiratory and expiratory neuronal activity, appears to be quite unusual in otherwise normal infants and children during non-REM/quiet sleep. Brief central apnea is normal during REM/active sleep. When prolonged central apneas occur during quiet sleep, central hypoventilation syndrome or a primary underlying central nervous system or brainstem abnormality may be present.

Mixed apnea contains polysomnographic components of both central and obstructive respiratory pauses (see Figure 3). There is some evidence, however, that the "central" component of a mixed apnea is either prolonged expiration or an expiratory apnea (20). It may also represent a combination of the two.

Expiratory apnea, which has received little attention in the medical literature, is defined as absence of polysomnographically recorded nasal and oral airflow in the presence of continued expiratory effort against an occluded or partially obstructed upper airway. A prolonged expiratory phase of breathing can be demonstrated (see Figure 4). Almost all expiratory apneas are preceded by an augmented breath or sigh (21).

Upper-airway occlusion may occur at any level, from the nasopharynx to the larynx. There is preliminary evidence that in some children there may be reflex glottic adduction occurring in the presence of continued diaphragmatic contraction. Increased parasympathetic tone may be present and affect the diaphragm via the vagus nerve, as well as increasing vocal cord adduction via the recurrent laryngeal nerve. A significant decrease in the heart rate seems to occur during the first third of the respiratory pause in a manner similar to that seen during the Valsalva maneuver. There is little change in the SaO_2, notwithstanding the length of the apnea. This might be explained by a temporary increase in lung

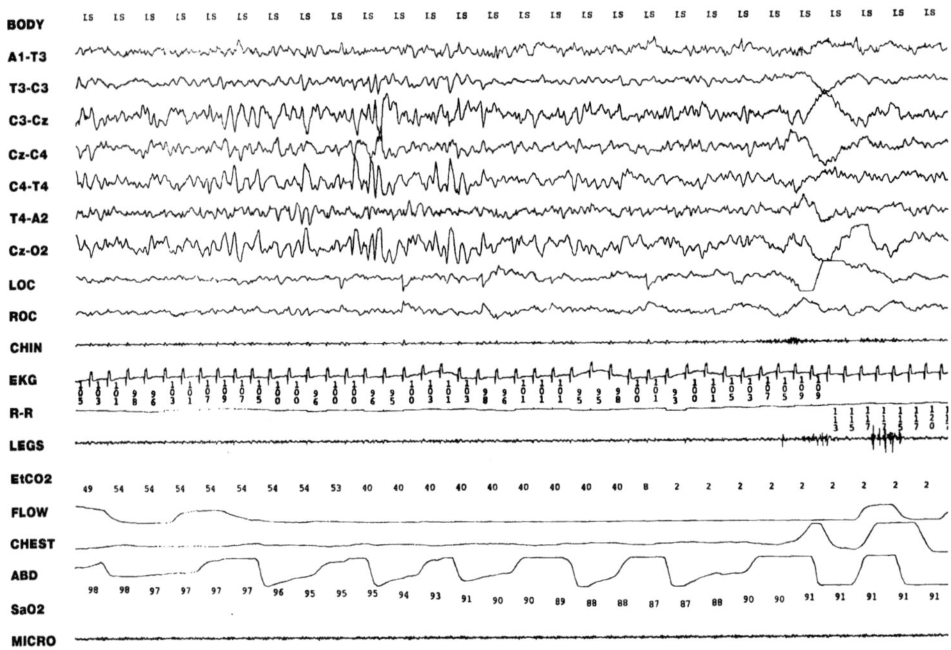

Figure 1 Obstructive apnea. This 30-second polysonmographic epoch was recorded from a 3-year-old boy during REM sleep. Note absence of nasal/oral airflow lasting approximately 20 seconds, oxygen desaturation to a nadir of 87%. EEG arousal occurs, but there are no significant changes in cardiac rhythm. ECO_2 maximum of 54 torr at the beginning of the apnea represents recovery from a previous occlusive respiratory event. E_tCO_2 digital printout represents an average of E_tCO_2 sampled over the previous 10 seconds.

volume and positive expiratory pressure. Potential importance and recognition of expiratory apnea is evident when assessing apnea/bradycardia during infant home monitoring, and in some patients with underlying CNS or autonomic nervous system abnormalities.

Postsigh apneas seem to be associated with little to no upper airway obstruction (see Figure 5). An augmented breath is followed by a central-appearing apnea. There is little change in heart rate, almost no oxygen desaturation, and absence of hypercarbia during and after the event. In certain cases, a continued rise in E_tCO_2 can be demonstrated. Identification of these respiratory pauses are also important in evaluating infants with apnea and in follow-up of infants being monitored at home.

Periodic breathing is a pattern of respiration characterized by three or more respiratory pauses of 3 seconds or longer separated by normal breathing for less than 20 seconds (22). Periodic breathing is a normal pattern of respiration in premature infants during active/REM and quiet/non-REM sleep (see Figure 6). Proportion of the total sleep time occupied by periodic breathing decreases as the youngster matures. Periodic breathing is most often confined to active/REM sleep in the term newborn. Persistence later in infancy and childhood may be abnormal and reflect immaturity or an abnormality in brainstem respiratory control. Unfortunately, clear norms regarding appropriate percentages of periodic breathing across age groups are not yet available.

Obstructive hypoventilation occurs when there is chronic upper airway obstruction associated with high-upper-airway resistance. Overt apnea may not be present (see Figure 7). If obstructive apneas and hypopneas occur, they tend to be most significant during REM sleep. Often, however, the number of apneas and or hypopneas per hour of sleep is within age-appropriate normal limits. Respiratory rate during sleep is often increased and oxygen saturation may be normal. E_tCO_2, however, is significantly elevated and remains high because of upper-airway occlusion. It has been recommended that obstructive hypoventilation be considered when E_tCO_2 measurements remain above 46 mm Hg for more than 60% of the total sleep time or when E_tCO_2 rises above 53 mm Hg (23).

Alveolar hypoventilation is the percentage of time spent asleep with CO_2 >50 mm Hg. If this percentage exceeds 8% of total sleep time, a diagnosis of alveolar hypoventilation is made. In the premature infant, respiratory abnormalities are often more severe and associated with bradycardia (24).

Key to all figures in this chapter
BODY: Body position as recorded by accelerometry.
EEG (A1 to O2): EEG electrode array conforms with the International 1020 System of electrode placement.
LOC: Left outer canthus (electro-oculogram).
ROC: Right outer canthus (electro-oculogram).
CHIN: Chin muscle EMG.
EKG: Lead II.
R-R: Digital representation of the instantaneous heart rate.
LEGS: Bilaterally linked anterior tibialis EMG.
EtCO2: Digital recording of sidestream end-tidal CO_2 measurement. Numerical output is depicted every second; however, each depiction represents an average E_tCO_2 over the previous 10 seconds of data acquisition.
FLOW: Flow tracing is obtained by graphic representation of E_tCO_2. Because of sampling time there is a 3-second skewing of flow when compared to chest and abdominal effort (i.e., the flow appears 3 seconds after the respiratory effort) associated with the airflow.
CHEST: Chest respiratory effort as measured by piezo crystal belt.
ABD: Abdominal respiratory effort as measured by piezo crystal belt.
SaO2: Oxygen saturation as measured by pulse oximetry.
MICRO: Sonogram of respiratory sounds recorded from a microphone placed on the anteriolateral aspect of the patient's neck.

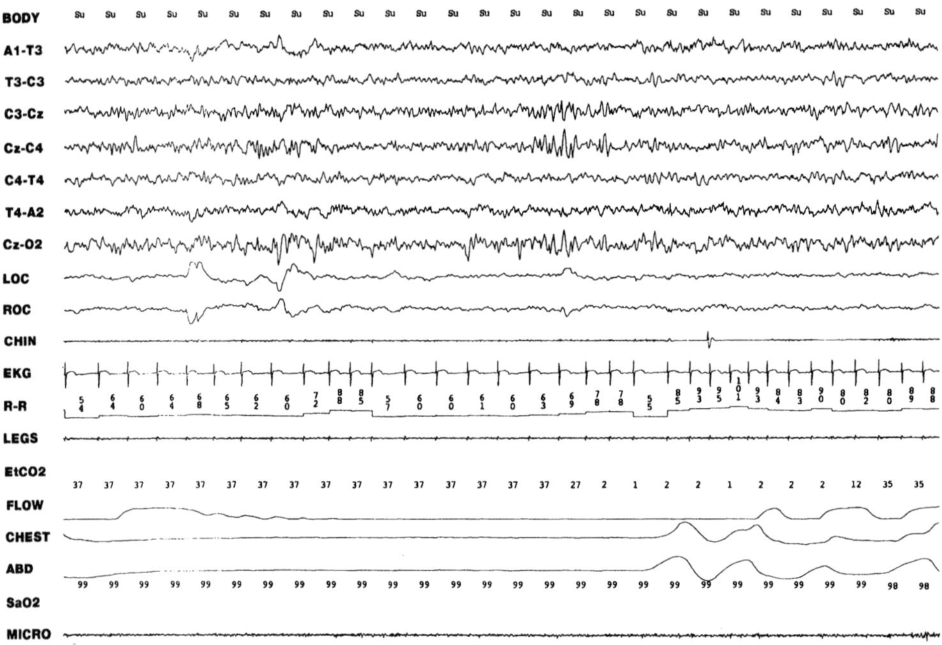

Figure 2 Central apnea. This 30-second polysomnographic segment was recorded during REM sleep from a 1½-year-old girl. Note the cessation of nasal and oral airflow associated with absence of respiratory effort. There is no EEG state change, significant oxygen desaturation, or EKG dysrhythmias. Despite lasting about 17 seconds, this is most likely a normal phenomenon related to REM respiratory instability. Abnormality may exist if these central apneas appear frequently, are associated with significant gas-exchange abnormalities, are frequent, or occur during non-REM sleep.

The above values are used by convention; it is expected that they will be modified in the future pending more research.

Sleep-Apnea Syndromes in Childhood

The upper airway serves a variety of functions during the respiratory cycle, including protection of the lower airway and phonation. Little is known regarding the physiological function and reflex activity of the upper airway and larynx in breathing during sleep in neonates, and there is a paucity of studies regarding normal and abnormal pharyngeal and laryngeal respiratory function in prepubertal children. During the normal respiratory cycle, the laryngeal airway is widely

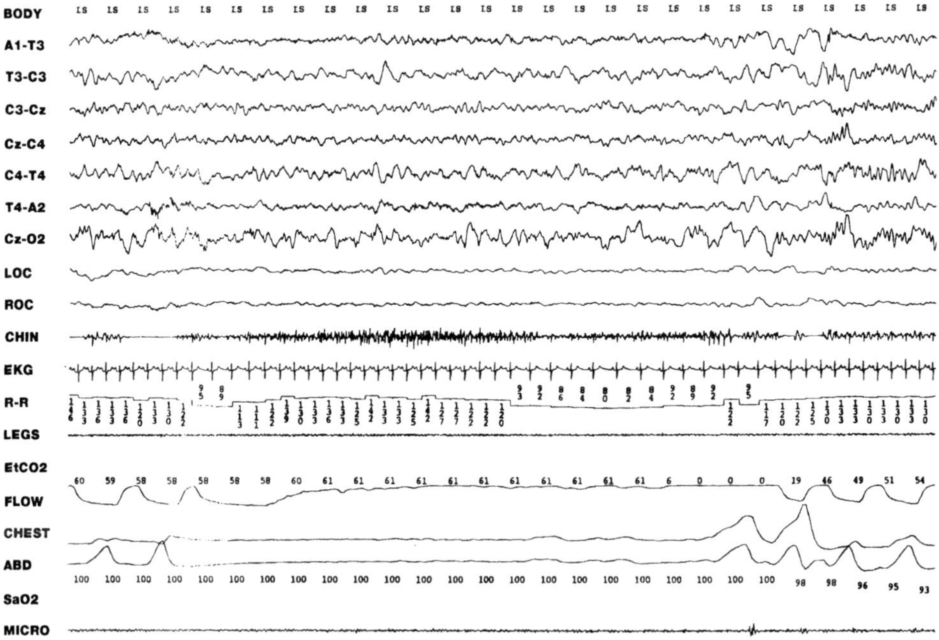

Figure 3 Mixed apnea. This 30-second polysomnographic segment was recorded during non-REM sleep from a 5-year-old boy being studied for obstructive sleep apnea. Note the elevated endtidal CO_2 prior to the apnea and absence of nasal/oral airflow. Approximately 7 seconds prior to resumption of airflow, there are three brief respiratory efforts without resumption of airflow, characteristic of a mixed apnea.

patent during inspiration and narrows during expiration (25). Changes in glottic aperture during the respiratory cycle result from phasic activity of the posterior cricoarytenoid (PCA) and pharyngeal constrictor (PC) muscles (26). PCA muscles widen the glottis and are the principal abductors of the vocal cords. Along with the PC muscles, the lateral cricoarytenoid, the oblique and transverse arytenoid, and the thyroarytenoid (TA) muscles, they close the glottis by adduction of the vocal cords. Controlled decline in PCA muscle activity acts in consort with a decrease in activity of thoracic inspiratory muscles to cause expiratory braking, a reflexly controlled regulation of expiratory airflow and end-expiratory volume (27). Appropriate function of the upper airway in regulating the respiratory cycle is critical. There is increasing evidence that the upper airway must dilate before the diaphragm can initiate inspiration. Children with neurological deficits and/or autonomic nervous system abnormality may be at high risk of

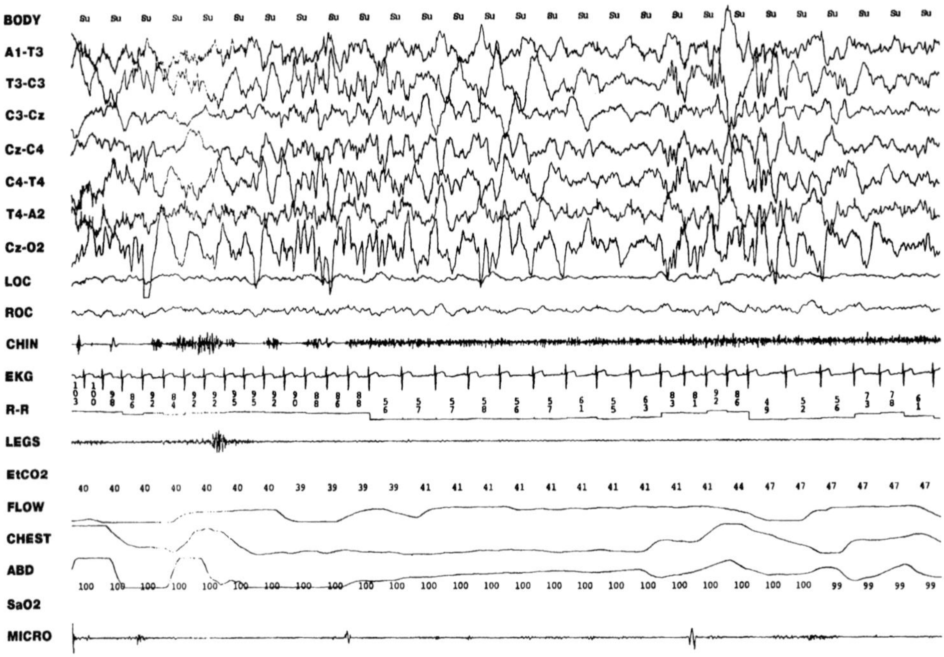

Figure 4 Expiratory apnea. This 30-second polysomnographic epoch was recorded from a 6-year-old boy being studied for noisy breathing during sleep. Note the augmented breath immediately prior to the respiratory pause, and continued elevation of E_tCO_2 during the absence of graphic airflow indicating prolonged expiration against an occluded upper airway. There is a significant fall in heart rate during the first third of the apnea, similar to that seen during a Valsalva maneuver.

abnormalities of respiration (Table 2). Obstructive apnea predominates in children with neurological abnormalities, but other types of apnea often occur (Table 3).

Apneas are classified as obstructive, central, or mixed.

In *obstructive apnea*, airflow is absent (or less than 30% of baseline ventilation), and respiratory effort (chest and abdomen) is present. This is the most common form.

In *central apnea*, airflow is absent, respiratory effort absent.

Mixed apnea is initially central, followed by an obstructive component. Mixed apneas are rarely seen in children and often represent pure obstructive apneas, in which respiratory effort is not recorded during the "central" component because of insufficient sensitivity of the respiratory belts.

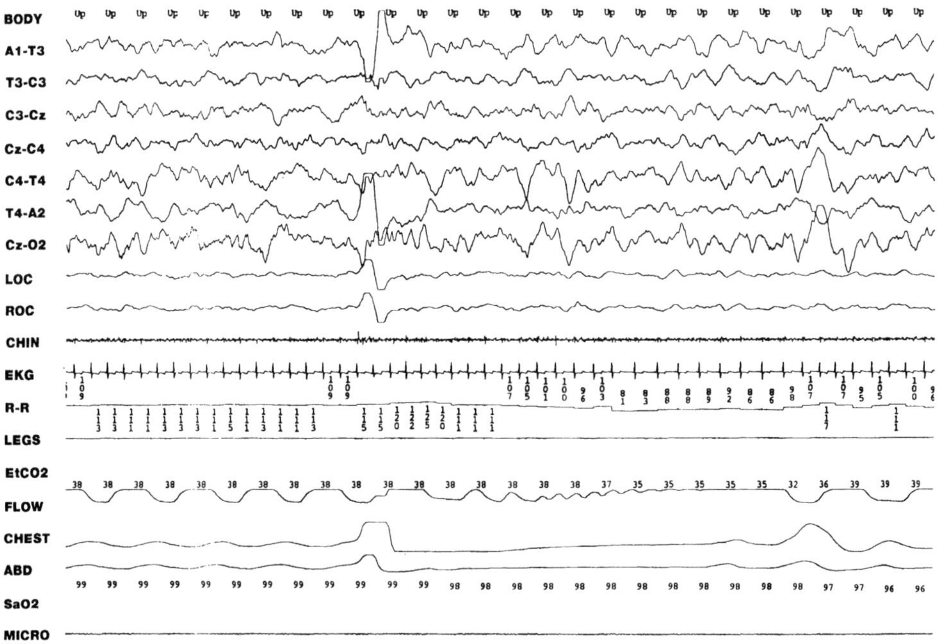

Figure 5 Postsigh apnea. This 30-second epoch was recorded from an 11-month-old girl. Note the augmented breath immediately prior to the respiratory pause, absence of nasal/oral airflow, pulse artifact in the graphic representation of airflow, and minimal fall in oxygen saturation. E_tCO_2 falls during this event, the pulse artifact indicates an open upper airway, and the gradual cardiac deceleration with the nadir during the last third of the pause suggests a physiological postsigh apnea.

Obstructive Apneas

The hallmark of obstructive sleep apnea (OSA) in children is snoring, although it can be absent even in severe OSA. Breathing is often punctuated with pauses and snorts. Difficulty in breathing during sleep, restless sleep, diaphoresis, morning headaches, excessive morning thirst, nightmares, sleep terrors, and enuresis may be associated symptoms (Table 4).

Daytime abnormalities (Table 5) include sleepiness, hyperactivity, poor school performance, abnormal behavior, aggressiveness, pathological shyness, and social withdrawal. Learning problems, frequent upper-airway infections, failure to thrive, or obesity may occur. In severe cases, pulmonary hypertension and cor pulmonale can develop.

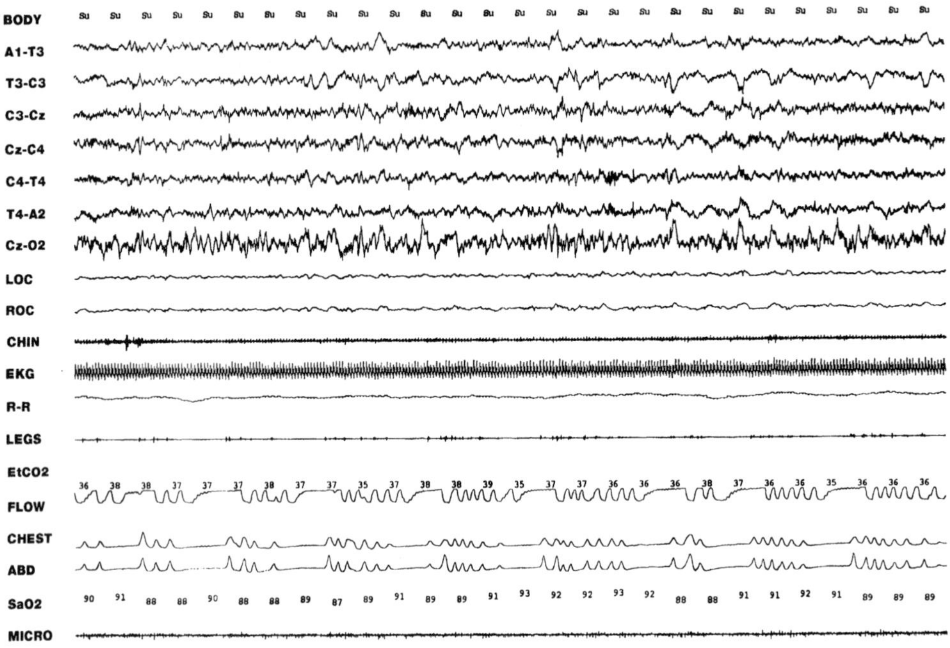

Figure 6 Periodic breathing. This 120-second epoch was recorded during active sleep in a 32-week-old premature infant. Note pauses of more than 3 seconds separated by normal-appearing respiration lasting less than 20 seconds. Also note that there is periodic oxygen desaturation associated with the respiratory pauses.

Patients with neuromuscular disease often have abnormal muscle tone of the bulbar musculature, which includes upper-airway dilator muscles such as the geniohyoid, tensor veli palatini, and myohyoid. During sleep, especially during REM sleep, muscle tone decreases physiologically, and there is a partial collapse of the upper airway from the negative pressure generated during inspiration. Patients with any condition compromising bulbar muscle tone, bulk, and strength are at an additional disadvantage and will be at risk for obstructive sleep apnea syndrome. If pharyngeal muscles are more severely affected than the diaphragm or the ancillary inspiratory muscles, the usual reduction of upper-airway muscle tone can precipitate obstructive sleep apnea through the negative pressure generated during inspiration (32).

In a recent study (33), patients visiting a neuromuscular clinic were randomly selected for evaluation of sleep-disordered breathing. Forty-two percent had a respiratory disturbance index (RDI) of 15 or more (up to 5 is normal), and most patients had symptoms of daytime dysfunction.

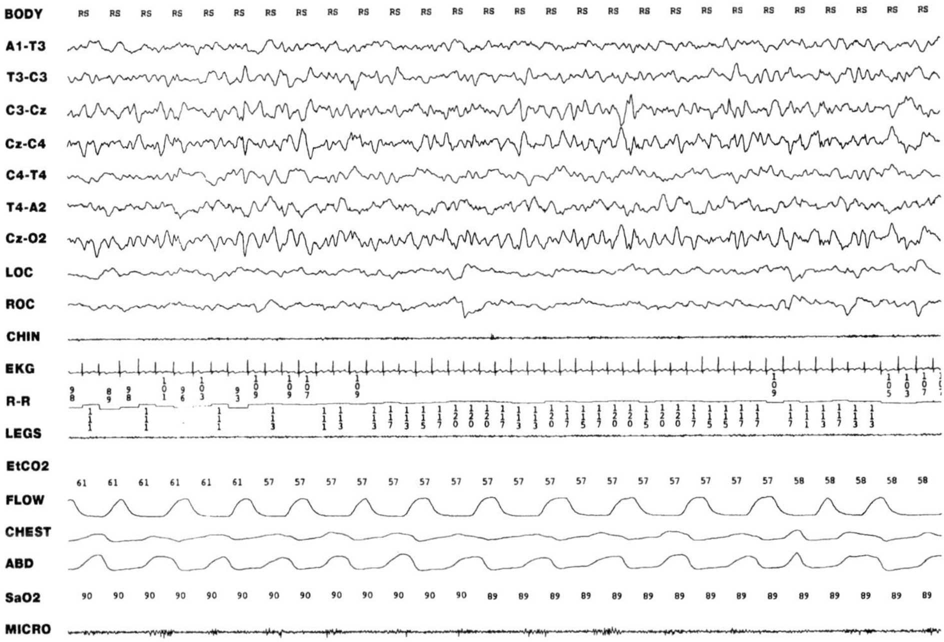

Figure 7 Obstructive hypoventilation. This 30-second epoch was recorded during REM sleep from an 8-year-old youngster with Down's syndrome. Parents reported loud snoring associated with pauses and snorts. Although there is normal-appearing respiratory effort and airflow, oxygen saturation is low, E_tCO_2 is elevated, and there are periodic decelerations in heart rate. in association with paradoxical breathing, loud snoring, and normal gas exchange during wakefulness, this segment suggests obstructive hypoventilation.

Table 2 Neurological Disorders Underlying Obstructive Sleep Apnea Syndrome

Syringomyelia-syringobulbia
Myotonic dystrophy (29)
Arnold-Chiari malformation
Poliomyelitis (30)
Duchenne muscular dystrophy (31)

Table 3 Nonneurological Conditions Underlying Obstructive Sleep Apnea Syndrome

Hypertrophied tonsils and adenoids, most common cause of OSAS (35)
Craniofacial abnormalities
Micrognathia
Retrognathia
Long soft palate
Macroglossia (Down's syndrome)
Obesity with fatty infiltration of the upper airway
Idiopathic conditions such as hypopharyngeal collapsibility

Table 4 Nocturnal Symptoms of Obstructive Sleep Apnea

Loud snoring
Respiratory pauses
Snorts
Gasping and gurgling sounds
Restless sleep
Nocturnal diaphoresis
Waking up frightened (in a child)

Table 5 Diurnal Symptoms of Obstructive Sleep Apnea Syndrome

Hyperactivity
Excessive daytime sleepiness
Behavioral difficulties
Failure to thrive
Morning headaches
Symptoms of cor pulmonale
Elevated hematocrit (28)

Table 6 Treatment Options for Obstructive Sleep Apnea Syndrome

Tonsillectomy/adenoidectomy—most common procedure
Nasal CPAP/BiPAP
Noninvasive intermittent positive pressure ventilation (nIPPV)
Tracheostomy—cures OSAS, but is invasive
Uvulopalatopharyngoplasty (UPPP)—consists of removal of the uvula, posterior part of the soft palate, and tissue from the tonsillar fossa; results are inconsistent (38)
Weight loss if child is obese
Surgical correction of craniofacial abnormalities
Positional training (avoid sleeping on back) if apneas occur predominantly when patient is sleeping supine

OSA during childhood is often associated with an anatomical abnormality of the upper airway. The most common cause of upper-airway obstruction in children is hypertrophy of the tonsils and adenoids (34). Malformations of the mandible and maxillae can also causes upper-airway obstruction during sleep. Central and peripheral neurological abnormalities can also result in OSA due to dysfunction of pharyngeal muscular movements.

As treatment for obstructive sleep apnea syndrome in children (Table 6), surgical removal of enlarged tonsils and adenoids is usually sufficient. In rhinitis with nasal obstruction, antihistamines, nasal cromolyn, or nasal steroids have been used successfully. With symptoms that persist despite surgery, or if surgery is not an option, noninvasive ventilation such as nasal CPAP or bilevel positive airway pressure (BiPAP) should be considered. Possible problems with noninvasive ventilation are noncompliance, air leaks around the mask leading to persistence of symptoms and eye irritation, midface deformities, and an allergic reaction to the mask (36). For patients with neuromuscular disease, noninvasive intermittent positive pressure ventilation (nIPPV) has been used successfully (37).

In summary, obstructive sleep apnea syndrome is common in children, and often caused by hypertrophied tonsils and adenoids. Surgical correction is usually sufficient. Noninvasive nasal positive pressure ventilation may be indicated in the neuromuscular patient.

Central Apneas

Control of breathing during wakefulness is due mostly to metabolic factors. Peripheral chemoreceptors (carotid and aortic bodies) and central chemoreceptors in the pons and medulla sense blood gas and acid–base status. In addition, the waking neural drive provides tonic, nonspecific excitation to the respiratory neurons and increases central drive to respiratory muscles.

Table 7 Symptoms of Central Sleep Apnea Syndrome

Respiratory failure with
Cyanosis
Apneas
Cardiac arrhythmias
Cardiac arrest
Morning headaches
Excessive daytime sleepiness
Polycythemia
Cor pulmonale

Control of breathing during sleep is different. The waking neural drive is absent, and in disorders affecting the central brainstem controller, a decline in ventilation to the point of an apnea can occur.

Congenital central hypoventilation syndrome (CCHS) is an uncommon disorder manifested by insufficient ventilatory effort due to inadequate output from brainstem centers that control breathing (Tables 7 and 8): namely, there is a failure of the automatic control of breathing. Hypoventilation in the absence of lung disease or dysfunction of respiratory muscles is exacerbated during sleep. Respiratory rate may appear normal, but tidal volume during sleep is low. On the other hand, some children with central hypoventilation have normal or increased tidal volumes but a significantly reduced respiratory rate. Hypoventilation may also occur during wakefulness. When mechanical ventilation is instituted, weaning is difficult. Blunted response to hypercapnea and hypoxemia is often demonstrable.

Usually CCHS is apparent at birth, with symptoms of respiratory failure as soon as the infant falls asleep. Since these patients have normal ventilatory

Table 8 Disorders Associated with Central Sleep Apnea Syndrome

Prematurity
Congenital central hypoventilation syndrome (CCHS)
Encephalitis
Cervical cordotomy
Brainstem infarction
Brainstem tumor
Bulbar poliomyelitis
Arnold-Chiari malformation

Table 9 Treatment of Central Sleep Apnea Syndrome

Tracheostomy and mechanical ventilatory support.
Diaphragmatic pacing. Unilateral pacing is sufficient in the older child. The young child with higher metabolic rates requires greater alveolar ventilation, and bilateral pacing may be neccessary. Potential problems with bilateral pacing are diaphragmatic fatigue and permanent injury to the phrenic nerve.
Intermittent positive pressure ventilation with a tightly fitting nasal mask. This modality has been used for central sleep apnea as well as hypoventilation (40).

function while awake, in many cases mechanical ventilatory support only at night is sufficient (39).

However, symptoms may be manifested later in infancy, including cyanosis and/or pulmonary hypertension. The clinical course is chronic, and lifelong ventilatory support is often required, particularly during sleep. Some infants improve with time and may be able to support ventilation during wakefulness. Others may deteriorate and require 24-hour mechanical ventilatory support.

In summary, central sleep apnea syndrome is due to impaired ventilatory drive, and is seen in conditions affecting the brainstem or with diffuse brain dysfunction. Treatment options are tracheostomy and mechanical ventilation, diaphragmatic pacing, and nasal intermittent positive pressure ventilation (Table 9).

SUDDEN INFANT DEATH SYNDROME

The incidence of sudden infant death syndrome (SIDS) is approximately 1.5 per 1000 infants. It generally occurs between ages 1 month and 1 year; the peak incidence is at 2–3 months of age.

Siblings of SIDS victims have a risk five times higher than infants without such siblings (41). Infants who had an ALTE (acute life-threatening event, or "near-miss" event) are at more than twice the risk. An ALTE is characterized by pallor, bradycardia, and hypo- or hypertonia (Tables 10 and 11).

Increased periodic breathing and decreased responsiveness to hypercarbia may be associated with an ALTE (42). However, these findings could not be confirmed in subsequent studies (43,44).

Gastroesophageal reflux can lead to apnea and bradycardia through the laryngeal chemoreceptor reflex (45), but Rosen et al. (46) were unable to find a correlation between gastroesophageal reflux and apnea on polysomnographic tracings (Table 12). In the majority of patients, no cause is found despite extensive work-up and there are no neurological sequelae after an ALTE.

Most prospective cardiorespiratory studies on patients who later died of SIDS have not shown any physiological differences in such variables as heart-

Table 10 Conditions That Have Been Associated with SIDS

Young mother
Low birth weight
Maternal smoking
Placement of infant in prone position
No breastfeeding
Low socioeconomic class
Overheated sleeping environment
Winter months
Preceding upper-respiratory-tract infection
Preceding gastrointestinal symptoms
Infection wih *Campylobacter jejuni*

Table 11 Conditions Associated with an ALTE

Acute infections (sepsis, meningitis, RTI)
Aspiration
Seizures
Cardiac and metabolic disorders
Breath-holding spells
Congenital central hypoventilation syndrome
CNS tumors
Upper-airway obstruction
Child abuse
Poisoning
Prematurity
Idiopathic apnea

Table 12 Polysomnographic Findings of Future SIDS Victims

Less artifact-contaminated periods during sleep, which may reflect fewer body movements
More REM sleep, and less wake time in the early morning, which may indicate an abnormally high arousal threshold (49)
More obstructive apneas than in controls—however, it has never been demonstrated that obstructive apneas were the direct cause of SIDS (50)

Table 13 Possible Indications for Apnea Monitors

Congenital central hypoventilation syndrome (CCHS)
Two SIDS-victim siblings
Tracheostomy
Severe bronchopulmonary dysplasia

rate variability, breath-to-breath interval, breath-to-breath variability, or increased apneic pauses or periodic breathing, except for significantly higher heart rates (47,48).

The usefulness of apnea monitors is controversial, as they have not been shown to affect mortality (Table 13).

In summary, infants who succumb to SIDS are more likely than controls to have had an ALTE and/or a sibling who died of SIDS, and to have higher heart rates, less artifact-contaminated time during sleep studies (which may represent fewer body movements), increased amounts of REM sleep, and less waking time in the early morning.

The role of apnea monitors is unclear, as they have not been shown to affect mortality. Their use should be reserved for high-risk patients.

PEDIATRIC POLYSOMNOGRAPHY

Indications for Sleep Studies in Children

Accurate diagnosis of respiratory pauses during sleep is based on continuous monitoring of respiratory, cardiovascular, and electroencephalographic parameters across the child's habitual sleep period (Table 14). Severity of breathing

Table 14 Indications for Polysomnography as a Diagnostic Tool for Sleep-Disordered Breathing

Observed apneas
Heavy snoring and gasping
Excessive daytime sleepiness
Hyperactivity
Failure to thrive
Polycythemia
Cor pulmonale
Chest-wall retractions
Paradoxical respiratory effort
Preoperatively in children with only mild symptoms
Postoperatively if symptoms persist (53)

disorders during sleep often varies in a circadian manner. the highest incidence of pathological apnea, even in very young infants, occurs during early morning hours (51). Polysomnographic monitoring is most reliable when attended by a technician and performed during the major sleep period at night. Premature newborns and term neonates may be evaluated adequately during daytime hours if several continuous sleep–wake cycles are monitored. The most common referral diagnosis for performance of overnight polysomnography is obstructive sleep apnea syndrome, which is usually due to adenotonsillar hypertrophy. It has been estimated that 7 to 9% of children snore regularly, with the prevalence of OSAS being 0.7% in 4- to 5-year-old children (52).

Children with neuromuscular disease often have a combination of obstructive apneas, central apneas, and alveolar hypoventilation.

The initial work-up should include examination of the upper airway to assess the size of tonsils and adenoids and patency of nasal passages. Pulmonary-function testing may be neccessary in patients with neuromuscular disease.

Guidelines for Performing Polysomnography in Children

Laboratory Conditions and Timing

The child should arrive at the sleep laboratory early in the day to get acquainted with the unusual situation. One parent is usually asked to stay with the child overnight. The laboratory should resemble a typical child's home environment, with appropriate wallpaper, artwork, and toys. It is helpful to allow the child to be actively involved with the placement of the chestbands and electrodes. Computer games can be made available on the sleep computer for older children to play during the daytime. Home studies—when performed as full-montage polysomnography—have been well accepted.

Parameters continuously monitored during polysomnography include nasal and oral airflow by capnography, thermistor, or airflow pressure gauge and measurement of chest and abdominal respiratory effort, oxygen saturation, and, usually, E_tCO_2. Oxygen saturation is monitored using pulse oximetry. Continuous EKG is also recorded. This provides feedback of the cardiovascular effects of respiratory pauses. Continuous EEG monitoring with an expanded electrode array, chin muscle EMG, electro-oculogram, anterior tibialis EMG, and objective recording of patient behavior during the sleep study are essential. When indicated, esophageal pH may also be monitored. Recording multiple physiological variables provides accurate identification of sleep state–related respiratory changes as well as identification of apneas associated with other significant sleep-related disorders (e.g., sleep-related seizure activity, gastroesophageal reflux).

Pneumography (respiratory-effort monitoring by thoracic impedance and heart-rate monitoring) should be avoided as a diagnostic method (22). Pneumograms have been widely used for screening in asymptomatic premature and term infants. Unfortunately, integrity of respiration during sleep can be significantly underestimated by this type of recording. Sensitivity and specificity of pneumography are poor. False-positive and false-negative results are common. Partial airway obstruction may cause false breath detection, and breaths immediately following a sigh or biphasic augmented breaths are often missed (54). In addition, unless nasal and oral airflow are recorded, only central apneas can be detected. Monitoring only thoracic impedance may result in failure to detect obstructive apnea, can confuse cardiac pulse artifact with respiratory effort, and cannot detect abdominal respiratory efforts. Impedance pneumography done in the home is almost as costly as comprehensive technician-attended polysomnography conducted in the laboratory. Pneumograms should be reserved for evaluation of infants who trigger frequent home monitor alarms. Pneumography may help by differentiating true from false activation of the monitor.

Technician-attended polysomnography is still considered the most reliable and effective method available for describing respiration during sleep and for identification of normal vs. abnormal upper-airway function during sleep.

Montage for Overnight Polysomnography

In older children (above age 8), at least 11 channels should be recorded (Table 15). In infants and young children, oxygen desaturations may not occur, but hypoventilation can still be present with resulting retention of carbon dioxide. It is thus obligatory that at least one capnometry channel be recorded. End-tidal capnometry involves an additional probe placed in the infant's or child's nose, which may be difficult to fit together with the nasal/oral airflow sensor. Another disadvantage of E_tCO_2 measurement is the need for ''flushing,'' a recalibration process that has to be performed by the sleep technician every few hours.

Table 15 Montage for Polysomnography in Children Above Age 8

1. Centroparietal EEG C4/A1 (optional: a ''spare'' C3/A2)
2. Occipital EEG O1/A2 (optional: a ''spare'' O2/A1)
3. Electro-oculogram—right outer canthus (ROC)
4. Electro-oculogram—left outer canthus (LOC)
5. Nasal/oral airflow
6. Submental surface EMG
7. EKG rhythm strip
8. Respiratory effort—chest
9. Respiratory effort—abdomen
10. Anterior tibialis surface EMG (right and left combined)
11. Oximeter—ear or finger

Alternatively, transcutaneous CO_2 monitoring can be used effectively in infants and young children, and has become routine. The older child, however, has thicker skin, which may impair the accuracy of transcutaneous CO_2 measurements. In addition, the technician needs to change the site of the probe every 2 or 3 hours to ensure a fresh and clean site for accurate measurements, and to avoid overheating at the site of the probe.

Thus, the twelfth obligatory channel for pediatric polysomnography is capnometry (transcutaneous or end-tidal).

Summary

In summary, full technician-attended polysomnography is the gold-standard diagnostic tool for evaluation of sleep-disordered breathing. Because respiratory impairment and hypoventilation in infants and children may manifest only through CO_2 retention and not oxygen desaturation, capnometry should be performed routinely. Transcutaneous capnometry is recommended for infants and young children, end-tidal capnometry for older children.

OUTLOOK ON FUTURE RESEARCH

Age-specific normal values for all polysomnographic parameters should be generated in large multicenter studies. The correlation of polysomnographic abnormalities with morbidity could be better defined. The natural history of sleep apnea (e.g., does OSAS resolve with natural involution of tonsils and adenoids?) needs to be more closely studied. The neurological, psychological, cognitive, and social consequences of sleep disorders should undergo more extensive evaluation.

REFERENCES

1. Parmelee AH, Stern E. Development of states in infants. In: Clements CD, Purpura DP, eds. Sleep and the Maturing Nervous System. New York: Academic Press, 1972: 199–228.
2. Stern E, Parmelee AH, Akiyama Y, Schultz MA, Wenner WH. Sleep cycle characteristics in infants. Pediatrics 1969; 43:65–70.
3. Knill R, Andrews W, Bryan AC, Bryan MH. Respiratory load compensation in infants. J Appl Physiol 1976; 40:357–361.
4. Muller N, Gulston G, Cade D, Whitton J, Froese AB, Bryan MH, et al. Diaphragmatic muscle fatigue in the newborn. J Appl Physiol: Resp Env Exercise Physiol 1979; 46:688–695.
5. Bosma JF. Postnatal ontogeny of performances of the pharynx, larynx, and mouth. Am Rev Respir Dis 1985; 131:10–15.
6. Sankaran K, Wiebe H, Seshia MM, Boychuk RB, Cates D, Rigatto H. Immediate

and late ventilatory response to high and low O_2 in preterm infants and adult subjects. Pediatr Res 1979; 13:875–878.
7. Remmers JE, Bartlett D Jr, Putnam MD. Changes in the respiratory cycle associated with sleep. Respir Physiol 1976; 28:227–238.
8. Bouterline-Young HJ, Smith CA. Respiration of full-term and premature infants. Am J Dis Child 1953; 80:753.
9. Dransfield DA, Spiter AR, Fox WW. Episodic airway obstruction in premature infants. Am J Dis Child 1983; 137:441–443.
10. Milner AD, Boon AW, Saunders RA, Hopkin IE. Upper airway obstruction and apnoea in preterm babies. Arch Dis Child 1980; 55:22–25.
11. Kelly DH, Shannon DC. Treatment of apnea and excessive periodic breathing in the full-term infant. Pediatrics 1981; 68:183–186.
12. Bairam A, Boutroy MJ, Badonnel Y, Vert P. Theophylline versus caffeine: comparative effects in treatment of idiopathic apnea in the preterm infant. J Pediatr 1987; 110:636–639.
13. Sims ME, Yau G, Rambhatla S. Cabal L, Wu PY. Limitations of theophylline in the treatment of apnea of prematurity. Am J Dis Child 1985; 139:567–570.
14. Rosenkrantz TS, Oh W. Aminophylline reduces cerebral blood flow velocity in low birth weight infants. Am J Dis Child 1984; 138:489–491.
15. Miller MJ, Carlo WA, Martin RJ. Continuous positive airway pressure selectively reduces obstructive apnea in preterm infants. J Pediatr 1985; 106:91–94.
16. Jones RAK. Apnoea of prematurity. I. A controlled trial of theophylline and face mask continuous positive airway presure. Arch Dis Child 1982; 57:761–765.
17. Hirsch K, Wang SC. Selective respiratory stimulating action of doxapram compared to pethylene-tetrazol. J Pharmacol Exp Ther 1974; 189:1–11.
18. Barringion KJ, Finer NN, Peters KL, Barton J. Physiologic effects of doxapram in idiopathic apnea of prematurity. J Pediatr 1986; 108:124–129.
19. Brouillette RT, Fernbach SK, Hunt CE. Obstructive sleep apnea in infants and children. J Pediatr 1982; 100:31–40.
20. Sanders MH, Rogers RM, Pennock BE. Prolonged expiratory phase in sleep apnea: a unifying hypothesis. Am Rev Respir Dis 1985; 131:401–408.
21. Sheldon SH, Oenal E, Lillie J, Spire JP. Sleep-related post-inspiratory upper airway obstruction in children. Sleep Res 1993; 22:270.
22. National Institutes of Health Consensus Development Conference. Infantile Apnea and Home Monitoring. Bethesda, MD: US Department of Health and Human Services, October 1, 1987, NIH Pub 87–2950.
23. Marcus CL, Omlin KJ, Basinki DJ, Bailey SL, Rachal AB, Von Pechmann D, et al. Normal polysomnographic values for children and adolescents. Am Rev Respir Dis 1992; 146:1235–1239.
24. Kahn A, Dan B, Groswasser J, Franco P, Sottiaux M. Normal sleep architecture in infants and children. J Clin Neurophysiol 1996; 13:184–197.
25. Mathew OP, Remmers JE. Respiratory function of the upper airway. In: Saunders NA, Sullivan CE, eds. Sleep and Breathing. New York: Marcel Dekker, 1984:163–200.
26. Bartlett D Jr. Effects of hypercapnia and hypoxia on laryngeal resistance to airflow. Respir Physiol 1979; 37:293–302.

27. Remmers JE, Bartlett D Jr. Reflex control of expiratory airflow and duration. J Appl Physiol 1977; 42:80–87.
28. Lamm C. Sleep-disordered breathing in children. Mt Sinai J Med 1994; 61:131–138.
29. Begin R, Bureau MA, Lupien L, Lemieux B. Control and modulation of respiration in Steinert's myotonic dystrophy. Am Rev Respir Dis 1980; 121:281–289.
30. Bye PT, Ellis ER, Issa FG, Donnelly PM, Sullivan CE. Respiratory failure and sleep in neuromuscular disease. Thorax 1990; 45:241–247.
31. Smith PE, Calverley PM, Edwards RH. Hypoxemia during sleep in Duchenne muscular dystrophy. Am Rev Respir Dis 1988; 137:884–888.
32. Skatrud J, Iber C, McHugh W, Rasmussen H, Nichols D. Determinants of hypoventilation during wakefulness and sleep in diaphragmatic paralysis. Am Rev Respir Dis 1980; 121:587–593.
33. Labanowski M, Schmidt-Nowara W, Guilleminault C. Sleep and neuromuscular disease: frequency of sleep-disordered breathing in a neuromuscular disease clinic population. Neurology 1996; 47:1173–1180.
34. Sheldon SH, Spire JP, Levy HB. Pediatric Sleep Medicine. Philadelphia: WB Saunders, 1992:142.
35. Ward SL, Marcus CL. Obstructive sleep apnea in infants and young children. J Clin Neurophysiol 1996; 13:198–207.
36. Guilleminault C, Nino-Murcia G, Heldt G, Baldwin R, Hutchinson D. Alternative treatment to tracheostomy in obstructive sleep apnea syndrome: nasal continuous positive airway pressure in young children. Pediatrics 1986; 78:797–802.
37. Barthlen GM. Nocturnal respiratory failure as an indication of non-invasive ventilation in the patient with neuromuscular disease. Respiration 1997; 64(suppl 1):35–39.
38. Guilleminault C. Obstructive sleep apnea syndrome and its treatment in children: areas of agreement and controversy. Pediatr Pulmonol 1987; 3:429–436.
39. Rodman T, Close HP. The primary hypoventilation syndrome. Am J Med 1959; 26: 808–817.
40. Bach JR, Alba AS. Management of chronic alveolar hypoventilation by nasal ventilation. Chest 1990; 97:52–57.
41. Guntheroth WG, Lohmann R, Spiers PS. Risk of sudden infant death syndrome in subsequent siblings. J Pediatr 1990; 116:520–524.
42. Kelly DH, Shannon DC. Periodic breathing in infants with near-miss sudden infant death syndrome. Pediatrics 1979; 63:355–360.
43. Hodgman JE, Hoppenbrouwers T, Geidel S, Hadeed A, Sterman MB, Harper R, et al. Respiratory behavior in near-miss sudden infant death syndrome. Pediatrics 1982; 69:785–792.
44. Williams AL, Uren EC, Bretherton L. Respiratory viruses and sudden infant death. Br Med J (Clin Res Ed) 1984; 288:1491–1493.
45. Downing SE, Lee JC. Laryngeal chemosensitivity: a possible mechanism for sudden infant death. Pediatrics 1975; 55:640–649.
46. Rosen CL, Frost JD Jr, Harrison GM. Infant apnea: polygraphic studies and follow-up monitoring. Pediatrics 1983; 71:731–736.
47. Southall DP, Richards JM, Rhoden KJ, Alexander JR, Shinebourne EA, Arrowsmith

WA, et al. Prolonged apnea and cardiac arrhythmias in infants discharged from neonatal intensive care units: failure to predict an increased risk for sudden infant death syndrome. Pediatrics 1982; 70:844–851.

48. Wilson AJ, Stevens V, Franks CI, Alexander J, Southall DP. Respiratory and heart rate patterns in infants destined to be victims of sudden infant death syndrome: average rates and their variability measured over 24 hours. Br Med J (Clin Res Ed) 1985; 290:497–501.
49. Schechtman VL, Harper RM, Wilson AJ, Southall DP. Sleep state organization in normal infants and victims of the sudden infant death syndrome. Pediatrics 1992; 89:865–870.
50. Groswasser J, Scaillet T, Franco P, Kahn A. Obstructive sleep apneas in infancy as a risk for SIDS. Somnologie 1997; 1(suppl 2):18.
51. Guilleminault C. Sleep apnea in infancy. In: Guilleminault C, ed. Sleep and Its Disorders in Children. New York: Raven Press, 1987:213–224.
52. Corbo GM, Fuciarelli F, Foresi A, De Benedetto F. Snoring in children: association with respiratory symptoms and passive smoking. Br Med J 1989; 299:1491–1494.
53. American Thoracic Society. Standards and indications for cardiopulmonary sleep studies in children. Am J Respir Crit Care Med 1996; 153:866–878.
54. Brouillette RT, Morrow AS, Weese-Mayer DE, Hunt CF. Comparison of respiratory inductive plethysmography and thoracic impedance for apnea monitoring. J Pediatr 1987; 111:377–383.

5

Dissociated States of Brain and Mind

Mark W. Mahowald and Carlos H. Schenck
Hennepin County Medical Center
and University of Minnesota Medical School
Minneapolis, Minnesota

The state of a system at a given instant is the set of numerical values which its variables have at that instant (1).

INTRODUCTION

Over the centuries, the presentations and concepts of dissociated or automatic behaviors have changed dramatically—ranging from demon possession, witchcraft, shamanism, hysteria, various psychiatric conditions, and frank malingering to the current notion of psychobiological phenomena. The purpose of this chapter is to present such behaviors from the perspective of their state-dependent nature. To convey a better understanding of these fascinating conditions, there is a brief look at the states of human existence, with a review of the currently known spectrum of dissociated and automatic behaviors—both nonpsychological (sleep-related and neurological) and psychological. This will enable the placing of sleep-related phenomena and neurological and psychiatric conditions into the more global perspective of dissociation in general.

The following case example of a 24-year-old man with complex sleepwalking demonstrates one form of state dissociation—a mixed state of wakefulness and sleep, resulting in the appearance of complex behaviors in the absence of conscious awareness or recollection for the events.

> The patient had a history of complex behaviors arising from the sleep period since he was 5 years old. As a child, he sleepwalked downstairs from his bedroom, went into the bathroom, took the toilet paper off the spindle, put it on the kitchen table, and went back up to bed. He never said a word about it to anybody, and did not remember it the next day. He often "wakes up" thinking there is something wrong with his wife or that there is something threatening in the house. He gets up very suddenly and sometimes goes to the bedroom door and feels it to see if it is hot (he is a fireman). At other times, he kicks his legs quickly and lunges forward, thinking someone is on the other side of the room, or thinks there is a noise and tells his wife to "be quiet and shut up." His wife cannot "get him awake enough to tell him it's okay." Once when their dog was sleeping in the bed with them, he picked it up and threw it against the wall. On another occasion, when his wife came to bed, he suddenly sat up and punched her in the face, thinking she was a threatening person in his dream. His wife reported that "he always looks awake," but is almost impossible to awaken during these episodes.

NORMAL STATE DETERMINATION

State determination—wakefulness (W), rapid eye movement (REM) sleep, and non-REM sleep—may be made using various criteria: behavioral (eyes open or closed, body position, movements, reactivity to the environment), electrographic (electroencephalogram [EEG], electro-oculogram [EOG], electromyogram [EMG]), or neuronal state (brain neuronal activity). The state-determining properties of each state usually cycle in a predictable and uniform manner, resulting in the behavioral appearance of a single prevailing state. However, even in normal subjects, the electrographic and neuronal activity transition among states is gradual and variable, with the simultaneous occurrence or rapid oscillation of multiple state-determining markers. Within each state, there is ongoing variability and fluctuation of central nervous system (CNS) activity (2,3).

As discussed in other chapters in this volume, wakefulness, non-REM, and REM sleep are very complex phenomena. There is compelling evidence of extensive reorganization of CNS activity as it moves across these three states of being. Factors involved in state generation are complex, and include a wide variety of neurotransmitters, neuromodulators, neurohormones, and a vast array of "sleep factors" that act upon the multiple neural networks. These facts lead to the conclusion that sleep is a fundamental property of numerous neuronal groups, rather than a phenomenon that requires the whole brain (4,5). Therefore, state determination is the result of a dynamic interaction among many variables, including circadian, neural network, neurotransmitter, and myriad sleep-promoting substances. Some identical neuronal groups are extremely active in more than one state, with differing state-dependent effects; i.e., many REM-sleep phenomena are similar to the alerting response seen in wakefulness (6–8). Some brainstem regions effect motor suppression in REM sleep but motor facilitation in W (9,10).

The state-determining variables of REM sleep have been the most extensively studied. REM sleep comprises both tonic (occurring throughout the entire REM cycle) and phasic (occurring intermittently during the REM cycle) components. Each of these elements is generated, modulated, and executed by different neuronal groups located at multiple levels of the neuraxis—from cerebral cortex to spinal cord—orchestrated by the dorsomedial pontine region.

There are striking neurophysiological semblances between wakefulness and REM sleep. The ascending brainstem reticular system potentiates thalamic and cortical responses during both states. Although the EEG is said to be "desynchronized" during wakefulness and REM sleep (in contrast to being "synchronized" during non-REM sleep), there is fascinating and compelling evidence that during the two states of brain arousal (wakefulness and REM sleep), activation of the mesencephalic reticular formation facilitates oscillatory activity in the gamma frequency band (>30 Hz), which enhances synchronization of cortical responses that may play a role in the processing of sensory signals. The waking and REM-sleep "desynchronized" EEG pattern is more apparent than real—it is actually highly synchronized (11,12). This synchronization may be important for information processing by facilitating the establishment of synchrony over large distances in the cortex, linking remote neurons into functional groups (13).

THE EVOLUTION OF THE CONCEPT OF STATE

The clinical concept of states of being has changed dramatically over the past few decades. It was formerly thought that human existence encompassed only two states: wakefulness and sleep, with sleep being considered simply the passive absence of wakefulness. With the discovery of REM sleep in 1953, it became apparent that sleep is not a unitary phenomenon but consists of two completely different states, and each state is an active, rather than a quiescent, process (14). Each state consists of a number of physiological variables, which, under normal circumstances, tend to occur in concert, resulting in the appearance of one of the three conventional states of being: W, REM sleep, and non-REM sleep (2,15). Animal experiments and evaluation of humans in the sleep laboratory indicate that the "three states of being" concept must be further expanded to include the observations that the physiological event markers of one state may intrude into other states, and that the states may oscillate rapidly, resulting in the appearance of bizarre, previously difficult-to-explain, and occasionally extraordinary animal and human behaviors, which can occur in diverse naturalistic and clinical settings—with important treatment implications (16,17). Recent animal experiments support the concept of state dissociation as a normal manifestation of state transition, suggesting the staggered appearance of state-determining physiological variables. One found suppression of the cortical auditory evoked response shortly before the onset of REM sleep (18); the other demonstrated that sleep develops asynchronously in different cortical areas (19).

EXPERIMENTAL STATE DISSOCIATION (ANIMAL)

The recurrent recruitment of state-determining parameters is amazingly consistent. However, multiple experimental examples of state component dissociation exist (20). These fall into three categories.

Lesion/stimulation: Hypothalamic, thalamic, and brainstem manipulation/stimulation induces state dissociation (21–27). Recent studies in molecular biology may add a fascinating new dimension to such dissociation. For example, 6-hydroxydopamine (6-OHDA) lesions of the locus coeruleus inhibit the expected immediate early gene (c-Fos) expression (normally expected during wakefulness) in the cortex and hippocampus without changing the EEG. Therefore, following such lesions, the cortex may be at least partially functionally asleep, without a sleep EEG pattern (28).

Pharmacological: Manipulation of the cholinergic/glutamate neurotransmitter systems results in a variety of state dissociations (29–38).

Sleep Deprivation: REM-sleep deprivation in cats results in the appearance of PGO spikes during non-REM sleep (39).

In addition to these experimental dissociations, there is evidence in the animal kingdom for the natural occurrence of clinically wakeful behavior during physiological sleep. Two examples that dispel the concept of "all or none" state declaration are: 1) the concurrence of swimming or flight during sleep in birds (40) and 2) the phenomenon of unihemispheric sleep in some aquatic mammals (bottle-nosed dolphin, common porpoise, and northern fur seal) guaranteeing continued respiration while "sleeping" (41). Another naturally occurring dissociated state is seen during the arousal from torpor in hibernating ground squirrels, when there is an "uncoupling between thalamic, EMG, and cortical REM correlates" (42). It is conceivable that sleep may not be necessary in the setting of schooling of fish or flight in flocks by birds, in which case the functional process of sleep occurs during wakefulness (43).

Both experimentally induced and naturally occurring state dissociations in animals serve to predict spontaneously occurring "experiments of nature" and drug-induced state dissociation in humans, which undoubtedly exist on a broad spectrum of expression. Such state dissociations are the consequence of timing or switching errors in the normal process of the dynamic reorganization of the CNS as it moves from one state (or mode) to another. Elements of one state persist, or are recruited, erroneously into another state, often with fascinating and dramatic consequences.

CLINICAL STATE DISSOCIATION—NEUROLOGICAL (HUMAN)

A number of well-documented state dissociations in humans occur spontaneously, or as the result of neurological dysfunction or medication administration. It is practical to designate each as a variant of the predominant or prevailing parent state (W/non-REM/REM), rather than identify each possible dissociated state as an independent entity.

Wakefulness Variations

Narcolepsy

Narcolepsy is the prototypical dissociated state arising from the background of wakefulness, and may best be thought of as a disorder of "state boundary control." The symptom of cataplexy (sudden loss of muscle tone, usually in response to an emotion-laden event) simply represents the isolated "boundary-crossing" of REM sleep atonia into wakefulness. The element of surprise in triggering cataplexy supports the described similarity between the alerting response and REM sleep (7). Similarly, the symptom of sleep paralysis is the persistence of REM atonia into wakefulness. The hypnagogic (occurring at sleep onset) and hypnopompic (occurring upon awakening) hallucinations are dream mentation occurring during wakefulness. These "hallucinations" (dreams) may be particularly frightening if accompanied by sleep paralysis (44). Narcoleptic patients may experience waking dreams, particularly during drowsiness, and be misdiagnosed and even treated as having schizophrenia (45,46). The occurrence of ambiguous or dissociated sleep is well documented in the untreated narcoleptic (47). The induction of dissociated states in narcolepsy by tricyclic antidepressant administration indicates that genetically determined and pharmacologically potentiated state-disrupting factors may act in concert (48–50). Normal individuals may experience sleep paralysis (51).

Hallucinations as a State Dissociation Phenomenon (Wakeful Dreaming)

Historically, there has been a perceived dichotomy between dreams and hallucinations. The former, although occasionally unpleasant, have been held to be normal phenomena, whereas the latter have been considered a hallmark of, if not a defining factor for, certain major psychiatric disorders. Experience in clinical sleep-disorder centers, on psychiatric and internal-medicine wards, and in intensive care units raises questions as to the wisdom of perpetuating this dichotomous concept.

Consciousness is now considered a primary function and activity of the brain itself. If so, then consciousness is simply the brain's interpretation and integration of all information being made available to it at any given point in time. It is clear that the brain is active across all states of being: wakefulness, REM sleep, and non-REM sleep. Under certain circumstances, it is likely that dreaming and hallucinations represent variations on the same theme. Under usual circumstances, during wakefulness the brain is ignoring internally generated activity and attending to environmental sensory stimulation. This may reflect alterations in neuromodulation between wake and sleep (52,53). During sleep, dreaming occurs because the brain attends to endogenously generated activity. In unusual settings, such as sleep deprivation, sensory deprivation, or medication or drug ingestion, the brain has the opportunity to attend to exogenous and endogenous activities simultaneously, resulting in hallucinations, or wakeful dreaming. This concept is supported by numerous neurological conditions and syndromes associated with "hallucinations."

Dream experiences are generated by the brain during sleep (54). The ongoing activity of the brain, devoid of sensory input (during non-REM sleep) or with inattention to sensory input (during REM sleep), is the origin of dreams. The brain is much more active during REM sleep than during non-REM sleep, possibly explaining one advantage of another hallmark of REM sleep: the active paralysis of all somatic musculature (sparing the diaphragm). This paralysis possibly protects us from the ability to act on the REM dream mentation (55).

Although dreaming was initially thought to be a marker of REM sleep, it has recently been established that dreaming can occur during all stages of sleep, and may even occur during relaxed wakefulness, when alpha activity is present on the electroencephalogram (56–61). Further support of this is the fact that dreaming is frequently reported following non-REM sleep occurring during multiple sleep latency test naps (59).

In contrast to dreams, hallucinations are believed to be abnormal experiences, and are often presumed to indicate the presence of underlying psychiatric conditions. The term from which *hallucination* is derived means "to wander in the mind," and refers to waking sensory experiences having no apparent external physical stimulus (62).

All theories on the nature of hallucinations share the concept of misperception and misinterpretation of endogenously generated brain activity occurring in the setting of relative preservation of consciousness, supporting an organic neurophysiological explanation for many hallucinatory phenomena. The concept of state dissociation permits the thinking of some hallucinations as wakeful dreams (63).

The incidence of occasional hallucinations in the nonpsychiatric population is far greater than generally acknowledged (64–66). Hallucinations occur spontaneously, albeit infrequently, in the normal, presumably nonpsychiatric population: between 10% and 27% of the general population report having had a hallucinatory experience (62). Furthermore, hallucinations may be readily induced in normal individuals under a number of circumstances, such as sensory deprivation, drug administration, and deprivation of food or sleep (67).

Moreover, didactic dogma promulgates the myth that auditory hallucinations are indicative of psychiatric disease, whereas visual hallucinations are more suggestive of organic neurological conditions. Closer analysis of the data regarding the relationship between any specific type of hallucination and an underlying "organic" or "psychiatric" condition indicates that the overlap is extremely great, precluding use of the nature of the hallucination as a reliable predictor of neurological vs. psychiatric disease. In fact, hallucinations are *never* pathognomonic for any given disorder (68,69).

Hallucinations in Nonpsychiatric, Nonneurological Conditions

As mentioned above, under a number of different circumstances, hallucinations can readily be induced in individuals without psychiatric or neurological disease. Examples include:

1. Sensory deprivation (66,70–80)
2. Drugs and medications (for review, see Ref. 63)
3. Food deprivation (81)
4. Sleep deprivation (82,83)—sleep deprivation probably plays a role in the hallucinations seen in "intensive care unit psychosis" (84)

These hallucination-inducing situations have been used alone or in combination by mystics, prophets, ascetics, and religious figures to potentiate visual and/or auditory communications with the supernatural or to receive prophecies (85,86).

Hallucinations in Neurological Disorders

Hallucinations may be seen in a wide variety of neurological disorders, often in the setting of sensory deprivation and/or diffuse CNS dysfunction (87,88). In some (if not many) cases, the hallucinations may represent a release of REM (or non-REM) dreamlike mentation into wakefulness, supporting the concept of dream-hallucination isomorphism. Examples include the following.

Charles Bonnet syndrome This syndrome refers to visual hallucinations occurring in patients with reduced visual input to the CNS—at any level, usually ocular (89–92). In some series, these hallucinations occurred in slightly over 13–29% of patients with diminution of visual acuity (93,94). In primary lesions of the CNS, visual hallucinations may be seen in the hemianopic field (95).

The fact that precollicular blindness acquired in utero, in infancy, or in early childhood may result in permanent EEG changes (slowing and spike foci) in the occipital regions suggests that these hallucinatory experiences represent acquired changes or reorganization in brain function. It is well known that isolated cortex develops hypersensitivity (96).

Brainstem lesions and musical hallucinations Both formed and unformed auditory hallucinations have been well described in a variety of peripheral and central lesions resulting in impaired auditory acuity (97,98).

Phantom-limb phenomenon Phantom-limb hallucinations are reported in patients who have lost extremities or have lost sensory information coming from portions of the body (99). They have been reported to occur in up to 100% of patients following spinal-cord injury (100). Contrary to popular opinion, these hallucinations may involve midline structures (bladder and genitalia) (100,101). Breast phantoms are reported in 23% of postmastectomy patients (102). Interestingly, phantom limb perceptions may be present during dreaming, and may persist in dreams after resolving during wakefulness (103).

Amputation of an extremity is not necessary for the development of phantom limb sensations (i.e., the phantom limb phenomenon may follow brachial plexus injury without the loss of the arm). Subsequent surgical removal of the deafferented arm will have no effect on the hallucinations. It is clear that these sensations are arising from the higher levels of the CNS, because lesions of the peripheral nerves, spinal rootlets, pathways within the spinal cord, and areas of the thalamus, and even extirpation of the primary sensory cortex receiving information from the "phantom," will not predictably alleviate the symptom. Therefore, the brain generates the experience of the body, and sensory information simply modulates that experience. Supporting this concept is the fact that people born without limbs may experience phantoms (99,104).

There is now overwhelming evidence that the nervous system is far more plastic than previously thought (105,106). There are rapid changes in cortical organization following both deafferentation and deefferentation of peripheral structures (107). Deafferentation of an extremity by local anesthesia may result in increased excitability of cortical neurons, again indicating organic plasticity changes in the CNS as a response to absence of peripheral sensory stimulation (108).

Visual, auditory, and phantom limb hallucinations are all excellent examples of "deafferentation" hallucinations, resulting from distortions in the normal processing of sensory information, so that abnormal perceptions occur centrally. The fact that these hallucinations can arise from peripheral pathology (ocular, auditory, limb sensory) clearly indicates that primary brain lesions are not necessary (109). Rather, the normally functioning brain is generating false information by attending to internally generated phenomena that are "released" in the absence of competing external sensory information. Recent studies suggesting that tinnitus is centrally generated support the concept of cortical plasticity resulting in the generation of a sensation that is perceived as originating peripherally (110).

Peduncular hallucinosis Waking hallucinations have been well described in deep, midline lesions involving the thalamic, midbrain, hypothalamic, and third ventricular regions of the brain (111–113). The possibility that these hallucinations represent the release of REM- (or non-REM-) sleep dreamlike mentation is supported by the fact that lesions in the same brain regions may result in symptomatic narcolepsy and cataplexy, another condition associated with the intrusion of REM-sleep phenomena into the waking state (114).

Neurodegenerative disorders Hallucinations are often seen in a variety of neurodegenerative disorders such as Parkinson's disease, Alzheimer's disease, and related conditions such as corticobasilar degeneration and dementia with Lewy bodies (115–118). Fatal familial insomnia, a prion disease associated with thalamic degeneration, is often accompanied by hallucinatory behavior and shares some features with the REM-sleep behavior disorder, suggesting the admixture of states (119). The phenomenon of "sundowning" (agitation associated with darkness seen in patients with diffuse neurological dysfunction) may be related to reduced sensory input (120).

Miscellaneous Hallucinations have been reported in a number of other neurological conditions, including migraine (121), a paroxysmal olfactory nerve syndrome (122), following anterior cingulectomy (123), and a variety of cerebrovascular syndromes (124–130). It is likely that close observation will reveal many other neurological conditions associated with hallucinations, therefore expanding the concept of hallucinations as "wakeful dreaming."

It is abundantly apparent that hallucinatory phenomena occur in a wide variety of settings: in normal individuals (particularly in the setting of sleep or sensory deprivation, or exposure to medications/drugs), in patients with psychiatric disorders, and in patients with CNS abnormalities. The nature (auditory, visual, or somesthetic) of the hallucinatory experience is not specific for any of these groups. The unifying theme appears to be the rise (or intrusion) of internally generated brain activity into waking consciousness—the result of a mixed state of being: the waking brain attending *both* to the real environment *and* to internally generated brain activity that is usually suppressed by, or ignored due to, environmental stimulation. During all stages of sleep, attending to such internally generated brain activity is the norm, resulting in dreaming. The spectrum of dreams and hallucinations in various conditions is schematically shown in Figure 1.

REM-Sleep Variations

The REM-sleep behavior disorder (RBD) is the premier example of a dissociated state arising from the background of REM sleep. In retrospect, RBD was predicted in 1965 by animal experiments (25) but not formally recognized in humans until 1986 (55). During normal REM sleep, there is background atonia involving

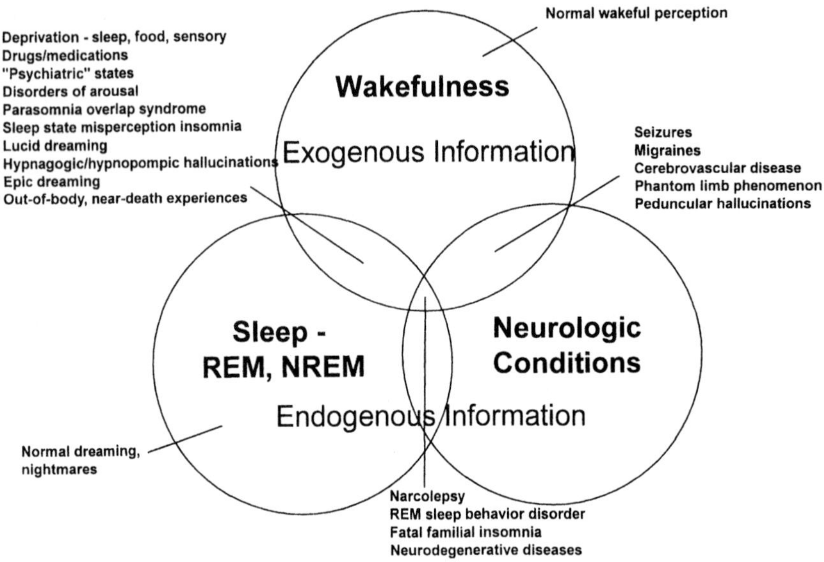

Figure 1 Consciousness working with available information. A schematic representation of the spectrum of dreams and hallucinations across the states of being and in various neurological and psychiatric conditions. (From Ref. 63.)

all somatic musculature (sparing the diaphragm and extraocular muscles). Although this generalized atonia may be briefly interrupted by excitatory inputs resulting in muscle jerks and twitches (131), the prevailing atonia prevents motor activity associated with dream mentation. RBD results from incomplete declaration of REM sleep: all elements of REM sleep are present except the atonia. In RBD, motor behavior attendant with dream imagery may be vigorous, occasionally with injurious results.

The acute, transient form of RBD is seen most frequently in the setting of drug intoxication or withdrawal states. There is also a chronic form of RBD, most often affecting older men. Nearly half of subjects with chronic RBD have identifiable underlying neurological disorders (55). The fact that over half of cases are idiopathic and tend to occur in the elderly suggests that RBD may be the reverse of sleep ontogeny (see ''Comment and Perspectives'' below). The absence of identifiable peri–locus coeruleus lesions in the ''symptomatic'' subgroup is of interest, and confirms animal experimental data that indicate that suprapontine lesions may also affect REM-sleep atonia (132). In the animal model, chloramphenicol administration can reverse the peri–locus coeruleus lesion-induced REM without atonia, indicating that other structures are capable of inducing REM-sleep atonia (133). An analogous situation during W is the contribution of cortical, rubral, and pontine neurons to anterior horn cell phasic excitation, indicating that motor activity may be initiated at several levels of the CNS (15).

Electrographic dissociation of REM sleep (absence of muscle atonia during REM sleep) and full-blown RBD may be induced in humans by the commonly prescribed tricyclic antidepressants, selective serotonin-reuptake inhibitors (SSRIs), and venlafaxine (134–137). Spontaneously occurring RBD has also been reported in dogs and cats (138).

A number of other sleep–dream phenomena have been attributed to mixed states of being, including the hypnagogic/hypnopompic hallucinations of narcolepsy and out-of-body and near-death experiences (and even "alien abductions"?) (17,139,140). It should be mentioned that hypnagogic and hypnopompic hallucinations occur in over one-third of the normal population (141). Lucid dreaming is another example of a mixed W/REM state, during which the dreamer is both aware of the fact that he or she is dreaming and able to influence the course of the dream. REM sleep is the parent state during lucid dreaming, yet there is sufficient persisting wakefulness that a subject has the ability to physically signal the presence of such a dream by means of voluntary eye and digit movements. Suppression of the H-reflex, a characteristic of REM sleep, persists during such dreaming (142). One recently described condition, "epic dreaming," may also represent a mixed state of being, with relatively complete preservation of the memory systems during sleep—resulting in the remembering of the continuous sleep-mentation that occurs in all normal individuals (143,144). It is also conceivable that some cases of "sleep-state misperception" (145) insomnia may represent an admixture of states.

Non-REM Sleep Variations

Disorders of arousal are the most impressive and most frequent of the non-REM sleep-state dissociation/admixture phenomena. Disorders of arousal occur on a broad spectrum ranging from confusional arousals, through somnambulism (sleepwalking), to sleep terrors (also called pavor nocturnus). Some take the form of "specialized" behaviors such as sleep-related eating and sleep-related sexual activity—without conscious awareness (146,147).

The disorders of arousal are prevalent (and perfectly normal) in childhood (1–17%), peaking at 11–12 years of age, and are far more common in adults (4–10%) than generally acknowledged (148–151). Although it has been commonly thought that persistence of these behaviors beyond childhood or their development in adulthood is an indication of significant psychopathology (152,153), numerous studies have dispelled this myth, indicating that significant psychopathology in adults with disorders of arousal is usually *not* present (154–157). The clinical features, laboratory evaluation, and treatment of disorders of arousal have been extensively reviewed elsewhere (158).

The recently described cyclic alternating pattern (CAP) may play a role in the etiology of the disorders of arousal. The CAP is a physiological component of non-REM sleep and is functionally correlated with long-lasting arousal oscillations. The CAP is a measure of non-REM instability with high level of arousal oscillation (159). There is no difference in the macrostructural sleep parameters between patients with disorders of arousal and controls (160). However, patients with disorders of arousal have been found to have increases in CAP rate, number of CAP cycles, and arousals with EEG synchronization.

A common thread linking RBD and the disorders of arousal is the appearance of motor activity that is dissociated from waking consciousness. In RBD, the motor behavior closely correlates with dream imagery, and in disorders of arousal, it often occurs in the absence of (remembered) mentation. This dissociation of behavior from consciousness may be explained by the presence of locomotor centers (LMCs), from the mesencephalon to the medulla, that are capable of generating complex behaviors without cortical input (161–164). These areas project to the central pattern generator of the spinal cord, which itself is able to produce complex stepping movements in the absence of supraspinal influence (165). This accounts for the fact that decorticate experimental and barnyard animals are capable of performing very complex, integrated motor acts.

It is likely that during non-REM sleep, the LMCs are not activated. The thesis that LMCs are actively inhibited during REM sleep is supported by the observations that in cats, smaller peri–locus coeruleus lesions result in REM sleep without atonia—without any behavioral manifestations—but larger lesions are necessary to produce active motor movements. Clearly, the isolated loss of REM-sleep atonia is insufficient to explain complex REM-sleep motor activity in the experimental animal (166), suggesting a release of LMCs during the parent state, just as is seen in the loss of REM-sleep atonia. Dissociation of the LMCs from the parent state of REM or non-REM sleep would explain the presence of complex motor behavior seen in RBD and disorders of arousal. It is likely that the complex motor activity associated with amnesia characteristic of alcohol-induced "blackouts" (167) and with "unconscious" behavior during partial complex seizures represents dissociation between LMCs and waking consciousness and/or memory (168). Such dissociation between behavior and consciousness may be related to inactivation of attentional or memory systems (4).

The recently described "parasomnia overlap" syndrome, further linking RBD with disorders of arousal, may serve to expand the concept of state-dependent motor dyscontrol. In this syndrome, the patients have both clinical and PSG evidence of both disorders of arousal and RBD, suggesting that motor dyscontrol during sleep is the primary abnormality. If this occurs during non-REM sleep, the result is disorders of arousal; if during REM sleep, the result is RBD (169).

A condition called status dissociatus, the most extreme form of RBD, appears to represent a complete breakdown of state-determining boundaries. Clinically, these patients, by behavioral observation, appear to be either awake or "asleep." Clinically, however, their behavioral "sleep" is very atypical, characterized by frequent muscle-twitching, vocalization, and reports of dreamlike mentation upon spontaneous or forced awakening. Polygraphically, there are few, if any, features of either conventional REM or non-REM sleep; rather, there is the simultaneous admixture of elements of wakefulness, REM sleep and non-REM sleep. Conditions associated with status dissociatus include protracted withdrawal from alcohol abuse, narcolepsy, olivopontocerebellar degeneration, and prior open-heart surgery. Clonazepam may be effective in treating the sleep-related motor and verbal behaviors (16,17). The clinical features of fatal familial insomnia, a prion disease closely related to Creutzfeldt-Jakob disease, are highly reminiscent of status dissociatus (170,171).

The Significance of State Dissociation

The multiple-component concept of state determination is a most important notion to consider when pharmacological or lesion studies are employed to "suppress" one or another state. Such manipulation may suppress some of the commonly used markers for that state (i.e., polygraphic)—without affecting other variables of that state. The naturally occurring (172) and drug-induced dissociation between REM-sleep-related penile tumescence and conventional polygraphic features of REM sleep attest to this fact (173–176).

CLINICAL STATE DISSOCIATION—PSYCHOGENIC (HUMAN)

It is now apparent that psychogenic dissociative disorders may arise exclusively or predominately from the sleep period (177,178). Virtually all patients with nocturnal dissociative disorders evaluated at our center were victims of repeated physical and/or sexual abuse—which is often remembered incompletely, if at all—beginning in childhood (178). There is now overwhelming neurophysiological evidence in animal models that such physical or psychic trauma may lead to permanent alterations in functioning of the central nervous system (16,17), predisposing to clinical dissociative disorders. This suggests that these disorders also have a neuro(psycho)biological basis, and may not be "functional" in the psychiatric sense. These conditions include psychogenic dissociative disorder and multiple-personality disorder, and have been reviewed elsewhere (178).

CLINICAL AND LABORATORY EVALUATION OF STATE-DISSOCIATION DISORDERS

The above discussion indicates that all types of automatic/dissociated behaviors may be the manifestation of either organic or psychiatric conditions. Thorough evaluation should be conducted to rule out organic conditions. Our experience with over 300 adult cases of sleep-related complex behavior has indicated that clinical differentiation among the various dissociative disorders is often impossible (178–180). Clinical evaluation should include a complete review of sleep–wake complaints from both the patient and his or her bedpartner (if available). This should be followed by a thorough general physical, neurological, and psychiatric examination. The diagnosis may only be suspected clinically. Extensive polygraphic study employing an extensive scalp EEG at a paper speed of 15 mm/sec, electromyographic monitoring of all four extremities, and continuous audiovisual recording are mandatory for correct diagnosis in atypical cases (179,181–188). Establishing the diagnosis of nocturnal seizures may be particularly difficult (189).

COMMENT AND PERSPECTIVES

Review of the ontogeny of state appearance facilitates the analysis of observed experimental and clinical state dissociations. During embryogenesis, there are no clear-cut states but rather the simultaneous admixture of all states, which gradually coalesce to form the three recognizable states of W, REM sleep, and non-REM sleep (190–194). This ontogeny of state development is supported by phylogenetic studies (195,196). The mechanisms of complex synchronization/recruitment of the state-specific variables are unknown. Basic-science neurophysiologists have long known that state dissociation in animals occurs frequently, under many circumstances (197). The inability of animals to report or indicate mentation and consciousness (i.e., waking hallucinations, mental imagery with disorders of arousal, dream-mentation-associated motor behavior in RBD) has been a significant limitation on the evaluation of animal state dissociation and its application to the human clinical experience.

Many endogenous and exogenous factors can affect state cycling/synchronization, including (198–200):

1. Age
2. Sleep deprivation
3. Shiftwork or rapid travel across time zones
4. Endogenous humoral factors (hormonal)
5. Drugs/medication
6. Affective disorders
7. Environmental stress

With the multiplicity of state markers, and the relatively rapid normal cycling of states requiring recruitment of these numerous physiological markers, there are innumerable theoretically possible state combinations. It is likely that major psychic or neural insults can result in an acquired functional restructuring of the

CNS, which may then interfere with conventional state determination (201). There is strong evidence that environmentally mediated events can and do affect the structure and function of the CNS (200,202–204) and that the CNS displays learning of new neural behaviors (205–207)—i.e., the development of secondary epileptogenesis [''mirror foci''] (208) or acquired sensory synesthesia (209,210). Such dissociated states may play a role in the appearance of psychogenic dissociative states. Indeed, given the genetic variability of CNS development and its plasticity (201,211–213), the relentless cycling, and the ever-present multiplicity of endogenous and environmental influences on both CNS plasticity and cycling, it is actually surprising that state-component timing errors do not occur more frequently. Truly, the drive for complete state determination must be very powerful. Striking sleep abnormalities have been reported in a wide variety of degenerative (171,214–219) and acquired (220–223) neurological conditions. This patient population should serve as a rich source of ''high risk for state-dissociation'' subjects.

As mentioned above, the multiple-component concept of state determination must be remembered when pharmacological or lesion studies are employed to ''suppress'' one or another state. Such manipulation may suppress some of the commonly used markers for that state (i.e., polygraphic) without affecting other variables of that state. Recent molecular biological studies mentioned above underscore the complexity of state determination (28). Nielsen's concept of ''phantom REM'' to explain the confusion of REM sleep vs. non-REM sleep dreaming lends clinical relevance to the concept of part of one state manifesting itself during polygraphic trappings of another state (224).

SUMMARY

The concept of state dissociation in humans was made possible only by applying information obtained from basic-science animal research studies to the human condition—without which these often dramatic, and treatable, conditions would have remained in the mystical or psychiatric arena, without appropriate or effective treatment options. Continued study of state dissociation by both basic scientists and clinicians will undoubtedly identify and explain even more of these fascinating conditions, with important therapeutic implications. The reciprocal benefits of close collaboration between basic scientists and clinicians will continue to be appreciated.

REFERENCES

1. Ashby WR. Design for a brain: the origin of adaptive behavior. London: Chapman Hall, 1960:16.

2. Hobson JA, Scheibel AB. The brainstem core: sensorimotor integration and behavioral state control. Neurosci Res Program Bull 1980; 18.
3. Terzano MG, Parrino L, Spaggiari MC. The cyclic alternating pattern sequences in the dynamic organization of sleep. EEG Clin Neurophysiol 1988; 69:437–447.
4. Hobson JA, Schmajuk NA. Brain state and plasticity: an integration of the reciprocal interaction model of sleep cycle oscillation with attentional models of hippocampal function. Arch Italiennes de Biologie 1988; 126:209–224.
5. Krueger JM, Obal F Jr, Kapas L, Fang J. Brain organization and sleep function. Behav Brain Res 1995; 69:177–185.
6. Bowker RM, Morrison AR. The startle reflex and PGO spikes. Brain Res 1976; 102:185–190.
7. Glenn LL. Brainstem and spinal control of lower limb motoneurons with special reference to phasic events and startle reflexes. In: McGinty DJ, Drucker-Colin R, Morrison A, Parmeggiani PL, eds. Brain Mechanisms of Sleep. New York: Raven Press, 1985:81–95.
8. Morrison AR. Paradoxical sleep and alert wakefulness: variations on a theme. In: Chase MH, Weitzman ED, eds. Sleep Disorders: Basic and Clinical Research. New York: Spectrum, 1983:95–122.
9. Wills N, Chase MH. Brain stem control of masseteric reflex activity during sleep and wakefulness: mesencephalon and pons. Exp Neurol 1979; 64:98–117.
10. Chase MH. The motor functions of the reticular formation are multifaceted and state-determined. In: Hobson JA, Brazier MAB, eds. The Reticular Formation Revisited. New York: Raven Press, 1980: 449–472.
11. Munk MHJ, Roelfsema PR, Konig P, Engel AK, Singer W. Role of reticular activation in the modulation of intracortical synchronization. Science 1996; 272:271–274.
12. Steriade M, Amzica F, Contreras D. Synchronization of fast (30–40 Hz) spontaneous rhythms during brain activation. J Neurosci 1996; 16:392–417.
13. Konig P, Engel AK, Singer W. Relation between oscillatory activity and long-range synchronization in cat visual cortex. Proc Nat Acad Sci USA 1995; 92:290–294.
14. Jones B. Basic mechanisms of sleep-wake states. In: Kryger MH, Roth R, Dement WC, eds. Principles and Practice of Sleep Medicine. Philadelphia: WB Saunders, 1994:145–162.
15. Hobson JA, Lydic R, Baghdoyan HA. Evolving concepts of sleep cycle generation: from brain centers to neuronal populations. Behav Brain Sci 1986; 9:371–448.
16. Mahowald MW, Schenck CH. Status dissociatus—a perspective on states of being. Sleep 1991; 14:69–79.
17. Mahowald MW, Schenck CH. Dissociated states of wakefulness and sleep. Neurology 1992; 42:44–52.
18. Niiyama Y, Sekine A, Fushimi M, Hishikawa Y. Marked suppression of cortical auditory evoked response shortly before the onset of REM sleep. NeuroReport 1997; 8:3303–3308.
19. Pigarev IN, Nothdurft H-C, Kastner S. Evidence for asynchronous development of sleep in cortical areas. NeuroReport 1997; 8:2557–2560.
20. McGinty DJ, Drucker-Colin RR. Sleep mechanisms: biology and control of REM sleep. Int Rev Neurobiol 1982; 23:391–436.

21. McGinty DJ. Somnolence, recovery and hyposomnia following ventro-medial diencephalic lesions in the rat. EEG Clin Neurophysiol 1969; 26:70–79.
22. Villablanca J, Salinas-Zeballos ME. Sleep-wakefulness, EEG and behavioral studies of chronic cats without the thalamus: the ''athalamic'' cat. Arch Italiennes de Biologie 1972; 110:383–411.
23. Feldman SM, Waller HJ. Dissociation of electrocortical activation and behavioral arousal. Nature 1962; 196:1320–1322.
24. Hendricks JC, Morrison AR, Mann GL. Different behaviors during paradoxical sleep without atonia depend upon lesion site. Brain Res 1982; 239:81–105.
25. Jouvet M, Delorme F. Locus coeruleus et sommeil paradoxal. C Roy Soc Biol 1965; 159:895–899.
26. Pompeiano O. The Neurophysiological Mechanisms of the Postural and Motor Events During REM Sleep. Research Publication: Association for Research in Nervous and Mental Disease 1967:351–423.
27. Webster HH, Jones BE. Neurotoxic lesions of the dorsolateral pontomesencephalic tegmentum-cholinergic cell area in the cat. II. Effects on sleep-waking states. Brain Res 1988; 458:285–302.
28. Cirelli C, Pompeiano M, Tononi G. Neuronal gene expression in the waking state: a role for the locus coeruleus. Science 1996; 274:1211–1215.
29. Delorme F, Froment J, Jouvet M. Suppression du sommeil par la p-chloromethamphetamine et la p-chlorophenylalanine. C Roy Soc Biol (Paris) 1966; 160:2347.
30. Vivaldi E, McCarley RW, Hobson JA. Evocation of desynchronized sleep signs by chemical microstimulation of the pontine brainstem. In: Hobson JA, Brazier MAB, eds. The Reticular Formation Revisited. New York: Raven Press, 1980.
31. Delinger SL, Patarca R, Hobson JA. Differential enhancement of rapid eye movement sleep signs in the cat: a comparison of microinjection of the cholinergic agonist carbachol and the beta-adrenergic antagonist propranolol on pontogeniculo-occipital wave clusters. Brain Res 1988; 473:116–126.
32. Domino EF, Yamamoto K, Dren AT. Role of cholinergic mechanisms in states of wakefulness and sleep. Progress Brain Res 1968; 128:113–133.
33. Hazra J. Effect of hemicholinium-3 on slow wave and paradoxical sleep of cat. Eur J Pharmacol 1970; 11:395–397.
34. Mitler MM, Dement WC. Cataplectic-like behavior in cats after microinjection of carbachol in the pontine reticular formation. Brain Res 1974; 69:335–343.
35. Baghdoyan HA, Rodrigo-Angulo ML, McCarley RW, Hobson JA. Cholinergic induction of desynchronized sleep signs by carbachol microinjection shows intrapontine site differentiation. Sleep Res 1982; 11:51.
36. Harper RM. Relationship of neuronal activity to EEG waves during sleep and wakefulness. In: Phillips MI, ed. Brain Unit Activity During Behavior. Springfield, IL: Charles C Thomas, 1973: 130–154.
37. Irmis F. ''Dissociation'' between EEG and spontaneous behavior of rats after atropine. Actvitas Nervosa Superior 1971; 13:217–218.
38. Lai YY, Siegel JM. Medullary regions mediating atonia. J Neurosci 1988; 8:4790–4796.
39. Dement WC. The biological role of REM sleep (circa 1968). In: Kales A, ed. Sleep Physiology and Pathology. Philadelphia: Lippincott, 1969: 245–265.

40. Amlander CJJ, Ball NJ. Avian sleep. In: Kryger MH, Roth T, Dement WC, eds. Principles and Practice of Sleep Medicine. Philadelphia: WB Saunders, 1989:30–49.
41. Zeplin H. Mammalian sleep. In: Kryger MH, Roth T, Dement WC, eds. Principles and Practice of Sleep Medicine. Philadelphia: WB Saunders, 1989:30–49.
42. Krilowicz BL, Glotzbach SF, Heller HC. Neuronal activity during sleep and completed bouts of hibernation. Am J Physiol 1988; 255:R1008–R1019.
43. Kavanau JL. Vertebrates that never sleep. Brain Res Bull 1998; 46:269–279.
44. Van Den Hoed J, Lucas EA, Dement WC. Hallucinatory experiences during cataplexy in patients with narcolepsy. Am J Psychiatry 1979; 136:1210–1211.
45. Shapiro B, Spitz H. Problems in the differential diagnosis of narcolepsy versus schizophrenia. Am J Psychiatry 1976; 133:1321–1323.
46. Douglass AB, Hays P, Pazderka F, Russell JM. A schizophrenic variant of narcolepsy. Sleep Res 1989; 18:173.
47. DeBarros-Ferreria M, Lairy GC. Ambiguous sleep in narcolepsy. In: Guilleminault C, Dement WC, Passouant P, eds, Narcolepsy. Advances in Sleep Research. Vol 3. New York: Spectrum, 1976:57–75.
48. Bental E, Lavie P, Sharf B. Severe hypermotility during sleep in treatment of cataplexy with clomipramine. Isr J Med Sci 1979; 15:607–609.
49. Guilleminault C, Raynal D, Takahashi S, Carskadon M, Dement W. Evaluation of short-term and long-term treatment of the narcolepsy syndrome with clomipramine hydrochloride. Acta Neurol Scand 1976; 54:71–87.
50. Cadilhac J. Tricyclics and REM sleep. In: Guilleminault C, Dement WC, Passouant P, eds. Narcolepsy. Advances in Sleep Research. Vol 3. New York: Spectrum, 1976:605–623.
51. Takeuchi T, Miyasita A, Sasaki Y, Inugami M, Fukuda K. Isolated sleep paralysis elicited by sleep interruption. Sleep 1992; 15:217–225.
52. Kahn D, Pace-Schott EF, Hobson JA. Consciousness in waking and dreaming: the roles of neuronal oscillation and neuromodulation in determining similarities and differences. Neuroscience 1997; 78:13–38.
53. Hobson JA. Dreaming as delirium: a mental status analysis of our nightly madness. Sem Neurol 1997; 17:121–128.
54. Hobson JA, McCarley RW. The brain as a dream state generator: an activation-synthesis hypothesis of the dream process. Am J Psychiatry 1977; 134:1335–1348.
55. Mahowald MW, Schenck CH. REM sleep behavior disorder. In: Kryger MH, Dement W, Roth T, eds. Principles and Practice of Sleep Medicine. Philadelphia: WB Saunders, 1994:574–588.
56. Cavallero C, Cicogna P, Natale V, Occhionero M, Zito A. Slow wave sleep dreaming. Sleep 1992; 15:562–566.
57. Bosinelli M. Mind and consciousness during sleep. Behav Brain Res 1995; 69: 195–201.
58. Cicogna P. Dreaming during sleep onset and awakening. Perceptual and Motor Skills 1994; 78:1041–1042.
59. Benbadis SR, Wolgamuth BR, Perry MC, Dinner DS. Dreams and rapid eye movement sleep in the multiple sleep latency test. Sleep 1995; 18:105–108.

60. Rosenlicht N, Maloney T, Feinberg I. Dream report length is more dependent on arousal level than prior REM duration. Brain Res Bull 1994; 34:99–101.
61. Foulkes D. Dreaming and REM sleep. J Sleep Res 1993; 2:199–202.
62. Stevenson I. Do we need a new word to supplement "hallucination"? Am J Psychiatry 1983; 140:1609–1611.
63. Mahowald MW, Woods SR, Schenck CH. Sleeping dreams, waking hallucinations, and the central nervous system. Dreaming 1998; 8:89–102.
64. Rees WD. The hallucinations of widowhood. Br Med J 1971; 4:37–41.
65. Matchett WF. Repeated hallucinatory experiences as a part of the mourning process among Hopi Indian women. Psychiatry 1972; 35:185–194.
66. Siegel RK. Hostage hallucinations: visual imagery induced by isolation and life-threatening stress. J Nerv Ment Dis 1984; 172:264–271.
67. Slade P. Hallucinations. Psycholog Med 1976; 6:7–13.
68. Asaad G, Shapiro B. Hallucinations: theoretical and clinical overview. Am J Psychiatry 1986; 143:1088–1097.
69. Goodwin DW, Alderson P, Rosenthal R. Clinical significance of hallucinations in psychiatric disorders. Arch Gen Psychiatry 1971; 24:76–80.
70. Freedman SJ, Grunebaum HU, Stare FA, Greenblatt M. Imagery in sensory deprivation. In: West L, ed. Hallucinations. New York: Grune & Stratton, 1962:108–117.
71. Myers TI. Reported visual sensation during brief exposure to reduced sensory input. In: West L, ed. Hallucinations. New York: Grune & Stratton, 1962:118–125.
72. Solomon P, Mendelson J. Hallucinations in sensory deprivation. In: West L, ed. Hallucinations. New York: Grune & Stratton, 1962:125–134.
73. Vernon JA, McGill RE. Sensory deprivation and hallucinations. In: West L, ed. Hallucinations. New York: Grune & Stratton, 1962:146–152.
74. Mendelson J, Solomon P, Lindemann E. Hallucinations of poliomyelitis patients during treatment in a respirator. J Nerv Ment Dis 1958; 126:421–428.
75. Heron W. The pathology of boredom. Scientific American 1957; 196:52–56.
76. Mullaney DJ, Kripke DF, Fleck PA. Effects of sustained continuous performance on subjects working alone and in pairs. Perceptual and Motor Skills 1983; 57:819–832.
77. Ziskind E, Augsburg T. Hallucinations in sensory deprivation. Dis Nerv System 1967; 28:721–726.
78. Hayashi M, Morikawa T, Hori T. EEG alpha activity and hallucinatory experiences during sensory deprivation. Perceptual and Motor Skills 1992; 75:403–412.
79. Schultz DP. Sensory Restriction: Effects on Behavior. New York: Academic Press, 1965:93–95.
80. Newberg AB. Changes in the central nervous system and their clinical correlates during long-term space flight. Aviation Space Environmental Med 1994; 65:562–572.
81. Phillips RW. Religious revelations and bovine ketosis (a nonsacred cow). Perspect Biol Med 1978; 21:398–405.
82. Babkoff H, Sing HC, Thorne DR, Genser SG, Hegge FW. Perceptual distortions and hallucinations reported during the course of sleep deprivation. Perceptual and Motor Skills 1989; 68:787–798.

83. Belenky GL. Unusual visual experiences reported by subjects in the British army study of sustained operations, exercise early call. Military Med 1979; 144:695–696.
84. Weber RJ, Oszko MA, Bolender BJ, Grysiak DL. Intensive care unit syndrome: causes, treatment, and prevention. Drug Intell Clin Pharm 1985; 19:13–20.
85. Bennett BM. Vision and audition in biblical prophecy. Parapsychol Rev 1978; 9: 1–12.
86. Kroll J, Bachrach B. Visions and psychopathology in the middle ages. J Nerv Ment Dis 1982; 170:41–49.
87. Carter JL. Visual, somatosensory, olfactory, and gustatory hallucinations. Psychiatr Clin North Am 1992; 15:347–359.
88. Benson DF, Gorman DG. The neural basis of hallucinations. Curr Neurol 1993; 13:265–288.
89. Teunisse RJ, Cruysberg JR, Hoefnagels WH, Verbeek AL, Zitman FG. Visual hallucinations in psychologically normal people: Charles Bonnet's syndrome. Lancet 1996; 347:794–797.
90. Gold K, Rabins PV. Isolated visual hallucinations and the Charles Bonnet syndrome: a review of the literature and presentation of six cases. Comprehen Psychiatry 1989; 30:90–98.
91. Cole MG. Charles Bonnet hallucinations: a case series. Can J Psychiatry 1992; 37: 267–270.
92. Bhatia MS, Khastgir U, Malik SC. Charles Bonnet syndrome. Br J Psychiatry 1992; 161:409–410.
93. Holroyd S, Rabins PV. A three-year follow-up study of visual hallucinations in patients with macular degeneration. J Nerv Ment Dis 1966; 184:188–189.
94. Berrios GE, Brook P. Visual hallucinations and sensory delusions in the elderly. Br J Psychiatry 1984; 144:662–664.
95. Kolmel HW. Complex visual hallucinations in the hemianopic field. J Neurol Neurosurg Psychiatry 1985; 48:29–38.
96. Chattha AS, Lombroso CT. Electroencephalographic changes in childhood optic neuritis. Electroencephalog Clin Neurophysiol 1972; 33:81–88.
97. Murata S, Naritomi H, Sawada T. Musical auditory hallucinations caused by a brainstem lesion. Neurology 1994; 44:156–158.
98. Fenton GW, McRae DA. Musical hallucinations in a deaf elderly woman. Br J Psychiatry 1989; 155:401–403.
99. Melzak R. Phantom limbs. Scientific American 1992:120–126.
100. Bors E. Phantom limbs of patients with spinal cord injury. Arch Neurol Psychiatry 1951; 66:610–631.
101. Heusner AP. Phantom genitalia. Transactions Am Neurolog Assn 1950:128–131.
102. Jarvis JH. Post-mastectomy breast phantoms. In: Keup W, ed. Origin and Mechanisms of Hallucinations. New York: Plenum Press, 1970:457–459.
103. Frank B, Lorenzoni E. Experiences of phantom limbs in dreams. Psychopathology 1989; 22:182–187.
104. Kolb LC. Phantom sensations, hallucinations and the body image. In: West L, ed. Hallucinations. New York: Grune & Stratton, 1962:239–249.

105. Kilgard MP, Merzenich MM. Cortical map reorganization enabled by nucleus basalis activity. Science 1998; 279:1714–1718.
106. Merzenich MM, Recanzone GH, Jenkins WM, Grajski KA. Adaptive mechanisms in cortical networks underlying cortical contributions to learning and nondeclarative memory. Cold Spring Harbor Symposium on Quantitative Biology 1990; LV: 873–887.
107. Rijntjes M, Tegenthoff M, Liepert J, Leonhardt G, Kotterba S, Muller S, Keibel S, Malin J-P, Diener H-C, Weiller C. Cortical reorganization in patients with facial palsy. Ann Neurol 1997; 41:621–630.
108. Sadato N, Zeffiro TA, Campbell G, Konishi J, Shibasaki H, Hallett M. Regional cerebral blood flow changes in motor cortical areas after transient anesthesia of the forearm. Ann Neurol 1995; 37:74–81.
109. Ross ED, Jossman PB, Bell B, Sabin T, Geschwind N. Musical hallucinations in deafness. J Am Med Assn 1975; 231:620–621.
110. Lockwood AH, Slavi RJ, Coad ML, Towsley ML, Wack DS, Murphy BW. The functional neuroanatomy of tinnitus: evidence for limbic system links and neural plasticity. Neurology 1998; 50:114–120.
111. Matthews MK Jr, Alter M, Sirken DH. MRI and electrophysiological findings in a case of peduncular hallucinosis associated with a thalamic-midbrain infarction. Neurology 1992; 42(suppl 3):165.
112. Feinberg WM. "Peduncular hallucinosis" following paramedian thalamic infarction. Neurology 1989; 39:1535–1536.
113. McKee AC. Peduncular hallucinosis associated with isolated infarction of the substantia nigra pars reticulata. Ann Neurol 1990; 27:500–504.
114. Aldrich MS, Naylor MW. Narcolepsy associated with lesions of the diencephalon. Neurology 1989; 39:1505–1508.
115. Schneider JA, Watts RL, Gearing M, Brewer RP, Mirra SS. Corticobasal degeneration: neuropathologic and clinical heterogeneity. Neurology 1997; 48:959–969.
116. Lerner AJ, Koss E, Patterson MB, Ownby RL, Hedera P, Friedland RP, Whitehouse PJ. Concomitants of visual hallucinations in Alzheimer's disease. Neurology 1994; 44:523–527.
117. Klatka LA, Louis ED, Schiffer RB. Psychiatric features in diffuse Lewy body disease: a clinicopathologic study using Alzheimer's disease and Parkinson's disease comparison groups. Neurology 1996; 47:1148–1152.
118. Sanchez-Ramos JR, Ortoll R, Paulson GW. Visual hallucinations associated with parkinson disease. Arch Neurol 1966; 53:1265–1268.
119. Reder AT, Mednick AS, Brown P, Spire JP, Van Cauter E, Wollmann RL, Cervenakova L, Goldfarb LG, Garay A, Ovsiew F, Gajdusek DC, Roos RP. Clinical and genetic studies of fatal familial insomnia. Neurology 1995; 45:1068–1075.
120. Bliwise D. What is sundowning? JAGS 1994; 42:1009–1011.
121. Panayiotopoulos CP. Elementary visual hallucinations in migraine and epilepsy. J Neurol Neurosurg Psychiatry 1994; 57:1371–1374.
122. Kaufman MD, Lassiter KRL, Shenoy BV. Paroxysmal unilateral dysosmia: a cured patient. Ann Neurol 1988; 24:450–451.
123. Whitty CWM, Lewin W. Vivid day-dreaming: an unusual form of confusion following anterior cingulectomy. Brain 1957; 80:72–76.

124. Peroutka SJ, Sohmer BH, Kumar AJ, Folstein M, Robinson RG. Hallucinations and delusions following a right temporoparietooccipital infarction. Johns Hopkins Med J 1982; 151:181–185.
125. Chamorro A, Sacco RL, Ciecierski K, Binder JR, Tatemichi TK, Mohr JP. Visual hemineglect and hemihallucinations in a patient with a subcortical infarction. Neurology 1990; 40:1463–1464.
126. Rousseaux M, Cebrock D, Cabaret M, Steinling M. Visual hallucinations with written words in a case of left parietotemporal lesion. J Neurol Neurosurg Psychiatry 1994; 57:1268–1271.
127. Caplan LR. ''Top of the basilar'' syndrome. Neurology 1980; 30:72–79.
128. Schmidley JW, Messing RO. Agitated confusional states in patients with right hemisphere infarctions. Stroke 1984; 15:883–885.
129. Devinsky O, Bear D, Volpe BT. Confusional states following posterior cerebral artery infarction. Arch Neurol 1988; 45:160–163.
130. Mori E, Yamadori A. Acute confusional state and acute delirium: occurrence after infarction in the right middle cerebral artery territory. Arch Neurol 1987; 44:1139–1143.
131. Chase MH, Morales FR. Subthreshold excitatory activity and motoneurone discharge during REM periods of active sleep. Science 1983; 221:1195–1198.
132. Culebras A, Moore JT. Magnetic resonance findings in REM sleep behavior disorder. Neurology 1989; 39:1519–1523.
133. Aguilar-Roblero R, Arankowsky G, Drucker-Colin R, Morrison AR, Bayon A. Reversal of rapid eye movement sleep without atonia by chloramphenicol. Brain Res 1984; 305:19–26.
134. Passouant P, Cadilhac J, Ribstein M. Les privations de sommeil avec mouvements oculaires par les anti-depresseurs. Rev Neurologique 1972; 127:173–192.
135. Besset A. Effect of antidepressants on human sleep. Adv Biosci 1978; 21:141–148.
136. Schutte S, Doghramji K. REM behavior disorder seen with venlafaxine (Effexor). Sleep Res 1996; 25:364.
137. Schenck CH, Mahowald MW. Does REM sleep behavior disorder protect against obstructive sleep apnea? Sleep Res 1992; 21:257.
138. Hendricks JC, Lager A, O'Brien D, Morrison AR. Movement disorders during sleep in cats and dogs. J Am Vet Med Assn 1989; 194:686–689.
139. Olson M. The out-of-body experience and other states of consciousness. Arch Psychiatr Nursing 1987; 1:201–207.
140. Greyson B. Varieties of near-death experience. Psychiatry 1993; 56:390–399.
141. Ohayon MM, Priest RG, Caulet M, Guilleminault C. Hypnagogic and hypnopompic hallucinations: pathological phenomena? Br J Psychiatry 1996; 169:459–467.
142. Brylowski A, Levitan L, LaBerge S. H-reflex suppression and autonomic activation during lucid REM sleep: a case study. Sleep 1989; 12:374–378.
143. Schenck CH, Mahowald MW. A disorder of epic dreaming with daytime fatigue, usually without polysomnographic abnormalities, that predominately affects women. Sleep Res 1995; 24:137.
144. Zadra AL, Nielsen TA. Epic dreaming: a case report. Sleep Res 1996; 25:148.
145. Salin-Pascual RJ, Roehrs TA, Merlotti LA, Zorick F, Roth T. Long-term study of

the sleep of insomnia patients with sleep state misperception and other insomnia patients. Am J Psychiatry 1992; 149:904–908.
146. Schenck CH, Mahowald MW. Review of nocturnal sleep-related eating disorders. Int J Eating Disord 1994; 15:343–356.
147. Rosenfeld DS, Elhajjar AJ. Sleepsex: a variant of sleepwalking. Arch Sexual Behav 1998; 27:269–278.
148. Klackenberg G. Somnambulism in childhood—prevalence, course and behavior correlates: a prospective longitudinal study (6–16 years). Acta Paediatr Scand 1982; 71:495–499.
149. Bixler EO, Kales A, Soldatos CR, Healey S. Prevalence of sleep disorders in the Los Angeles metropolitan area. Am J Psychiatry 1979; 136:1257–1262.
150. Goldin PR, Rosen RC. Epidemiology of nine parasomnias in young adults. Sleep Res 1997; 26:367.
151. Hublin C, Kaprio J, Partinen M, Heikkila K, Koskenvuo M. Prevalence and genetics of sleepwalking: a population-based twin study. Neurology 1997; 48:177–181.
152. Kales A, Soldatos C, Bixler EO, Ladda RL, Charney DS, Weber G, Schweitzer PK. Hereditary factors in sleepwalking and night terrors. Br J Psychiatry 1980; 137:111–118.
153. Soldatos CR, Kales A. Sleep disorders: research in psychopathology and its practical implications. Acta Psychiatr Scand 1982; 65:381–387.
154. Schenck CH, Hurwitz TD, Bundlie SR, Mahowald MW. Sleep-related injury in 100 adult patients: a polysomnographic and clinical report. Am J Psychiatry 1989; 146:1166–1173.
155. Moldofsky H, Gilbert R, Lue FA, MacLean AW. Sleep-related violence. Sleep 1995; 18:731–739.
156. Guilleminault C, Kushida C, Leger D. Forensic sleep medicine and nocturnal wanderings. Sleep 1995; 18:721–723.
157. Llorente MD, Currier MB, Norman S, Mellman TA. Night terrors in adults: phenomenology and relationship to psychopathology. J Clin Psychiatry 1992; 53:392–394.
158. Mahowald MW, Schenck CH. NREM parasomnias. Neurolog Clinics 1996; 14: 675–696.
159. Zuccone M, Oldani A, Ferini-Strambi L, Smirne S. Arousal fluctuations in non-rapid eye movement parasomnias: the role of cyclic alternating pattern as a measure of sleep instability. J Clin Neurophysiol 1995; 12:147–154.
160. Schenck CH, Pareja JA, Patterson AL, Mahowald MW. An analysis of polysomnographic events surrounding 252 slow-wave sleep arousals in 38 adults with injurious sleepwalking and sleep terrors. J Clin Neurophysiol 1998; 15:159–166.
161. Mori SH. Integration of posture and locomotion in acute decerebrate cats and in awake, freely moving cats. Progress Neurobiol 1987; 28:161–195.
162. Grillner S, Dubic R. Control of locomotion in vertebrates: spinal and supraspinal mechanisms. Adv Neurol 1988; 47:425–453.
163. Berntson GG, Micco DJ. Organization of brainstem behavioral systems. Brain Res Bull 1976; 1:471–483.
164. Mogenson GJ. Limbic-motor integration. Progr Psychobiol Physiolog Psychol 1986; 12:117–170.

165. Mori S, Nishimura H, Aoki M. Brain stem activation of the spinal stepping generator. In: Hobson JA, Brazier MAB, eds. The Reticular Formation Revisited. New York: Raven Press, 1980:241–259.
166. Morrison AR. Paradoxical sleep without atonia. Arch Italiennes de Biologie 1988; 126:275–289.
167. Zucker DK, Austin FM, Branchey L. Variables associated with alcoholic blackouts in men. Am J Drug Alcohol Abuse 1985; 11:295–302.
168. Penfield W, Jasper H. Epilepsy and the Functional Anatomy of the Brain. Boston: Little, Brown, 1954:116–126, 452–469.
169. Schenck CH, Mahowald MW. A parasomnia overlap disorder involving sleepwalking, sleep terrors and REM sleep behavior disorder: report in 33 polysomnographically confirmed cases. Sleep 1997; 20:972–981.
170. Gambetti P. Fatal familial insomnia and familial Creutzfeldt-Jakob disease: a tale of two diseases with the same genetic mutation. Curr Topics Microbiol Immunol 1996; 207:19–25.
171. Lugaresi E, Medori R, Montagna P, Baruzzi A, Cortelli P, Lugaresi A, Tinuper P, Zucconi M, Gambetti P. Fatal familial insomnia and dysautonomia with selective degeneration of thalamic nuclei. N Engl J Med 1986; 315:997–1003.
172. Lavie P, Pratt H, Sharf B, Peled R, Brown J. Localized pontine lesion: nearly total absence of REM sleep. Neurology 1984; 34:118–120.
173. Karacan I, Salis PJ, Thornby JI, Williams RL. The ontogeny of nocturnal penile tumescence. Waking and Sleeping 1976; 1:27–44.
174. Steiger A, Holsboer F, Benkert O. Dissociation of REM sleep and nocturnal penile tumescence in volunteers treated with brofaremine. Psychiatry Res 1987; 20:177–179.
175. Steiger A, Holboer F, Benkert O. Effects of brofaramine (CGP 11 305A), a short-acting, reversible, and selective inhibitor of MAO-A on sleep, nocturnal penile tumescence and nocturnal hormonal secretion in three healthy volunteers. Psychopharmacology 1987; 92:110–114.
176. Steiger A. Effects of clomipramine on sleep EEG and nocturnal penile tumescence: a long-term study in a healthy man. J Clin Psychopharmacol 1988; 8:349–354.
177. Fleming J. Dissociative episodes presenting as somnambulism. Sleep Res 1987; 16:263.
178. Schenck CS, Milner DM, Hurwitz TD, Bundlie SR, Mahowald MW. Dissociative disorders presenting as somnambulism: polysomnographic, video, and clinical documentation (8 cases). Dissociation 1989; 4:194–204.
179. Mahowald MW, Schenck CH. Parasomnia purgatory—the epileptic/non-epileptic interface. In: Rowan AJ, Gates JR, eds. Non-Epileptic Seizures. Boston: Butterworth-Heinemann, 1993:123–139.
180. Rosen G, Mahowald MW, Ferber R. Sleepwalking, confusional arousals, and sleep terrors in the child. In: Ferber R, Kryger M, eds. Principles and Practice of Sleep Medicine in the Child. Philadelphia: WB Saunders, 1995:99–106.
181. Pedley TA, Guilleminault C. Episodic nocturnal wanderings responsive to anticonvulsant drug therapy. Ann Neurol 1977; 2:30–35.
182. Soldatos CR, Vela-Bueno A, Bixler EO, Schweitzer P, Kales A. Sleepwalking and

night terrors in adulthood, clinical and EEG findings. Clinical EEG 1980; 11:136–139.

183. Halbreich U, Assael M. Electroencephalogram with spheniodal needles in sleepwalkers. Psychiatria Clin 1978; 11:213–218.
184. Popoviciu L, Szabo L, Corfariu O, et al. A study of the relationships of certain pavor nocturnus (PN) attacks with nocturnal epilepsy. In: Popoviciu L, Asgian B, Badiu G, eds. Sleep 1978. Fourth European Congress on Sleep Research, Tirgu-Mures. Basel: S Karger, 1980:599–605.
185. Dervent A, Karacan I, Ware JC, Williams RL. Somnambulism: a case report. Sleep Res 1978; 7:220.
186. Amir N, Navon P, Silverberg-Shalev R. Interictal electroencephalography in night terrors and somnambulism. Isr J Med Sci 1985; 21:22–26.
187. Broughton R. Pathophysiology of enuresis nocturna, sleep terrors and sleepwalking: current status and the Marseilles contribution. In: Broughton R, ed. Henri Gastaut and the Marseilles School's Contribution to the Neurosciences. Amsterdam: Elsevier, 1982:401–410.
188. Guilleminault C, Silvestri R. Disorders of arousal and epilepsy during sleep. In: Sterman MB, Shouse MN, Passouant PP, eds. Sleep and Epilepsy. New York: Academic Press, 1982:513–531.
189. Mahowald MW, Schenck CH. Sleep disorders. In: Engel J Jr, Pedley TA, eds. Epilepsy: A Comprehensive Textbook. Philadelphia: Lippincott-Raven, 1997: 2705–2715.
190. Corner MA. Sleep and the beginnings of behavior in the animal kingdom—studies in ultradian motility cycles in early life. Progress Neurobiol 1977; 8:279–295.
191. Corner MA, Bour HL. Postnatal development of spontaneous neuronal discharges in the pontine reticular formation of free-moving rats during sleep and wakefulness. Exp Brain Res 1984; 54:66–72.
192. Corner MA. Ontogeny of brain sleep mechanisms. In: McGinty DJ, Drucker-Colin R, Morrison AR, Parmeggiani PL, eds. Brain Mechanisms of Sleep. New York: Raven Press, 1985:175–197.
193. Corner MA. Maturation of sleep mechanism in the central nervous system. Exp Brain Res 1984; 54(suppl 8):50–66.
194. Corner MA. Brainstem control of behavior: ontogenetic aspects. In: Klemm R, Vertes RP, eds. Brainstem Mechanisms of Behavior. New York: John Wiley & Sons, 1990:239–266.
195. Siegel JM. Phylogeny and the function of REM sleep. Behav Brain Res 1995; 69: 29–34.
196. Siegel JM. The evolution of REM sleep. In: Lydic R, Baghdoyan HA, eds. Handbook of Behavioral State Control: Cellular and Molecular Mechanisms. Boca Raton, FL: CRC Press, 1999:87–100.
197. Steriade M, Ropert N, Kitsikis A, Oakson G. Ascending activating neuronal networks in midbrain core and related rostral systems. In: Hobson JA, Brazier MAB, eds. The Reticular Formation Revisited. New York: Raven Press, 1980:125–167.
198. Inoue S. Biology of Sleep Substances. Boca Raton, FL: CRC Press, 1989.
199. Anch AM, Browman CP, Mitler MM, Walsh JK. Sleep: A Scientific Perspective. Englewood Cliffs, NJ: Prentice Hall, 1988.

200. Hefez A, Metz L, Lavie P. Long-term effects of extreme situational stress on sleep and dreaming. Am J Psychiatry 1987; 144:344–347.
201. Edelman GM. Neural Darwinism. New York: Basic Books, 1987.
202. Gorman JM, Liebowitz MR, Fyer AJ, Stein J. A neuroanatomical hypothesis for panic disorder. Am J Psychiatry 1989; 146:148–161.
203. Oppenheim JS, Skerry JE, Tramo MJ, Gazzaniga MS. Magnetic resonance imaging morphology of the corpus collosum in monozygotic twins. Ann Neurol 1989; 26: 100–104.
204. McKee AC, Kowall NW, Kosik KS. Microtubular reorganization and dendritic growth response in Alzheimer's disease. Ann Neurol 1989; 20:652–659.
205. Reiser MF. Mind, Brain, Body—Toward a Convergence of Psychoanalysis and Neurobiology. New York: Basic Books, 1984:103–113.
206. Kandel ER. Environmental determinants of brain architecture and of behavior: early experience and learning. In: Kandel ER, Schwartz JH, eds. Principles of Neural Science. New York: Elsevier/North Holland, 1981:620–632.
207. Iriki A, Pavlides C, Keller A, Asanuma H. Long-term potentiation in the motor cortex. Science 1989; 245:1385–1387.
208. Morrell F. Varieties of human secondary epileptogenesis. J Clin Neurophysiol 1989; 6:227–275.
209. Rizzo M, Eslinger PJ. Colored hearing synesthesia: an investigation of neural factors. Neurology 1989; 39:781–784.
210. Cytowic RE. Synesthesia an mapping of subjective sensory dimensions [editorial]. Neurology 1989; 39:849–850.
211. Aoki C, Siekevitz P. Plasticity in brain development. Scientific American 1988; 259:56–64.
212. Lipton SA. Growth factors for neuronal survival and process regeneration: implications in the mammalian central nervous system. Arch Neurol 1989; 46:1241–1248.
213. Snider WD, Johnson EMJ. Neurotropic molecules. Ann Neurol 1989; 26:489–506.
214. Salva MAQ, Guilleminault C. Olivopontocerebellar degeneration, abnormal sleep, and REM sleep without atonia. Neurology 1986; 36:576–577.
215. Mina M, Autret A, Laffont F, Beillevaire T, Cathala HP, Castaigne P. A study on sleep in amyotrophic lateral sclerosis. Biomedicine 1979; 30:40–46.
216. Mouret J. Differences in sleep in patients with Parkinson's disease. EEG Clin Neurophysiol 1975; 38:653–657.
217. Osorio I, Daroff RB. Absence of REM and altered NREM sleep in patients with spinocerebellar degeneration and slow saccades. Ann Neurol 1980; 7:277–280.
218. Aldrich MS, Foster NL, White RF, Bluemlein L, Prokopowicz G. Sleep abnormalities in progressive supranuclear palsy. Ann Neurol 1989; 25:577–581.
219. Sasaki H, Sudoh K, Hamada K, Hamada T, Tashiro K. Skeletal myoclonus in olivopontocerebellar atrophy: treatment with trihexyphenidyl. Neurology 1987; 37: 1258–1262.
220. DeBarros-Ferreira M, Chodkiewicz J-P, Lairy GC, Salzarulo P. Disorganized relations of tonic and phasic events of REM sleep in a case of brain-stem tumor. EEG Clin Neurophysiol 1975; 38:203–207.
221. Hobson JA. Dreaming sleep attacks and desynchronized sleep enhancement. Arch Gen Psychiatry 1975; 32:1421–1424.

222. Autret A, Laffont F, de Toffol B, Cathala J-P. A syndrome of REM and non-REM sleep reduction and lateral gaze paresis after medial tegmental pontine stroke. Arch Neurol 1988; 45:1236–1242.
223. Little BW, Brown PW, Rodgers-Johnson P, Perl DP, Gajdusek DC. Familial myoclonic dementia masquerading as Creutzfeldt-Jakob disease. Ann Neurol 1986; 20:231–239.
224. Nielsen TA. Mentation during sleep: the NREM/REM distinction. In: Lydic R, Boghdoyan HA, eds. Handbook of Behavioral State Control: Cellular and Molecular Mechanisms. Boca Raton, FL:CRC Press, 1999:101–128.

6

The Role of Melatonin in Sleep and Sleep Disorders

Irina V. Zhdanova
Massachusetts Institute of Technology
Cambridge, Massachusetts

INTRODUCTION

The identification of melatonin as a pineal hormone was a 20th-century event. In 1915, studies performed by McCord and Allen showed that mammalian pineal tissue contains a substance that causes the skin of tadpoles to blanch. In 1958, Aaron Lerner, a dermatologist interested in a human skin pigmentation disorder, isolated and identified the pineal hormone responsible for the amphibian skin blanching effect as melatonin (N-acetyl-5-methoxytryptamine). Although melatonin proved to be without effect on distribution of human skin pigment, Lerner and Case (1) were the first to observe and report a sedative effect of the pineal hormone in humans. While research efforts in the last four decades of the 20th century have taught us much about melatonin and its role in the circadian and circannual organization of physiology and behavior in animals, many questions regarding its role in human and animal physiology remain either unanswered or, as yet, not addressed.

NORMAL PINEAL PHYSIOLOGY

Evolutionary Roots

In order to appreciate melatonin's role in human physiology, it may be useful to review some basics of the gland that secretes it, including its ontogeny and phylogeny. The pineal gland, or *epiphysis cerebri*, develops from the roof of the diencephalon, along with the lateral eyes and a major circadian ''clock,'' the suprachiasmatic nuclei (SCN) of the hypothalamus. All three structures are related to the perception and/or translation of photic information, and thereby facilitate an organism's adaptive adjustment to rhythmic changes in environmental illumination. The pineal complex of phylogenetically primitive vertebrates contains photoreceptor cells that share molecular features with retinal photoreceptors, including the presence of proteins that play an important role in the retinal phototransduction processes. In some of the lower vertebrate species, the distal segment of the pineal complex forms a functional parietal eye that is strikingly similar to the lateral eyes, having both a cornea and lens.

Another feature common to both the pineal gland and the lateral eyes is their ability to synthesize melatonin. While the lateral eyes apparently retain the melatonin they produce for local paracrine functions, the evolution of the epiphysis cerebri has transformed the organ into a neuroendocrine gland whose major output is the hormone melatonin. A significant relationship between the secretion of melatonin and environmental light is preserved through multiple changes in the course of evolution of the pineal gland. In species whose pineals have direct access to light, a light stimulus elicits an acute physiological response, inhibiting melatonin synthesis. In mammals, their enlarged cerebral hemispheres and/or opaque skull shields the pineal gland from a direct light input. In these species the pineal glands receive indirect information about environmental lighting via a complex neuronal pathway that involves the retinohypothalamic tract, the SCN, preganglionic elements in the spinal cord, and, finally, sympathetic fibers originating in the superior cervical ganglia. Such indirectly perceived light has been shown to acutely suppress melatonin synthesis in the pineal gland and to entrain its rhythmic production.

The earth's daily rotation under the sun makes it important for organisms to temporally organize adaptive functions within the 24-hour cycle. This circumstance necessitates an internal ''clock,'' a mechanism that provides for the prediction of changes in environmental temperature and lighting, and helps to structure an animal's physiology and behavior accordingly. To this end, those cells and organs that were specialized for direct or indirect photoreception developed the unique properties of spontaneous circadian oscillators. Intimate details of the mechanism underlying this phenomenon remain a mystery. Photoreceptor cells of the lateral eyes, pineal organs of many nonmammalian vertebrates, and SCN neurons of the hypothalamus are capable of sustaining a circadian pattern of activity even in the absence of a rhythmic environmental input. As far as we can tell, the mammalian pineal gland has lost this property with the loss of its capacity for photoreception. Human pinealocytes rely on the SCN neurons to deliver a circadian pattern of input that drives the nightly increase in melatonin production.

Thus, the mammalian pineal gland has come to represent a key component of the circadian photoneuroendocrine axis. It has evolved into a highly specialized endocrine organ—the main, if not the exclusive, source of circulating melatonin. By way of the cerebrospinal fluid and the general circulation, the lipid-soluble melatonin has ready access to every cell of the body. Our understanding of the mechanisms of action of melatonin at the cellular level has been substantially advanced over the last few years. Studies conducted in many laboratories demonstrate that melatonin has specific binding sites in various central and peripheral tissues of different animal species. Examples of these diverse binding sites include the SCN of the hypothalamus, the medial preoptic area, the pineal gland itself, the anterior pituitary, and the pars tuberalis of the adenohypophysis. Specific melatonin-binding sites have also been demonstrated in the retina, ovaries, testes, spleen, kidney, thymus, arteries, spermatozoa, blood platelets, and other tissues. The recent cloning of a family of G protein–coupled melatonin receptors (2) was an important advance that opened new possibilities for the understanding of melatonin's action in various target cells. Melatonin's high lipid solubility suggests that this hormone may well have some direct actions inside cells, independent of or in addition to its actions on cellular membrane receptors.

Melatonin Secretion in Humans

In 1975 Harry Lynch and colleagues (3) demonstrated that in humans, as in other animals, melatonin is secreted at night but not to a great extent in the daytime. Daytime melatonin levels in human adults do not normally exceed 2–4 pg/ml, while at night they rise to about 100 pg/ml, peaking in the early morning hours (1–5 A.M.). This rhythmic pattern of melatonin secretion persists in people maintained in constant darkness; however, the abrupt imposition of bright light has been shown to promptly suppress melatonin secretion. The human fetus and newborn infant do not produce their own melatonin but instead rely on hormone supplied via the placental blood and, postnatally, via the mother's milk. Rhythmic melatonin production increases rapidly in infants 9–12 weeks old, with the highest nocturnal melatonin levels observed in children under 5 years of age. Although no adequate longitudinal studies of human melatonin production have been conducted, cross-sectional studies suggest that melatonin levels decrease with physiological aging (Figure 1). Marked interindividual variation in nocturnal melatonin levels is observed in all age groups; however, the circulating melatonin pattern for a given individual tends to remain surprisingly constant if measured over several nights. Endogenous serum melatonin concentrations in healthy young adults typically fluctuate from about 0.5–3 pg/ml during the day to about 30–150 pg/ml at night. Some individuals may display nocturnal levels as high as 200 pg/ml, or as low as 5–7 pg/ml.

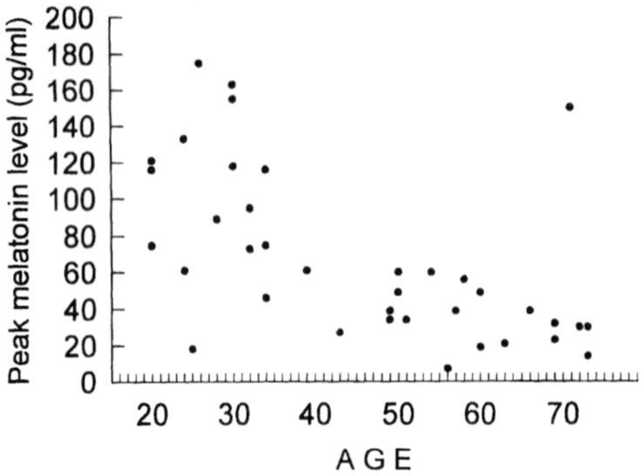

Figure 1 Peak endogenous serum melatonin levels in people of different ages ($n = 36$). (From Ref. 19.)

Circulating melatonin is inactivated in the liver, where it is converted to 6-hydroxymelatonin, conjugated with sulfate or glucuronide, and excreted in the urine.

MELATONIN AND SLEEP

Indirect Signs of a Melatonin–Sleep Relationship

The earliest observations of melatonin secretion in humans documented the concurrence of melatonin release from the pineal gland and the habitual hours of sleep. More recent reports from various laboratories confirm this temporal relationship and correlate the daily onset of melatonin secretion with the onset of nocturnal sleepiness. Observations in human babies reveal a correlation between the time of consolidation of nocturnal sleep and the normal onset of rhythmic melatonin secretion, both of which occur when the infant is about 3 months old.

The decline of both melatonin secretion and sleep efficiency with age are thought to be related phenomena. For example, middle-aged and elderly insomniacs are reported to exhibit lower melatonin production than that in good sleepers of the same age (4). Studies of circadian phase shifts in humans also show that a change in the timing of the onset of melatonin secretion correlates with the change in the timing of evening sleepiness, a phenomenon widely observed in shift workers and transmeridian jet travelers. Acute changes in circulating melatonin levels due to the suppression of melatonin production by, for example, treatment with β-adrenergic blockers, are reported to cause insomnia, while an increase in circulating melatonin induced by suppression of melatonin-metabolizing enzymes results in sleepiness. Although these correlational observations do not prove a causal relationship between melatonin secretion and sleep, they tend to substantiate direct experimental results.

Acute Sleep-Promoting Effects of Melatonin

Initial studies addressing melatonin's effects on sleep were conducted at a time when sensitive methods for measuring circulating melatonin levels were not available. In the absence of knowledge concerning normal melatonin levels, these studies employed what we now recognize were enormous doses of the hormone. The lack of an obvious acute toxic effect of even very high melatonin doses was another factor that encouraged overdosing with the hormone. Although doses employed in research studies did gradually decline over time, for many years the typical oral dose of melatonin remained in the milligram range. Table 1 summarizes some of the studies that tested sleep-promoting effects of melatonin in humans. It is not easy to compare individual entries or generalize from the results of these investigations because the melatonin doses, the subject populations, and the study designs were very dissimilar. With few exceptions, these studies reported subjective and/or objective sleep-promoting effects of melatonin treatment. Depending on the methods used in these studies and the baseline sleep patterns characteristic of the various populations tested, the effects of melatonin treatment were described as increased reaction time, diminished subject alertness, increased fatigue or sleepiness, increase in sleep propensity, reduction in latency to sleep onset, decrease in the number of nocturnal awakenings, and an increase in sleep efficiency.

The availability of new, sensitive assay methods that allow accurate measurement of circulating melatonin concentrations in the picogram-per-milliliter range has allowed the demonstration that oral melatonin doses in excess of about 0.3 mg elevate circulating melatonin to high, supraphysiological levels. Thus, the effects of melatonin treatment on sleep observed in earlier studies might merely represent side effects resulting from the very high pharmacological levels of the hormone. The recent finding that an increase in circulating melatonin concentration only within the normal nocturnal range of melatonin levels promotes sleep initiation in humans (5–7) (Figure 2) brought this phenomenon into the domain of normal physiology. These results led to the suggestion that the normal nocturnal surge in melatonin production may indeed be an important factor in human sleep regulation, and that a melatonin deficiency might contribute to an altered sleep pattern.

Acute Effects of Melatonin on Sleep Architecture

Compelling evidence exists regarding the effects of melatonin treatment on latency to sleep onset (5–11). Both physiological and pharmacological circulating melatonin levels shorten latency to sleep. There is no clear dose dependency of

Table 1 Acute Effects of Melatonin Treatment[a] on Human Sleepiness and Sleep

Author, year	Dose	Baseline sleep	Tests	Treatment results
Lerner and Case, 1960	200 mg, i.v.	Normal	Subjective	↑S
Anton-Tay et al., 1971	100 mg, i.v.	Normal	Subjective	↑S
Anton-Tay et al., 1974	250 mg	Normal	PSG	↑Stage 2; ↓stage 4; ↑REMs
Cramer et al., 1974	50 mg, i.v.	Normal	PSG	↓SL;
Vollrath et al., 1981	1.7 mg, i.n.	Normal	Subjective	↑Sedation; ↑tiredness
Lieberman et al., 1984	240 mg	Normal	Subjective	↑S
Arendt et al., 1984	2 mg	Normal	Subjective	↑Fatigue
James et al., 1987	1 mg, 5 mg	Normal	PSG	↑REM latency (5 mg)
Nickelsen et al., 1989	50 mg	Normal	Subjective	↑Fatigue
James et al., 1990	1 mg, 5 mg	*Insomnia*	PSG	↑REM latency (1 mg)
Waldhauser et al., 1990	80 mg	Normal	PSG	↓SL; ↓AW; ↑SE; ↑stage 2
MacFarlane et al., 1991	75 mg	*Insomnia*	Subjective	↑TST
Dahlitz et al., 1991	5 mg	*Insomnia*	Subj., PSG	←SO; ↓SL(2)
Dollins et al., 1994	0.1–10 mg	Normal	Subj., behavioral	↓SL; ↑S
Tzischinsky and Lavie, 1994	5 mg	Normal	PSG/MSLT	↑SP
Jan et al., 1994	2.5–10 mg	*Insomnia*	Parents' reports	↓SL; ↑SE
Zhdanova et al., 1995	0.3, 1 mg	Normal	PSG	↓SL; ↑SE; ↑S
Cajochen et al., 1995	5 mg	Normal	PSG	w:↑θ; s:↑REMs, ↑stage 2
Nave et al., 1995	3, 6 mg	Normal	PSG	↓SL; ↑TST
Attenburrow et al., 1996	0.3, 1 mg	Normal	PSG	↓SL; ↓stage 1; ↑SWS
Garfinkel et al., 1995	2 mg	*Insomnia*	Actigraph	↑SE; ↓WASO
Wurtman and Zhdanova, 1995	0.3 mg	*Insomnia*	Actigraph	↓SL; ↓M; ↓AW
Zhdanova, et al., 1996	0.3, 1 mg	Normal	PSG	↓SL; ↑2 stage
Hughes et al., 1997	1–40 mg	Normal	PSG	↓SL; ↑SE; ↑stage 2; ↓SWS
Hughes et al., 1998	0.5 mg	*Insomnia*	PSG	↓SL

[a] Oral administration, unless otherwise indicated (i.n. = intranasal).

AW = number of awakenings; M = number of movements per sleep period; MSLT = multiple sleep latency test; PSG = polysomnography; REMs = number of rapid eye movements in sleep; S = sleepiness; s = while asleep; SE = sleep efficiency; SL = sleep latency; SL(2) = sleep latency (sleep stage 2); ←SO = advanced sleep onset; SP = sleep propensity; stage no. = duration of a particular sleep stage; subjective/subj. = subjective reports; SWS = slow-wave sleep duration; θ = theta frequency; TST = total sleep time; w = while awake; WASO = time awake after sleep onset.

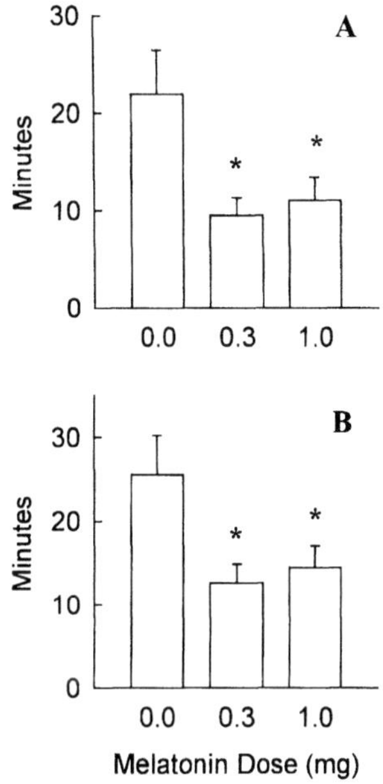

Figure 2 Effects of placebo (0.0) and melatonin (0.3 or 1.0 mg, p.o.) on mean (±SEM) latency to: (A) sleep onset and (B) stage 2 sleep ($n = 11$). * $p < 0.005$. (From Ref. 7.)

this effect with doses in excess of those that result in normal nocturnal melatonin levels, i.e., around 100 pg/ml. This phenomenon might be explained on the basis of the saturation levels of melatonin receptors, which are reported to be less than 100 pg/ml (12). Thus, if the hypnotic effect of melatonin is indeed receptor-mediated, a dose increase not only may fail to elicit an improved response but may even promote a down-regulation of receptors and a partial loss or modification of effect.

Melatonin's effect on sleep initiation is not accompanied by any dramatic changes in electrophysiological sleep architecture, a common complication encountered with many existing hypnotics. The tendencies observed in polysomnographic records after melatonin is administered in low "physiological" doses include a modest decrease in the duration of stage 4 and an increase in the duration of stage 2 sleep in some of the people studied (7). The lack of dramatic changes in the duration or relative amount of different sleep stages appears to be a general feature of the sleep-promoting effect of melatonin, independent of the dose used, as similar results are reported after administration of high pharmacological doses of the hormone (13,14).

Another intriguing aspect of the melatonin–sleep relationship is the effect of the pineal hormone on dream quality and content. Although Anton-Tay, in 1974 (15), reported that oral administration of 250 mg of melatonin facilitated subjects' dreaming and increased the number of rapid eye movements during REM sleep, this phenomenon has received little further attention. Some of our subjects, both young and old, described increases in dreaming or in the vividness of dreams after ingesting even a low—0.1 or 0.3 mg—dose of melatonin. This effect is especially striking among older people, some of whom report that as they aged, they experienced fewer dreams that were remembered in the morning than they had earlier in life. It is not clear whether these subjective reports reflect an increase in dreaming per se as a result of melatonin treatment, or simply better recall of dreams. Neither the effects of melatonin on memory function nor the objective parameters of REM sleep under treatment conditions has been adequately studied. What is repeatedly confirmed, however, is that, unlike some popular hypnotics, melatonin does not inhibit REM sleep.

The effect of melatonin on sleep is typically manifest within 30–60 minutes after the treatment is administered orally. Our observations suggest (7) that an increase in serum melatonin levels within the physiological range, occurring either during the daytime or late in the evening, is not an imperative signal for sleep but rather a gentle promoter of general relaxation and sedation, elements of sleepiness that, in favorable conditions, might significantly facilitate sleep onset and are typical of a period that is conventionally called "quiet wakefulness." Interestingly, when a person is adequately motivated, he can readily overcome these "feelings" and be both alert and productive for some time, regardless of his blood melatonin level.

Effects of Melatonin Treatment on Sleep in Children

As mentioned earlier, young children normally exhibit the highest circulating melatonin levels, and these gradually decline with age. This may or may not be a significant factor in the lower incidence of insomnia in the young population; however, it raises the interesting question as to whether children with chronic sleep disturbances may have abnormalities in their melatonin pattern. A Canadian clinical study showed that the administration of pharmacological oral doses of melatonin (2.5–5 mg) to multiply disabled children with severe sleep disorders caused substantial improvements in their sleep patterns and increased their sleep duration, as described by reports of their caregivers (16). We recently studied 13 children with Angelman syndrome (AS), a rare genetic disorder characterized by severe mental retardation, absent speech, seizures, ataxia, and disturbed sleep. For our study we obtained continuous actigraphic recordings of the patients' activity during several consecutive days prior to treatment, and also during the period in which each child received a daily 0.3-mg dose of melatonin half an hour before bedtime. The children's endogenous serum melatonin levels, as well

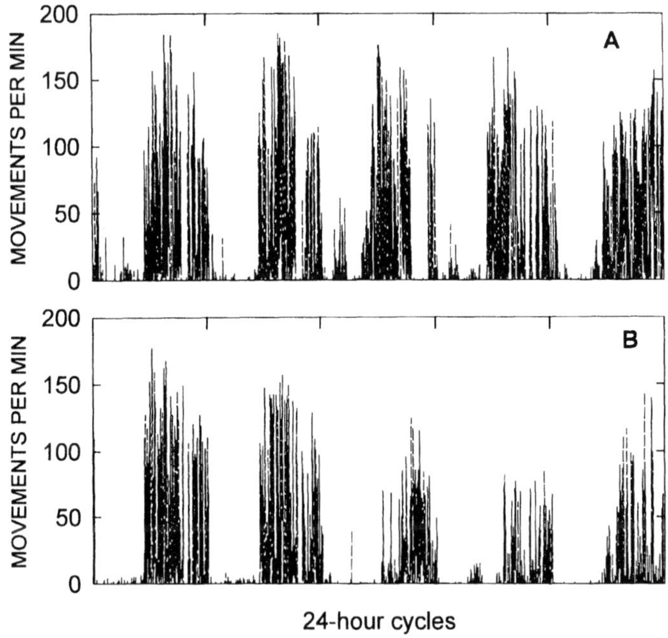

Figure 3 Motor activity of an 11-year-old child with Angelman syndrome over a baseline period (A) and (B) over 5 consecutive nights of melatonin treatment: 0.3 mg dose, a half hour before bedtime. Abscissa shows consecutive 24-hour cycles from 8 P.M. to 8 P.M.

as the levels induced by the hormone treatment, were measured. We found that AS children's peak melatonin levels tend to be lower than those reported in normal children of a similar age range, and four of our 13 subjects exhibited a phase delay in their nocturnal melatonin secretion. Analysis of group data revealed a significant decrease ($p < 0.001$) in motor activity during the total sleep period following melatonin treatment. No significant difference in total sleep time and no significant day-of-treatment effect was observed. After 1–2 days of treatment with a daily low dose of melatonin, the children's nighttime sleep was regularized and significantly less interrupted (Figure 3). Their daytime behavior was not significantly affected by the melatonin treatment; however, in some of the patients a decrease in hyperactivity was noticed by parents and teachers, and this effect correlated with an increase in their attention.

Effects of Melatonin Treatment in Older Populations

While only a few categories of children suffer from insomnia, many people over 50 years of age complain of an age-related decline in sleep quantity and quality.

There are certainly many factors that may contribute to this phenomenon of sleep deterioration; however, one of the factors may be a melatonin deficiency.

Actigraphic records indicate that sleep patterns in elderly insomniacs have been improved by melatonin treatment using a pharmacological 2-mg dose (17) or a physiological 0.3-mg dose of the hormone (18). Recent findings in our laboratory in a group of subjects over 50 years old showed positive effects of late-evening melatonin treatment (0.3 mg) on sleep parameters, as assessed polysomnographically, especially in subjects who had a nocturnal melatonin deficiency. However, we found a substantially higher variability in the sleep-promoting effect of melatonin in the older people than in young healthy adults. This phenomenon might be related to the differences in the mean serum melatonin levels that we observed following administration of the same dose of the hormone, 0.3 mg; postadministration levels tended to be higher in an older group of volunteers (254 ± 35.2 pg/ml compared to 170 ± 6.6 pg/ml in a younger group) (19). The range of interindividual variation was also significantly higher among the older subjects (76–423 pg/ml vs. 142–205 pg/ml in the younger group; $p < 0.0001$). Thus, in some individuals over 50 years old, even a low—0.3 mg—melatonin dose may induce supraphysiological circulating levels of the hormone. This finding bears on the important issue of whether, for therapeutic purposes, melatonin doses should be individualized, as discussed below.

Another factor that, perhaps, significantly influences the interindividual variability of melatonin's effect on human sleep is individual sensitivity to the pineal hormone. If melatonin's sleep-promoting effect depends on the activation of specific receptors, these individual differences in response might reflect individual differences in receptor sensitivity to activation or down-regulation induced by different melatonin concentrations. The investigation of these phenomena is at an early stage.

Mechanisms of Acute Effects of Melatonin on Sleep

The mechanisms underlying melatonin's hypnotic effect are not clear. Because melatonin is a lipid-soluble hormone, it has access to all cells of the body, and could act either at the membrane-receptor level or intracellularly. Thus, melatonin might acutely modulate the activity of many structures that are involved in sleep initiation and maintenance. The acute suppression of SCN activity by melatonin, discussed below, might also contribute to the sleep-promoting effect of the pineal hormone, relieving the mechanisms controlling sleep and wakefulness from the activating pressure of the circadian pacemaker during the day. Further studies are needed to elucidate the mechanisms of the acute sleep-promoting effect of melatonin, although they may remain obscure until more global mechanisms of sleep and wakefulness are clarified.

One of the well-tested ways to explore the mechanism of a physiological

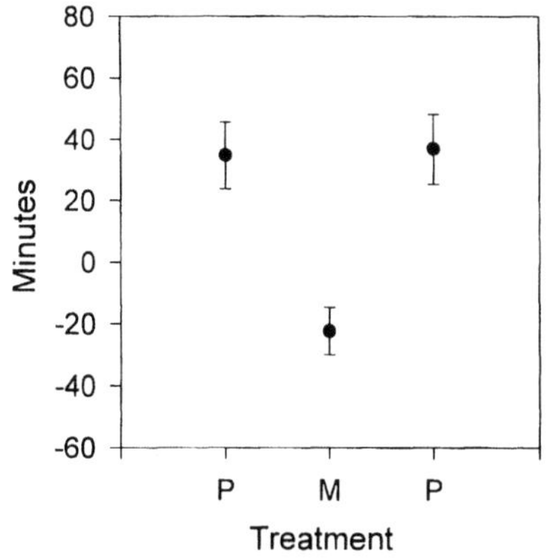

Figure 4 Timing of sleep onset relative to ''lights-out'' time in a 4-year-old *Macaca fascicularis* after the ingestion of placebo (P) or a 0.1-mg/kg dose of melatonin 2.5 hours before ''lights out.'' Each point represents the mean (±SEM) of 5 consecutive days of treatment. Sleep-onset estimate is based on a continuous actigraphic recording.

or pathophysiological process is through the development of an adequate animal model. While there is an extensive body of animal-based data regarding circadian effects of the pineal hormone, there are only a few animal studies of its acute effects, which has led to contradictory interpretations (see Ref. 20 for references). Inconsistencies may be explained by the extremely high, pharmacological concentrations of melatonin in blood, CSF, and brain tissue that were undoubtedly produced by the doses of the hormone that were used. Another major factor to be considered is differences in the temporal relationships of the sleep–wake cycles and the melatonin rhythms in the nocturnally active rats and the crepuscular cats that were studied, and the relationships characteristic of diurnally active humans. In nocturnal species the melatonin rhythm is similar to that in humans in that melatonin levels are higher at night. However, diurnal animals normally sleep at that time, while nocturnal animals are at the peak of their alertness and activity. Thus, melatonin may have a quite different biological significance in nocturnal and diurnal species.

A recently developed animal model for the acute sleep-promoting effects of melatonin administration involving nonhuman primates (20) might provide a means to further explore mechanisms involved in this phenomenon at the tissue, cellular, and molecular levels. We found that oral ingestion of melatonin affects sleep and behavior, as it does in humans, in three species of nonhuman primates: *Macaca nemestrina, Macaca mulatta*, and *Macaca fascicularis* (Figure 4). These observations suggest that the mechanisms of melatonin's effect on sleep might be preserved and similar among the different primate species, including humans.

CIRCADIAN EFFECTS OF MELATONIN

As discussed above, melatonin serves as an endocrine signal in the complex neuroendocrine machinery of a "biological clock." Thus, alterations in the timing of an increase in circulating melatonin concentrations may be perceived by different tissues and organs of the organism as a signal marking a particular circadian phase. What kinds of responses may follow is not well established. The effects of melatonin administration on the SCN, which is believed to be the site of a major circadian pacemaker in mammals, has been under intense investigation. Along with environmental stimuli (e.g., ambient light) or chemical agents (e.g., glutamate, neuropeptide Y, serotonin, substance P), melatonin has been shown to acutely alter neuronal activity and glucose metabolism in the SCN. A substantial stimulation or inhibition of SCN activity is typically accompanied by a shift in the phase of its timing mechanism, thereby modifying the temporal pattern of subsidiary physiological and behavioral rhythms, including the sleep–wake cycle. The magnitude and direction of such phase shifts depend on the quality of the alteration (stimulation or inhibition of SCN activity), its duration, and the circadian time at which the stimulus is administered. Application of melatonin in vitro can acutely suppress the metabolic activity and the firing rate of SCN neurons (21). Possibly, as a result, melatonin administration in the morning induces a delay in the circadian phase, while its administration in the afternoon causes a circadian phase advance in humans (22).

A phase shift in the circadian oscillation of SCN activity induced by melatonin treatment may thereby alter the physiological and behavioral rhythmicity of the entire organism. It has been shown that the human rest–activity cycle and the endogenous melatonin rhythm are subject to manipulation by treatment with exogenous melatonin and can be shifted to some extent by judicious timing of melatonin administration.

SHOULD MELATONIN BE USED THERAPEUTICALLY?

This simple question does not have a simple answer, owing mainly to the current lack of information on physiological functions of melatonin in humans, and the lack of a definition of "melatonin deficiency" and its symptoms. These gaps in our scientific and clinical knowledge are likely to be filled soon because of improved analytical methodology and the intensive research in this area that has recently been undertaken. Despite a relative lack of clinical data, we can rationally consider some possible benefits and anticipate some complications of melatonin treatment.

All available information from animal and human studies suggests that melatonin may participate in diverse physiological processes, including circadian rhythms, sleep, reproduction, temperature regulation, and immune responses. In dealing with something so multipurpose one must be very careful, especially if long-term administration of the hormone is considered, weighing the relative hazards of deficiency or excess. In the absence of a comprehensive picture of a melatonin-deficiency syndrome, let us discuss a hypothetical model case in which symptoms of insomnia can be related to low circulating-melatonin levels. It will allow us to consider possible therapeutic strategies.

Insomnia

Imagine that your patient is a 70-year-old woman who has suffered from insomnia for the past 20 years. Her symptoms include difficulty in falling asleep, several prolonged nocturnal awakenings, and a relatively early morning awakening. She takes a number of medications for her concurrent medical problems.

Endogenous Melatonin Level

After you measure your patient's nocturnal melatonin profile, you find that the maximum level of melatonin in her circulation at night is 12 pg/ml. Knowing that in healthy young adults the average peak melatonin levels are around 60–100 pg/ml, you hypothesize that your patient might have an age-related melatonin deficiency, and that it is likely to contribute to her insomnia. Eager to try a melatonin treatment, you must now choose a therapeutic melatonin dose and a time for its administration.

Time of Administration

In view of the fact that melatonin is normally secreted at night, and that it takes about half an hour for orally administered melatonin to substantially increase the hormone level in the general circulation, you are likely to advise your patient to take melatonin about half an hour prior to bedtime. In this way you coordinate the time of melatonin administration with the time of its normal increase in secretion, thus minimizing the possibility of a phase-shift complication of melatonin treatment.

Dose Range

In order to decide on an appropriate dose, you first have to decide whether to increase your patient's melatonin levels to a value within the "normal" physiological range or to exceed it. Even though you know that the "the more the better" strategy has limited utility and tends to be hazardous in most natural processes, the temptation to produce a robust and immediate effect is always great. Several known effects of melatonin might make you cautious in this situation. One is its clear hypothermic effect when the hormone is administered in pharmacological doses (23), reflecting acute changes in either energy metabolism or temperature regulation. Another possible effect of the pineal hormone is related to its potential alteration of the gonadal hormone levels and, in turn, their functions. A high dose of melatonin, especially using a continuous-release preparation of the hormone, is likely to increase daytime melatonin levels (13), blunting the circadian pattern of the melatonin signal and thereby altering the circadian pattern of other physiological functions. You may also be concerned by the lack of information on long-term effects of supraphysiological melatonin concentrations in humans, bearing in mind that the physiological levels are adaptive, having been established through natural selection.

Individualized Dose

If you choose a strategy of physiological replacement, the question you face next is exactly how much melatonin you should give your patient. Typically, capsules or tablets containing lactose, microcellulose, or similar filler ingredients have been shown to produce physiological serum melatonin levels (about 100 pg/ml) with doses around 0.1–0.3 mg (5). However, pronounced interindividual differences in induced melatonin levels have been observed after the same dose was administered to people of different ages, or even in the same age group (Figure 5). Perhaps the best way to identify an appropriate individual physiological dose is to measure the serum melatonin level in the patient's blood 1–2 hours after

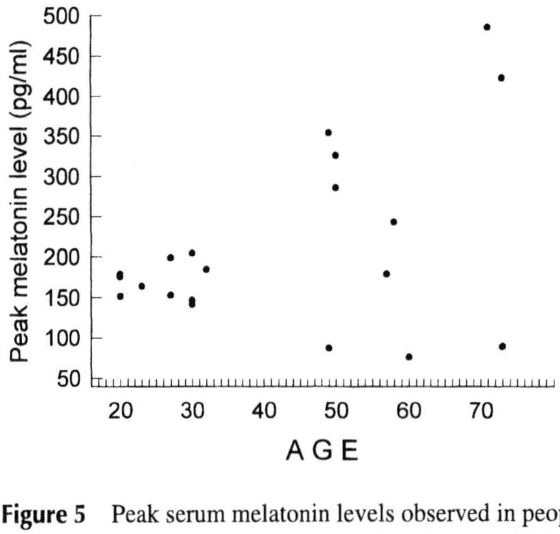

Figure 5 Peak serum melatonin levels observed in people of different ages an hour after the ingestion of a 0.3-mg dose of melatonin at 11.00 h ($n = 20$). (From Ref. 19.)

the daytime administration of a test dose. The circulating level observed at that time represents a value close to a maximum increase in circulating melatonin levels that will be produced by a given fast-release melatonin preparation. If a particular dose—for example, 0.2 mg—produces a blood level of around 100 pg/ml in your patient, it might represent a reasonable dose at which to start the treatment.

Expected Therapeutic Effects

First, it should be noted that the majority of, but not all, the individuals studied so far demonstrate a sleep-promoting effect of melatonin treatment. The observed variability in the responses of individuals to melatonin may simply represent individual sensitivity to a particular dose. No studies have attempted to finely titrate a dose dependency of melatonin's effect on human sleep, so the existence of a threshold effect or a narrow range of effective doses cannot be excluded.

In the clinical example discussed above, we chose a patient who has multiple symptoms of insomnia. While they all might result from a single pathological process, they may be affected by melatonin treatment to various extents, and require some modification of the therapeutic strategy. Shortening latency to sleep is the most commonly observed effect of melatonin treatment (6,7). However, you should warn your patient in advance that she will be unlikely to experience a sudden, dramatic increase in sleepiness or tiredness after melatonin ingestion. People who have previously been treated with the traditional hypnotics, including, for example, benzodiazepines, may expect a similar sensation when they are treated with melatonin. Those patients are likely to report a disappointing absence of any subjective effect, especially if they wait until they feel very sleepy before they retire. As mentioned above, melatonin usually acts as a gentle promoter of general relaxation and sedation that increases the probability of sleep initiation both in the evening and during nocturnal sleep interruptions, rather than being an imperative signal for sleep. This peculiarity of the effect of melatonin might reveal something of the normal context in which the pineal hormone acts in diurnal animals, i.e., the adaptive capacity for an emergency response while going to sleep is as basic to survival as a good night's sleep.

In this hypothetical example, your patient suffers from multiple nocturnal awakenings. Their number is likely to be diminished on melatonin treatment, but do not expect to eliminate them entirely. It is more typical for melatonin treatment to shorten the period of time your patient lies awake at night, allowing her to fall back to sleep more promptly. Is this a negative aspect of melatonin treatment? Probably not, if you consider that many metabolic processes in a 70-year-old are less "perfect" than in a 20-year-old. Thus, waking up at night for moderate water intake, for urination, or even for taking a medication for some concurrent condition might be a benefit if the patient can easily resume sleep.

Formulations to Use

The amount of melatonin that will enter a patient's bloodstream within a certain period of time following oral ingestion depends on several factors, including the amount of melatonin in the preparation and the diluent employed. Preparations that use oil as vehicle, for example, produce much higher concentrations of melatonin in blood due to rapid absorption, but for considerably shorter periods of time, than preparations containing lactose, microcellulose, or similar diluents. Within a 0.1–0.3-mg range of oral doses, the latter type of solid formulations are likely to induce physiological serum melatonin levels.

Until an ''ideal,'' perfectly predictable, melatonin preparation is available, it is important to consider differences in the pharmacokinetics of the so-called ''fast-'' and ''slow-release'' preparations, each of which has its benefits and drawbacks. Because of the high interindividual variability in melatonin pharmacokinetics, to evaluate the serum melatonin profile induced in the circulation after a ''slow-'' (''controlled-'') release preparation is used, you will need to analyze a set of blood samples collected at intervals over a 24-hour period in order to avoid induction of supraphysiological levels of the hormone at night or during the day (13). This complication does not occur if you are working with a ''physiological dose'' of a ''fast-release'' preparation. However, depending on an individual's characteristic rate of melatonin metabolism, a ''fast-release'' preparation may not be able to sustain a high enough level of the hormone in the second half of the night. If this is the case with your patient, you might recommend ingestion of an additional half dose of melatonin (e.g., 0.1 mg) when she wakes up early in the morning, if she finds it difficult to fall back asleep. She might need to use this strategy only occasionally.

Possible Interaction of Melatonin with Other Medications

It would perhaps be fair to say that interactions with other medications is one of the least-known aspects of the clinical application of melatonin. A possible complication may arise from the use of a common metabolic pathway by melatonin and other drugs. Melatonin inactivation occurs in the liver, where it is converted to 6-hydroxymelatonin by the P-450-dependent microsomal mixed-function oxidase enzyme system. Thus, any medication that might either slow down (e.g, methoxypsoralen) or facilitate (e.g., valproic acid) this pathway could significantly influence circulating melatonin levels. Similarly, the melatonin load may influence the rate of metabolism and therefore the circulating concentrations of other drugs taken concomitantly.

Melatonin is likely to exert various modulatory effects in addition to its direct functions. In a number of in vitro studies, a melatonin treatment that was inactive alone was shown to potentiate the effects of other agents, e.g., vasointestinal peptide or norepinephrine. Such potential modulatory effects of melatonin call for thoughtful use of the pineal hormone, careful consideration of the doses used, and the judicious timing of other treatments relative to the time of melatonin administration.

Circadian Sleep Disorders

The acute inhibitory effect of melatonin on the neuronal activity of the SCN, as mentioned above, promotes a shift in the phase of the major circadian pacemaker. In contrast to the time-independent acute sleep-promoting effect of melatonin, the timing of the hormone's administration is crucial for the exploitation of its phase-shifting effect. Melatonin tends to produce a phase advance when it is administered in the late afternoon, while early-morning treatment tends to cause a phase delay (22). This effect of melatonin is reported by some to be therapeutically useful with three major categories of people: ''free-running'' blind individuals, shift workers, and people experiencing the ''jet-lag'' syndrome after transmeridian flight.

Blindness

In totally blind individuals, a highly disrupted sleep–wake cycle is a common problem. It is explained by a lack of normal circadian entrainment by daily exposure to environmental illumination that results in a circadian rhythm with a period typically longer than 24 hours. Such a ''free-running'' rhythm results in a regular shift in the individual's physiological rhythms relative to environmental and social cues. Exogenous melatonin has been proposed as a device to entrain free-running rhythms. Although the phase-shifting phenomenon accomplished by melatonin administration in blind individuals has been repeatedly reported, the entrainment of their circadian rhythms through melatonin treatment is not easily achieved (24).

Shift Work

In undertaking the treatment of shift workers with melatonin, it is important to initially document the individual's endogenous melatonin pattern and its responsiveness to a change in the work schedule. The variability in the capacity of individuals to adapt to such changes is pronounced, and is influenced by many factors, including the subject's age, sex, and the magnitude and direction of the work schedule, as well as the intensity and timing of the individual's light exposure (24). Thus, the specific treatment of a circadian phase disorder in a particular shift worker requires substantial knowledge of his individual physiological responses.

Jet Lag

A number of studies have reported beneficial effects of melatonin treatment on the ''jet-lag'' syndrome. Utilizing the phase-shifting capacity of melatonin, some investigators seek to synchronize—prior to departure—subjects' circadian rhythms to the environmental conditions that prevail at the flight's destination. Others favor administering melatonin at an appropriate time while on the plane and again after arrival at the new location. It is not clear to what extent positive effects achieved by melatonin treatment in jet-lag syndrome are due to the phase-shifting of endogenous rhythms or to the acute sleep-promoting effect of the hormone, since most of the studies that have been described lack an objective evaluation of the subjects' circadian phases.

Our experience suggests that it is useful to administer melatonin (0.1–0.3 mg) at the local bedtime following a 3–6-hour eastward flight. Such treatment will restore the deficit in melatonin that the traveler will experience in his subjective afternoon, and might also promote a phase advance in his endogenous rhythmic pattern of melatonin secretion. In the case of a westward flight, it might be advisable not to ingest melatonin on the evening of arrival, when the endogenous level of the hormone during a subjective night is likely to be high. Instead, if the person wakes up at night, he might take a half dose to acutely facilitate resumption of sleep and its maintenance for the next several hours, and to support a phase delay of the circadian pacemaker by exploiting the phase-delaying effect of the hormone when administered in the subjective morning.

Historically, doses of melatonin used in jet-lag studies induced high pharmacological melatonin levels in the blood. More recent reports indicate that even physiological melatonin levels preserve the phase-shifting property. The magnitude of melatonin's effect on the circadian phase in humans is up to 60 minutes per day of treatment—comparable to the phase-shifting effect of exposure to bright light. The advantage of melatonin treatment in circadian phase disorders resides in the synergism of its acute sleep-promoting and phase-shifting effects and, of course, in the convenience of its administration.

POSSIBLE COMPLICATIONS OF MELATONIN TREATMENT IN DIFFERENT POPULATIONS

While all the issues considered above, and in our model case of melatonin treatment in an elderly person, are applicable to any age, gender, or race population, there are specific considerations that are population-dependent.

Children

As with any other treatment, children might be more sensitive not only to the primary effects of melatonin but also to possible untoward side effects. Children typically have the highest circulating melatonin levels of any age group. This fact might be very important for their normal development, and may contribute to their efficient sleep. While low melatonin levels may promote normal growth and development, reports suggest that an excess of the pineal hormone may correlate with the delay in the development of reproductive function. Until we know much more about the effects of melatonin on the growing human organism, melatonin treatment in children should be used very conservatively, in cases of documented and obvious melatonin deficiency or in special cases in which the benefits of melatonin treatment clearly outweigh any possible ill effects (16).

Women of Childbearing Age

Among the best-documented effects of exogenous melatonin is its antigonadal effect in seasonally breeding animals. The efficacy of the pineal hormone in modifying reproductive physiology has been found to vary markedly, depending on the species and age of the animal tested and the time of melatonin administration relative to the prevailing light–dark schedule. Animal studies show that in seasonal breeders melatonin normally mediates the effects of changes in photoperiod, and thus of season, on reproductive physiology. The effects of experimentally manipulated melatonin levels in animals that are adapted to fall–winter inhibition of reproductive activity (e.g., hamsters) appear to be the opposite of those in animals that are reproductively passive in the spring–summer season (e.g., goats and sheep). Whether pineal melatonin secretion influences, to any extent, reproductive physiology in nonseasonal mammals, including humans, is still not entirely clear. There are conflicting reports regarding serum melatonin levels during normal menstrual cycles in women. Some investigators report a transient decrease in nocturnal melatonin levels during the preovulatory phase; others failed to document any association between circulating melatonin concentrations and the phases of the menstrual cycle. Women during the second half of their pregnancy are reported to show increased levels of circulating melatonin, which might be the result of an increased secretion of the hormone or its slowed metabolism. Whether this circumstance bears importance for the preservation of pregnancy or fetal development is not known. On the basis of what we currently know, physiological melatonin levels are unlikely to negatively affect fetus development; however, induction of pharmacological melatonin levels should clearly be avoided.

Race

Melatonin research projects whose participants included mixed-race populations of volunteers have not revealed any significant dependency of circulating melatonin levels on race. However, direct studies of race- or nationality-dependent features of melatonin secretion and metabolism have not been conducted.

CONCLUSION

The fact that melatonin is a normal human hormone means that it is produced and utilized by the organism under specific circumstances and in specific concentrations. Available data on the sleep-promoting effects of changes in serum melatonin concentrations within the physiological range of levels suggest that the hormone may have a normal role in human sleep initiation and maintenance, perhaps serving as a humoral link between circadian and homeostatic sleep mechanisms. They further suggest that a melatonin deficiency might be expected to impair the integrity, quantity, and quality of nocturnal sleep, and that melatonin-replacement therapy might offer an effective and innocuous approach to the treatment of such insomnia, without disturbing normal sleep architecture. Melatonin therapy may also play a beneficial role in supporting other physiological functions that involve the hormone, including the entrainment and coordination of various biological rhythms.

The optimal use of melatonin in hormone-replacement therapy requires that the patient receive the correct dose of the hormone and at the proper time of day. A lack of documented negative side effects of melatonin treatment does not mean an absence of such effects. The notion that pharmacological doses are utterly safe rests on little research and on the common public experience of a lack of short-term toxic effects. However, biological and medical sciences teach us that subtle but important toxicities can take years to be expressed, and that it is very unusual for an extreme excess or deficit of any hormone (or vitamin, amino acid, mineral, etc.) not to result in an imbalance in the vital functions of an organism. Long-term clinical and experimental studies are needed to address these important questions.

The strategy for implementing melatonin-replacement therapy should consider the characteristic individual endogenous melatonin levels. It should also involve a melatonin dose that will increase the nocturnal hormone concentration only within the physiological range. The possible effects of concurrent medications should be taken into account, and so should any possible unique complications peculiar to a specific population.

REFERENCES

1. Lerner AB, Case JD. Melatonin. Fed Proc 1960; 19:590–592.
2. Ebisawa T, Karne S, Lerner MR, Reppert SM. Expression cloning of a high-affinity melatonin receptor from Xenopus dermal melanophores. Proc Natl Acad Sci USA 1994; 91:13:6133–6137.
3. Lynch HJ, Wurtman RJ, Moskowitz MA, Archer MC, Ho MH. Daily rhythm in human urinary melatonin. Science 1975; 187:169–171.
4. Haimov I, Laudon M, Zisapel N, Souroujon M, Nof D, Shlitner A, Herer P, Tzischinsky O, Lavie P. Sleep disorders and melatonin rhythms in elderly people. Br Med J 1994; 309:167.

5. Dollins AB, Zhdanova IV, Wurtman RJ, Lynch HJ, Deng MH. Effect of inducing nocturnal serum melatonin concentrations in daytime on sleep, mood, body temperature, and performance. Proc Natl Acad Sci USA 1994; 91:1824–1828.
6. Zhdanova IV, Wurtman RJ, Lynch HJ, Ives JR, Dollins AB, Morabito C, Matheson JK, Schomer DL. Sleep-inducing effects of low doses of melatonin ingested in the evening. Clin Pharm Ther 1995; 57:552–558.
7. Zhdanova IV, Wurtman RJ, Morabito C, Piotrovska VR, Lynch HJ. Effects of low oral doses of melatonin, given 2–4 hours before habitual bedtime, on sleep in normal young humans. Sleep 1996; 19(5):423–431.
8. Tzischinsky O, Lavie P Melatonin possesses a delayed hypnotic effect which is time dependent. Sleep 1994; 17(7):638–645.
9. Nave R, Peled R, Lavie P. Melatonin improves evening napping. Eur J Pharmacol 1995; 275:213–216.
10. Cramer H, Rudolph J, Consbruch U, Kendel K. On the effects of melatonin on sleep and behavior in man. Adv Biochem Psychopharmacol 1974; 11:187–191.
11. Attenburrow ME, Cowen PJ, Sharpley AL. Low dose melatonin improves sleep in healthy middle-aged subjects. Psychopharmacology 1996; 126(2):179–181.
12. Reppert SM. Melatonin receptors: molecular biology of a new family of G protein-coupled receptors. J Biol Rhythms 1997; 12(6):528–531.
13. Hughes RJ, Sack RL, Lewy AJ. The role of melatonin and circadian phase in age-related sleep-maintenance insomnia: assessment in a clinical trial of melatonin replacement. Sleep 1998; 21(1):52–68.
14. Waldhauser F, Saletu B, Trinchard-Lugan I. Sleep laboratory investigations on hypnotic properties of melatonin. Psychopharmacology 1990; 100:222–226.
15. Anton-Tay F. Melatonin: effects on brain function. In: Costa E, Gessa GL, Sandler M, eds. Serotonin—New Vistas: Biochemistry and Behavioral and Clinical Studies. Advances in Biochemical Pharmacology. Vol 11. New York: Raven Press, 1974:243–256.
16. Jan JE, Espezel H, Appleton RE. The treatment of sleep disorders with melatonin. Dev Med Child Neurol 1994; 36:97–107.
17. Garfinkel D, Laudon M, Nof D, Zisapel N. Improvement of sleep quality in elderly people by controlled-release melatonin. Lancet 1995; 346(8974):541–544.
18. Wurtman RJ, Zhdanova IV. Improvement of sleep quality by melatonin. Lancet 1995; 346(8988):1491.
19. Zhdanova IV, Wurtman RJ, Balcioglu A, Kartashov A, Lynch HJ. Endogenous melatonin levels and the fate of exogenous melatonin: age effects. J Gerontol July 1998; 53A(4):B293–B298.
20. Zhdanova IV, Cantor ML, Leclair OU, Kartashov A, Wurtman RJ. Behavioral effects of melatonin treatment in non-human primates. Sleep Research Online 1998; 1(3):114–118, *www.sro.org*
21. Shibata S, Cassone VM, Moore RY. Effects of melatonin on neuronal activity in the rat suprachiasmatic nucleus in vitro. Neurosci Lett 1989; 97:140–144.
22. Lewy AJ, Ahmed S, Jackson JM, Sack RL. Melatonin shifts human circadian rhythms according to a phase-response curve. Chronobiol Int 1992; 9(5):380–392.
23. Cagnacci A, Elliott JA, Yen SC. Melatonin: a major regulator of the circadian rhythm of core temperature in humans. J Clin Endocrinol Metab 1992; 75:447–452.
24. Sack RL, Lewy AJ. Melatonin as a chronobiotic: treatment of circadian desynchrony in night workers and the blind. J Biol Rhythms 1997; 12(6):595–603.

7

Delayed-Sleep-Phase Syndrome and Other Circadian-Rhythm Sleep Disorders

Charles P. Pollak
The Ohio State University Medical Center
Columbus, Ohio

OVERVIEW

J.B. is a 16-year-old high-school student who has been receiving failing grades because he cannot wake in time to attend morning classes. On the evening before a big test, he sets several alarms and reminds his mother to wake him at 7:00 A.M. He doesn't fall asleep until 2:30 A.M., which is typical for him. The next morning, he turns off both alarms without fully awakening. After much cajoling and scolding, his mother finally succeeds in getting him up at 7:30 A.M. He has to rush to get to the exam in time. Taking the exam is an ordeal: he finds it difficult to concentrate, and much of the material is unfamiliar because he was often not in class. He feels sleepy through much of the day and so goes to bed at 11 P.M.—much earlier than his usual bedtime between 1 and 3 A.M. Despite his sleepiness that day, he lies awake until 1:30 A.M.—not much earlier than his usual time of falling asleep. He has thus given up trying to go to bed earlier, because he then invariably lies awake for hours. Even the sleeping pills prescribed by a family physician have had little effect. The only time he has no problem with sleep is when he is on vacation, when he can indulge his preference to sleep from 4–5 A.M.

> to early afternoon. On such a schedule, he never awakens during the "night" and feels energetic and alert all "day." He has three musician friends who rehearse with him through the night, and he is thinking of becoming a professional musician. He is not confident, however, that he has the required talent.

This case illustrates several features of delayed-sleep-phase syndrome (DSPS): difficulty getting up in the morning at the hours most people consider appropriate, difficulty falling asleep, even when sleep-deprived, normal ability to sustain sleep once it has been initiated, and school or occupational disability. The syndrome was first described by Weitzman et al. (49).

Males appear to be affected more often than females (3). Patients may report onset of DSPS at almost any age, but onset during the first or second decades is most common (3,44,48). The overall prevalence is between 0.10% and 0.28%, with a small peak in the second and third decades, making DSPS more common than narcolepsy or multiple sclerosis and about as common as Parkinson's disease (41). Most affected individuals have not consulted a physician for their sleep disorder (42). The lifetime course of DSPS has not been ascertained in a population sample. One 3.9-year follow-up of 21 nonpsychiatric, treated cases showed reduced severity and improved social adaptation (29), but no evidence has been presented that DSPS spontaneously improves or remits. Disability is common, if not universal. In schoolchildren, DSPS causes tardiness and truancy (44) but has yet to be recognized as a common cause of school avoidance. In adults, DSPS may lead to acquiescence in undesired jobs and careers, job loss, and social isolation.

CLINICAL FEATURES AND DIAGNOSIS

History

Habitual oversleeping is the hallmark of DSPS. Even motivated teenagers require great effort to get up; they have literally had to be dragged out of bed, have cold water poured on them, and been driven to school by a parent at the last minute. They often describe a "zombie-like" state in the morning in which they turn off multiple alarms with no memory of doing so (automatic behavior). They may stumble out of bed and fall asleep while dressing (sleep drunkenness) (40). Teens with DSPS are often tardy to school, and they may fail to attend. Home tutoring may be needed for the morning classes that they are unable to attend. College-level students usually opt for classes taught late in the day and may fail courses that are taught only in the morning. Workers may suffer reprimands at or termination from day jobs and may prefer (select themselves for) evening or night shifts. Some patients with DSPS select occupations that provide flexible or nocturnal hours, such as freelance writing, entertaining, or bartending. Perhaps the recent increase of home-based employment will give DSPS patients greater latitude in their choice of occupation.

Most patients with DSPS experience frequent difficulty in falling asleep before 1–2 A.M., even under conditions of darkness, quiet, and warmth that are normally conducive to sleep. As described in the original case reports (49), patients often find themselves ruminating. Most of the nocturnal thoughts are mundane, but some may concern emotional topics, leading to an erroneous impression on the part of patients and their doctors that they have psychogenic insomnia. The true state of affairs will be understandable to anyone who has ever found himself engaged by an endless stream of thoughts while trying to fall a sleep at an unusually early time of night, for example, before an early plane trip. Medications or alcohol have often been tried without success by DSPS patients. Once asleep, the DSPS patient (and the early-morning traveler) typically has little further difficulty until it is time to get up.

A more variable feature of DSPS is daytime sleepiness. Some patients are sufficiently motivated to overcome their extreme morning sleepiness, interrupting sleep in time to meet their morning obligations. But this success is at the cost of truncating sleep that was initiated late in the night. The result is daytime sleepiness that persists for much of the day but does not facilitate sleep onset the following night. Indeed, nothing better illustrates the nature of DSPS as a disorder of sleep timing than this inability of extreme sleepiness to facilitate sleep onset. Patients who conscientiously force themselves to wake early in the morning rapidly become sleep-deprived, as shown by extended periods of weekend sleep. Patients are therefore faced with an unhappy choice between oversleeping and becoming sleep-deprived. Judging from the normal results of multiple sleep latency tests that have occasionally been performed (39), most oversleep.

Changes of sleep pattern in unusual situations may help in the diagnosis and assessment of severity of DSPS. The tendency to delay sleep on weekends and days off has already been mentioned. Longer periods that are free of schedules may result in the progressive delay of sleep periods through the entire 24-hour day, resembling the sleep patterns of normal subjects who are deprived of time cues in a temporal isolation laboratory (discussed below) or patients with the more severe hypernychthemeral syndrome (see below). Situations of the opposite type, in which rigid schedules are strongly enforced by group example (vacation camps, traveling parties) or threat of punishment (military), may either temporarily correct the problem or cause catastrophic failure (12).

Sleep Logs

When the diagnosis of DSPS is first considered, the patient should be asked to begin keeping a sleep log, or diary. A graphical log (1) should reveal the characteristic sleep–wake pattern: late sleep onsets, uninterrupted sleep periods, and late waketimes, especially on days off. The intervals from bedtime/lights-out to sleep onset may vary with the time of night. The greatest difficulty usually follows bedtimes before midnight. The intervals from waketime to time of arising are usually short (<15 minutes), especially on workdays, when sleep is likely to be forcibly interrupted. Sleep on weekends is not only late but often long in response to the sleep deficit that has accrued during the workweek (5). There may be a tendency to delay sleep during prolonged periods off work, but efforts made to maintain a 24-hour schedule are generally successful. Patients sometimes return to a workable sleep schedule by staying up all night. If medical management of DSPS is attempted (see below), the sleep log should continue to be kept to guide the clinician and the patient. Because workday/nonworkday changes in the sleep pattern are often marked, logs spanning less than 1 week may be misleading. Two-week logs are preferred for secure decision-making.

Wrist actigraphy has occasionally been used to corroborate the late timing of sleep in DSPS (39) and might eventually become a more accurate method of tracking sleep cycles. At present, there is no accepted criterion of sleep onset or offset based on motor activity alone. Not surprisingly, the delayed timing of sleep is associated with delays in the timing of other circadian rhythms, including those of plasma melatonin, body temperature (32), and serum cortisol (50).

Responses to Schedule Changes

Delays in the sleep period appear to be easily accommodated by patients with DSPS and are the basis for a therapeutic maneuver called "chronotherapy" (described below). This also appears to be true of delays caused by shift work (e.g., rotation from days to evenings or from evenings to nights) or rapid travel to a westward time zone. Shifts of sleep to earlier times, by contrast, cannot be accomplished unless they are very small (15 minutes or less) (36). Such shift asymmetries are also well known in normal travelers and shift workers and are presumed to result from the slowness with which the human biological clock "ticks." As will be seen, DSPS itself is thought to have a chronobiological basis.

Physical and Laboratory Examinations

One-night diagnostic sleep recordings (polysomnograms) are normal in DSPS, except for occasional prolonged latencies to sleep onset or short sleep durations if sleep is forcibly terminated (3). There are no consistent abnormalities on physical, neurological, psychiatric, or routine laboratory examination (3). Depression is a common but by no means universal feature of DSPS (37). Sleep recordings typically show normal sleep continuity and architecture but may confirm delayed sleep onset (3,9,48).

In summary, no single feature of DSPS is diagnostic. Diagnostic criteria therefore vary, and some reports include cases that can be considered mild or

Table 1 Essential Clinical Features of DSPS

1. Delayed timing of sleep on most days, independent of school attendance or workshifts.
2. Inability to correct the delay:
   a. Disabling inability to complete the night's sleep early enough to meet social obligations.
   and
   b. Inability to fall asleep early enough to fulfill daily sleep needs when sleep is terminated to meet social obligations.
3. Ability to maintain a 24-hour sleep pattern without incurring a sleep deficit.

doubtful. Alvarez et al. (3), for example, included cases with waketimes close to 8 A.M., which would not preclude most morning activities. By one definition of DSPS, symptoms must be present for 3 years or longer. This would preclude the disorder from being diagnosed near its onset—especially unfortunate in young students. Diagnostic criteria that avoid these problems are listed in Table 1.

DIFFERENTIAL DIAGNOSIS OF DSPS

Two conditions are so similar to DSPS that defining them is tantamount to defining DSPS. These are 1) the non-24-hour sleep–wake, or hypernychthemeral, syndrome and 2) eveningness.

Non-24-Hour-Day (Hypernychthemeral) Syndrome

DSPS patients are able to maintain a 24-hour day. Late and irregular as their sleep periods may be, they are spaced at intervals that average 24 hours, at least while the patient is attempting to follow a 24-hour schedule. There are rare patients, however, who are unable to maintain a mean 24-hour sleep pattern for more than a few days. The sleep period keeps shifting to later and later times even if it has already become delayed to daylight hours. The patient may explain that the shifts are made intentionally, to hasten the return to nocturnal hours of sleep. Because successive sleep periods occur ever later with respect to the 24-hour day, the mean interval between sleep periods exceeds 24 hours, often by several hours. This is termed the non-24-hour, or hypernychthemeral (longer than a day and night), syndrome (HNS) (23).

HNS is much less common than DSPS: no cases of HNS were found among 10,000 Norwegian adults surveyed for circadian-rhythm disorders (41).

The feature that distinguishes this severely disabling condition from DSPS is the long mean interval between sleep periods. DSPS patients often delay sleep onsets on days off, but they are able to reverse this early in the workweek. On vacations, the sleep period may shift around the clock, but the process halts with resumption of a 24-hour schedule. DSPS patients may occasionally attempt to return to sleeping at an early time of night by delaying sleep through an entire night and day. Presumably, the heavy "sleep debt" so incurred then enables them to sleep at an unusually early time of night. Alternatively, the maneuver may reset a biological clock, as explained later. Any multiday interval that happens to span such a marked delay of the sleep period would yield a mean interval between sleep periods that exceeds 24 hours. DSPS may therefore differ from HNS in degree rather than kind (48).

Eveningness

HNS is a diagnostic consideration for patients with severe DSPS. Milder cases must be distinguished from normal individuals who tend to go to bed and get up late ("owls," or evening types) (20). Such persons display many of the features of DSPS, but not to the degree that they have great difficulty meeting morning obligations. They sleep as late as possible, then rush to school or work. They also sleep late on weekends. They may feel more and more tired as the workweek progresses and recover by extending their sleep on weekends. They may have difficulty falling asleep, especially on Sunday evenings, just before resuming the work or school schedule.

This picture is widely familiar and is starting to be systematically investigated (22). DSPS is distinguished from it by degree: DSPS patients are tardy or miss morning obligations much more often and have greater difficulty falling asleep at bedtime. Evening types do not stay up all night in order to reschedule their sleep, nor are they likely to shift their hours of sleep around the clock on vacations, although such behaviors have not been systematically searched for.

Motivated Sleep-Phase Delay

Young people occasionally delay their hours of sleep to avoid school or to interact with peers who stay up very late. Such *motivated sleep-phase delay* has been distinguished from DSPS because the delay of sleep can be reversed during school breaks or at examination times (15,51).

Restless-Legs Syndrome

Chronic sleep-onset insomnia not associated with difficulty maintaining sleep has few causes other than DSPS and HNS. One alternative is the *restless-legs syndrome*—a peculiar, uncomfortable feeling in the calves that requires movement for relief. It may occur in the teen years, especially in familial cases, but is more common in midlife to adulthood.

Other Diagnostic Considerations

It has already been observed that attempts to sleep at an inappropriate time of day may result in a continuous stream of thoughts that may be blamed for the sleeplessness. On the other hand, anxious rumination may delay sleep, and patients with *psychophysiological insomnia* are anxious *because* they cannot sleep. Such difficulty may not be as consistent as the nightly sleep-onset insomnia of DSPS, and is more likely to be associated with difficulty maintaining sleep (frequent or prolonged awakenings). Similarly, insomnia associated with *major affective disorders* usually include difficulty in both initiating and maintaining sleep.

DSPS is usually easy to distinguish from sleep disorders that resemble it in one respect. *Nightshift* workers, whether voluntary or involuntary, may complain of difficulty in readjusting to the conventional day–wake schedule after shift rotations (17). We have seen patients with chronic sleep-onset insomnia dating to night shiftwork that was last performed years earlier. Some may have had pre-existing DSPS, of course, and may even have opted for nightshift work because of their propensity to delay sleep.

Little is known about individual variations in sleep need, but it appears that some *long sleepers* habitually obtain less sleep than they require. They may resemble DSPS patients if they truncate sleep in the morning for school or work. As a sleep deficit accrues, it becomes increasingly difficult to terminate sleep in the morning. The distinguishing feature of being a long sleeper is the ability to easily fall asleep at a conventional time in the evening. Sleep logs kept for at least 7 days should reveal mean sleep duration exceeding 8 hours.

Sleep apnea often causes sleepiness or lack of refreshment on awakening in the morning. Patients with sleep apnea are often sleepy all day and usually have little difficulty falling asleep at night. They also usually report loud snoring or nocturnal waking with a sensation of choking or gasping. Daytime sleepiness is also a symptom of *narcolepsy*, but such patients are often at their best on arising and do not have difficulty falling asleep. Features such as cataplexy, sleep paralysis, and multiple nocturnal awakenings also point to this diagnosis.

PATHOPHYSIOLOGY AND ETIOLOGY OF DSPS

The difficulty encountered by people with DSPS is not in sleeping per se but in sleeping at times that enable them to participate in morning activities, including school and work. DSPS is evidently a disorder of the *timing* of sleep, prompting consideration of the timing functions of the brain.

When normal humans are deprived of knowledge of the time of day, they sleep at intervals that are fairly regular but average slightly more than 24 hours (4). Body temperature, various hormones, electrolytes, blood pressure, performance ability, and many other functions fluctuate with similar rhythmicity. The significance of this non-24-hour periodicity is twofold. First, the rhythms cannot be the effects of subtle, environmental time cues, which are derived from the earth's period of rotation and therefore have periods of precisely 24 hours. Second, the closeness of the rhythms to 24 hours suggests that they nevertheless are an internal representation of the solar day, i.e., an evolutionary adaptation to the 24-hour rotation of the planet. Both features of the rhythms are embodied in the term *circadian* (''about daily'').

Because circadian rhythms approximate in period the solar day, they can be easily synchronized by environmental rhythms, especially the 24-hour alternation of daylight and darkness. A specialized mechanism exists for the transmission of photic information from the retina to the suprachiasmatic nuclei of the hypothalamus, where circadian rhythms are generated by a neural pacemaker, or ''clock.'' In particular, light–dark transitions at dawn and dusk reset the clock backward or forward by an amount that is dependent on the phase in the biological cycle at which they occur, i.e., their biological time of occurrence (35). Dawn resets the clock backward, so sleep thenceforth occurs earlier. Dusk retards the clock, delaying the next occurrence of sleep. The longer-than-24-hour period of most human clocks implies that events at dawn (increasing light, wakefulness, and motor activity) are the crucial ones for maintaining the synchrony of biological rhythms with events in the environment and thereby with one another and with society.

We now consider why patients with DSPS and HNS are unable to synchronize their sleep–wake cycles with the social schedules on which they depend for a living.

Abnormal Pacemaking (Long Intrinsic Period)

For the circadian clock to become synchronized with the environmental light–dark cycle, its intrinsic period must be fairly close to 24 hours. If its period is much longer, 24-hour environmental events will occur early in biological time. Because their resetting effects depend on their biological time of occurrence, environmental events then cannot exert their full effect, the biological clock will not be fully reset, and sleep and the other rhythms governed by the clock will also lag the environment (35). Direct testing of the hypothesis of a slow biological clock in DSPS will require measurement of the periods of the sleep–wake and other biological rhythms in patients living in isolation from environmental rhythms.

Unresponsiveness of the Pacemaker

In the absence of other environmental stimuli, a single light pulse may reset the circadian pacemaker to a new time of day. The direction and degree of resetting depends on the biological timing of the pulse. In humans, pulses near the onset of darkness and sleep retard the circadian pacemaker. Morning pulses have an advancing effect, and pulses during the waking portion of the day have no resetting effect. Evidence for such phase-resetting has been obtained in humans for both light and melatonin (reviewed in Ref. 25). The sleep–wake cycle loosely follows the circadian pacemaker, along with such additional factors as the duration of prior wakefulness and conditions conducive to sleep (recumbency, darkness, warmth) or wakefulness (upright posture, light, cold).

As originally proposed by Weitzman et al. (48) and Czeisler et al. (9), DSPS might be explained by deficient (but not absent) resetting of the pacemaker in the advance direction. The unopposed, delaying effects of evening light as well as the usually long period of the circadian pacemaker would then retard subsequent occurrences of sleep.

Deficient Time Cues

DSPS could also develop for reasons other than an abnormal circadian pacemaker. To synchronize biological clocks, environmental periodicities such as the light–dark cycle must have sufficient strength. In the absence of environmental timing signals, as found in a temporal isolation laboratory, the biological clock is free to express its own rhythmicity. Weak signals allow the biological clock to express some of its intrinsic, slow rhythmicity, causing sleep to lag but not escape the synchronizing influence of the 24-hour environment.

A relative lack of synchronizer strength can be explained in several ways. The environment itself may be deficient in time cues, as is the case in polar latitudes where the 24-hour light–dark cycle largely disappears near the summer and winter solstice. A single study of this question did not find north–south differences in the prevalence of DSPS (41). Another possibility is that people with DSPS may be insufficiently exposed to periodic environmental signals. DSPS is associated with a high rate of depression (37), which might cause patients to isolate themselves from their geophysical or social environments. There is, however, no direct evidence of this.

A third possibility is that sleep itself reduces the influence of environmental time cues, which may indeed not be necessary. It has been mentioned that normal sleep times are maintained by regular exposure to morning light. Oversleeping reduces morning light exposure, because the eyelids remain closed and the room often remains darkened. The tendency to delay waketime is thus self-reinforcing. This possibility is supported by the finding of a prolonged interval from the nadir of the circadian body-temperature rhythm (which is closely tied to the circadian pacemaker and therefore to its time-dependent ability to be reset to earlier times by light) to the termination of sleep (33). This finding is at variance, however, with an earlier study conducted in the absence of environmental time cues (46) and also with the ability of DSPS patients to maintain 24-hour sleep patterns, which implies that they do respond to the phase-advancing effect of morning light.

Deficient resetting might occur because of abnormal neural mechanisms of resetting rather than deficient stimuli. Resetting is mediated by specialized retinohypothalamic and geniculohypothalamic tracts that transmit environmental light–dark patterns to the pacemaking cells of the SCN (28). An abnormality might lie in those tracts, in their hypothalamic terminations, or in the pacemaking cells of the suprachiasmatic nuclei. Such a lesion, if present, would be only partial, since patients with DSPS are able to maintain 24-hour rhythms and therefore have some ability to phase-advance rhythms. As a result of such a lesion, they may be more dependent on nonphotic time cues, such as social cues, in the way some blind people are (30).

Deficient resetting of the circadian pacemaker by light underlies a form of HNS found in some blind people. It has been suggested that this is "true" HNS based on deficient pacemaker resetting, as distinct from cases in which sleep is delayed around the clock by "voluntary" efforts to avoid inconveniently late hours of sleep (38). However, this would not explain why such late hours of sleep develop in the first place. Furthermore, it is not unusual for patients to portray pathophysiological behaviors as voluntary (dyskinesias, as one example).

Behavioral Delays of Sleep

We have already mentioned "motivated sleep-phase delay." Both an immediate and an indirect effect of motivated changes in the hours of sleep have to be considered. The immediate effect is voluntary delay of sleep at bedtime, presumably via corticofugal activation of the reticular arousal system. This may be followed by delay of morning waketime as a result of a homeostatic effect of the extended period of wakefulness, plus the prolongation in the morning of conditions (darkness, repose, etc.) that are conducive to sleep. As a consequence of the delay of waking, the usual phase-resetting at dawn fails to occur, and the slow circadian pacemaker "drifts" toward a later setting, just as it does in the absence of environmental time cues. The interval during which the pacemaker is sensitive to resetting also becomes delayed. In this way, voluntary changes in the timing of sleep can have a lasting, adaptive effect.

The same mechanism of adaptation is presumably used by shiftworkers entering a new shift. It may also be used by some patients. Emens et al.(14) presented the case of a 31-year-old man who adopted a non-24-hour sleep–wake schedule to treat longstanding insomnia (presumably of the sleep-onset type). The patient scheduled sleep at intervals that averaged 25.17 hours—longer than the 24.51-hour period of his circadian pacemaker, which would otherwise have paced his sleep rhythm. The authors speculated that the self-selected schedule kept resetting the circadian pacemaker. This interpretation is supported by the finding, already mentioned, that the interval from the nadir of the circadian body-temperature rhythm (which marks the setting of the circadian pacemaker) to waking time is prolonged in some DSPS patients (33).

Is DSPS Psychogenic?

If behavior can delay the timing of sleep, a disabling syndrome of sleep delay might be psychogenic. This possibility has been considered from the time DSPS was first described (48). Patients sometimes report incessant rumination—inability to "turn off the mind"—as they are attempting to fall asleep. Furthermore, some cases of apparent DSPS can be reversed by voluntarily adhering to a conventional schedule, often when the school year has ended (15,51). For some adolescents, DSPS rationalizes academic or social failure ("secondary gain"). Psychiatric problems—chiefly depression—are also common among DSPS patients (5,37).

Despite the frequency of psychiatric problems in DSPS, no consistent psychiatric diagnosis has emerged. Furthermore, DSPS patients may be psychometrically normal (48). The most common diagnosis may be depression (37), but successful pharmacological treatment of depression has not alleviated the DSPS that it complicated (3). Depression is therefore not essential to the pathogenesis of DSPS. Furthermore, it may only appear to be common, because depressed DSPS patients are more likely to refer themselves for treatment (37,42). Finally, the association of depression with DSPS may be effect rather than cause: late sleep can be depressogenic (47), and the disabilities associated with DSPS would likely be depressing.

Two kinds of evidence favor abnormal biological timing systems as the basis of DSPS: resistance to correction of sleep phase and the success of treatments that do not have strong psychological meaning. The phase abnormality resists even strong efforts to correct it. This is indeed a defining feature of DSPS, because DSPS would otherwise blend too strongly into the circadian typology of eveningness. Even strong efforts to get up early do not hasten sleep onset the following night and only induce sleep deprivation. Investigator-imposed early sleep schedules have similarly failed within a few days (3). In one case, adherence to a conventional laboratory sleep schedule failed to phase-advance the delayed temperature rhythm of a patient with DSPS (18). On the other hand, resistance to correction of the late phase of sleep is not necessarily evidence against a motivational or psychopathological etiology. Because shifts of sleep (and coupled light exposure) can reset the circadian timing system, as we have just seen, the possibility exists that repeated shifts of sleep can result in retardation of the circadian timing system, which is then relatively resistant to correction. Given that phase delays can presumably be accomplished by most humans, although more easily by evening types (6), it would not be surprising if school refusal sometimes motivated a persisting delay of sleep.

Against psychogenicity is the effectiveness of several treatments, discussed below, that have no apparent psychological significance (chronotherapy, morning light, vitamin B_{12}, melatonin). Admittedly, the benefits have not been shown to persist and therefore do not neutralize the disease at its root. They may simply alleviate the symptomatic sleep delay, regardless of its etiology—psychogenic or organic.

Other Possible Etiologies of DSPS

Earlier, we alluded to the possibility that DSPS and HNS represent extremes of the expected human variation in circadian period. If such cases fell on the right tail of a bell-shaped distribution of circadian period, an equal number of short circadian periods should be found. Judging by the comparative rarity of patients with a counterpart *advanced* sleep-phase syndrome in which sleep occurs too early, this is not the case (41).

A genetic basis of DSPS is suggested by the occasional finding of families with multiple affected members (3). Eleven of 12 affected individuals serotyped for HLA had DQ1 (3). Several cases developed after a viral illness (3,5) or head trauma (5,34). Neoplastic or surgical lesions of the anterior hypothalamus can severely disrupt the temporal organization of sleep (8,16), but a focal abnormality specific for DSPS has not been described.

The etiology—or, more likely, etiologies—of DSPS therefore remain unknown. In many adolescent cases, psychopathology is prominent. In others, including adults who want to pursue a career during conventional hours, a chronobiological "pull" toward late phases of sleep seems inescapable.

TREATMENT

Treatment of DSPS may be divided into two aspects. One is correction of the abnormal sleep phase. The second is long-term maintenance of a normal sleep phase. The literature on this topic has been expanding, but a widely accepted countermeasure or clinical strategy remains lacking. The following is a personal view of how to approach such patients, although treatment success is often elusive.

Phase Correction

The first measure proposed for the correction of sleep timing in DSPS was chronotherapy (9,48). Its rationale is that DSPS patients are evidently unable to advance the phase of sleep to the desired position. Most patients report frequent, futile attempts to fall asleep early, and many have resorted to substances to force early sleep onset. Why not, then, have the patient *postpone* sleep to the desired time? Some patients have discovered this maneuver on their own, and DSPS patients do not complain of inability to stay up later than usual. The phase correction is carried out in a stepwise fashion, delaying bedtime and waketime by 2–3 hours per day, until a target schedule is reached. The patient is then instructed to maintain the target schedule.

Variable success has been reported with chronotherapy. In my experience with dozens of patients, chronotherapy can be effective. When it is not, failure is often explained by patients' lack of motivation, especially inability to accept the need for a regular sleep schedule. The lack of motivation is sometimes explained by covert benefits of going to sleep late, such as circles of friends who share an antipathy to school and to other conventional social behaviors. Failures are more likely in patients with major psychopathology (5). As in any clinical trial, information comes from the best-motivated patients.

The sleep log initially kept by the patient for diagnosis will also help assess suitability for treatment. Patients who are unable or unwilling to keep a daily record of sleep are also unlikely to conform to the chronotherapy schedule or, later, the long-term schedule. To define the patient's limits of compliance, a regular sleep schedule that approximates the complained-of delayed phase of sleep may be assigned before attempting to institute the stepwise delays of sleep that constitute chronotherapy. The initial sleep period should center on the hours of the 24-hour day when sleep is most frequent, and it should span as many hours as the patient sleeps on average. A surprising number of patients are unable to conform to such a schedule, even though it only regularizes what the patient is already doing. Some have perhaps been negatively conditioned to sleeping on a regular schedule by their nightly difficulty in falling asleep at a conventional bedtime. Others seem unable to accept any schedule. This does not bode well for maintaining the early schedule they profess to desire. Patients who succeed in following the preliminary schedule should be able to cooperate with chronotherapy.

The formulation of a chronotherapy regime has been given almost no attention in the literature. The starting phase of sleep can be taken as the midpoint of the hours of the 24-hour day during which the patient is most likely to be asleep and is easily calculated from a graphical sleep log (1). The patient should then be counseled regarding a realistic target schedule. The target schedule must be both physiologically feasible and compatible with the social change that can be accepted by the patient. Patients sometimes aim for unrealistically early schedules (bedtimes between 9 and 11 P.M., waketimes between 6 and 7 A.M.). We recommend getting up at the latest hour at which habitual social obligations can be met. To determine the target bedtime, the number of hours needed for sleep is calculated from a sleep log and subtracted from the target time of arising. The chronotherapy schedule should then be devised and written out for the patient.

From the starting phase of sleep, bedtimes and waketimes are scheduled 3 hours later each day until the target sleep time is reached (the last increment may be <3 hours). The total phase advance is typically 4 hours (4 A.M. bedtime → 12 midnight, for example) and will require about 7 days to complete. Because of the placement of several sleep periods during daylight hours, chronotherapy should be scheduled during a break from school or work. It has been suggested that chronotherapy may succeed best in patients with very late sleep phases; otherwise, the countervailing effects of daylight might be too strong (38). In our experience, completion of the stepwise delay of sleep can usually be completed. Difficulties are more likely to arise when it becomes necessary to adhere to the target schedule.

Patients have sometimes been hospitalized for chronotherapy (5), but we have not found this to be necessary. In a variant of chronotherapy, the sleep schedule is *set back* by 15 minutes a day or even less (36). While less disruptive to daytime activities, this strategy takes longer to complete: a 4-hour phase advance will require at least 16 days. Sudden imposition of a fixed, early sleep schedule (bedtime 11 P.M., arousal at 8 A.M.) was not successful (3).

In view of the time-dependent responsiveness of the human circadian timing system to light, it should not be surprising that light of sufficient strength and duration might help correct the timing of sleep in DSPS. Lewy et al. (24) used bright morning light to correct the sleep phase of a patient with DSPS in 3–4 days. Rosenthal et al. (39) used a 2-hour pulse of bright light between 6 A.M. and 9 A.M. combined with dark goggles worn in the evening to minimize any countervailing effects of evening light. The phase advance so achieved was quantified for the circadian body-temperature rhythm and amounted to only 1 hour, 25 minutes. Subjects felt more alert between 9 A.M. and 11 A.M., but no shift of sleep times was shown.

The validity of light's effects has not been established beyond doubt (13). An ideal placebo for perceptible light does not exist, and the use of light requires wakefulness with eyes open—a potential confound since wakefulness itself may affect the sleep–wake rhythm both through phase-resetting effects and by homeostatic responses to treatment-related deprivation of sleep. Artificial bright morning light has not been shown to be superior to morning sunlight (10).

Light may also have adverse effects. By truncating sleep, Terman et al. (43) point out, morning light may cause sleep deprivation before evening sleep onsets adjust. They therefore recommend that light be used to advance sleep in 10–30-minute daily steps. Paradoxical delay of sleep has occurred with morning light exposure (37). Light as an aid to correction of sleep phase in DSPS is therefore of limited effectiveness and may have adverse effects.

Partial phase correction has also been reported with vitamin B_{12} (32) and bedtime melatonin (3,11,45), but the phase advances have often been less than

1 hour. Melatonin can also prevent the repetitive insomnia of some blind people by halting the cycling of their sleep in and out of phase with the environment—a form of HNS (reviewed in Ref. 38). Vitamin B_{12} may shorten the longer-than-24-hour sleep–wake period in idiopathic HNS (21) but has not always been effective in DSPS, even when it advanced the timing of the nocturnal rise of melatonin (19). Little evidence for the clinical utility of these agents in correcting abnormal sleep phase has been presented. Elimination of caffeine may be helpful in phase correction (26).

Using various treatment methods, Regestein and Monk (37) achieved a treatment-response rate of less than 50% in DSPS patients and only 32% in depressed DSPS patients. They cited comparable discouraging rates in other case series.

Phase Maintenance

Few long-term follow-ups of any treatment for DSPS have been reported. Positive chronotherapy responses lasting 7 weeks to 20 months were obtained in the earliest described patients (48), and responses lasting 4–65 months have subsequently been reported (5). Success is more likely to be achieved in psychologically normal patients, perhaps because they adhere more consistently to their assigned schedules. Even well-motivated patients often notice that sleep tends to slip back into a late phase. One reason may be that their efforts to sleep at a conventional time failed to correct the phase of the circadian timing system (18). Relapses may be triggered by travel or late-night activities. Maintenance of the target sleep schedule may therefore require adjunctive treatments in addition to voluntary adherence to a schedule.

Despite the preeminent status of bright light as a resetter of the circadian pacemaker, there are few reports of its success in maintaining a serviceable sleep phase for longer than a few months. The effectiveness of morning sunlight—supplemented by occasional sleepless nights—was reportedly maintained for 3 months (10). Failures of light-maintenance therapy have been attributed to noncompliance (43), presumably because of the burden of spending several hours in front of bright lights in the morning—precisely the time of day at which these patients are incapacitated by oversleeping. Only one study has alluded to the ability of patients to maintain a normal sleep period with limited (1-hour) periods of morning light, but the duration of follow-up was not given (50). Terman et al. (43) suggested that an automatic, gradually increasing level of morning light simulating dawn may maximize therapeutic responsiveness, but this remains to be shown.

Relapses may occur within several days of discontinuing B_{12} or melatonin (3,11), and their long-term ability to maintain an improved sleep phase has not been shown.

Summary

The status of treatment for DSPS therefore remains unsatisfactory. Useful responses can nevertheless be obtained in carefully selected patients. Phase correction is most rapidly and surely achieved with chronotherapy. The starting phase of sleep should be calculated, and a realistic target phase must be chosen. In patients who are unable to follow a therapeutic schedule, phase correction with bright morning light, evening melatonin, and/or B_{12} may be tried. Maintaining a target schedule is the greatest challenge, and the literature is nearly devoid of useful information. It seems likely that long-term success will depend on adherence to a well-chosen target schedule supplemented by light, melatonin, or vitamin B_{12}. Unfortunately, success lasting longer than a few months may not have been achieved. The long-term outlook for DSPS patients is therefore unclear. Better social adaptation has been claimed (29), but the penalty for achieving it may be the adoption of occupations—and perhaps mates—suited to a late-night lifestyle.

OTHER CIRCADIAN-RHYTHM SLEEP DISORDERS

The International Classification of Sleep Disorders (ICSD) lists several circadian-rhythm sleep disorders in addition to DSPS (2). An *advanced-sleep-phase syndrome* (ASPS) with problems mirroring those of DSPS—inability to stay awake until a desired bedtime and inability to sleep late enough in the morning—was postulated on theoretical grounds but has rarely (if ever) been documented. Moldofsky et al. (27) described a 62-year-old man who slept from 6:30 P.M. to 3 A.M. subsequent to working alternating night–day shifts. An attempt to delay his sleep in the hospital did not succeed, but it was found possible to shift his sleep to earlier hours in daily steps, reversing the chronotherapy procedure. Five months later, he was found to be maintaining an 11-P.M.-to-7-A.M. sleep schedule. Although he was not clinically depressed at the time of study, he had been depressed 4 years earlier and continued to manifest an abnormally short latency from sleep onset to REM sleep. Major depression may be associated with both short REM latencies and early-morning awakening. Furthermore, progressive shifts of sleep to earlier times can have an antidepressant effect (47). It is therefore not easy to see how ASPS can be distinguished from depressive illness. Similarly, some elderly people fall asleep in the early evening, awaken before dawn, and have short REM-sleep latencies. No cases of ASPS meeting ICSD criteria (2) were detected among over 7600 Norwegian respondents to a survey of circadian-rhythm sleep disorders (41). We must conclude that ASPS is a rare entity if it exists as a separate entity at all.

Irregular sleep–wake patterns are found in patients whose time is not structured by work schedules and who indulge in daytime napping. Cumulative daytime sleep decreases the need for sleep at night, and nocturnal wakefulness reinforces the occurrence of daytime sleep. As a result, the circadian sleep–wake cycle may largely disappear. Promotion of napping in normal people can have a similar effect (7). Loss of circadian organization has also been described after removal of a pituitary tumor that involved the anterior hypothalamus, including the region of the suprachiasmatic nuclei (8).

REFERENCES

1. Metrodesign Inc. Homer, NY.
2. ICSD—International Classification of Sleep Disorders. Diagnostic and Coding Manual. Rochester, MN: American Sleep Disorders Association, 1990.
3. Alvarez B, Dahlitz MJ, Vignau J, Parkes JD. The delayed sleep phase syndrome: clinical and investigative findings in 14 subjects. J Biolog Rhythms 1992; 55:665–670.
4. Aschoff J. Circadian rhythms in man. Science 1965; 148:1427–1432.
5. Billiard M, Verge M, Touchon J, Carlander B, Besset A. Delayed sleep phase syndrome: subjective and objective data, chronotherapy and follow-up [abstr]. Sleep Res 1993; 22:172.
6. Breithaupt H, Hildebrandt G, Dohre D. Tolerance to shift of sleep as related to the individual circadian phase position. Ergonomics 1978; 21:767–774.
7. Campbell S, Zulley J. Napping as a biological rhythm: disentrainment of the human sleep/wake system. In: Visser P, ed. Sleep '86. Stuttgart: Gustav Fischer Verlag, 1988:3–10.
8. Cohen RA, Albers HE. Disruption of human circadian and cognitive regulation following a discrete hypothalamic lesion: a case study. Neurology 1991; 41:726–729.
9. Czeisler CA, Richardson GS, Coleman RM, Zimmerman JC, Moore-Ede MC, Dement WC, Weitzman, ED. Chronotherapy: resetting the circadian clocks of patients with delayed sleep phase insomnia. Sleep 1981; 4(1):1–21.
10. Dagan Y, Tzischinsky O, Lavie P. Sunlight treatment for delayed sleep-phase syndrome: case report [abstr]. Sleep Res 1991; 20:451.
11. Dahlitz M, Alvarez B, Vignau J, English J, Arendt J, Parkes JD. Delayed sleep phase syndrome response to melatonin. Lancet 1991; 337:1121–1124.
12. deBeck TW. Delayed sleep phase syndrome—criminal offense in the military? Milit Med 1990; 155:14–15.
13. Eastman CI. Does light treatment work? Is light treatment a placebo? Light Treat Biol Rhyth 1993; 5:30–31.
14. Emens JS, Brotman DJ, Czeisler CA. Evaluation of the intrinsic period of the circadian pacemaker in a patient with a non-24-hour sleep-wake schedule disorder [abstr]. Sleep Res 1994; 23:256.
15. Ferber R, Boyle MD. Delayed sleep phase syndrome versus motivated sleep phase delay in adolescents [abstr]. Sleep Res 1983; 12:239.
16. Fulton J, Bailey P. Tumors in the region of the third ventricle: their diagnosis and relation to pathological sleep. J Nerv Ment Dis 1929; 69:1–25, 145–164, 261–277.

17. Guilleminault C, Czeisler CA, Coleman RM, Miles L, Cobb WA, Okuma T. Circadian rhythm disturbances and sleep disorders in shift workers. In: Buser PA, ed. Kyoto Symposium (EEG Suppl 36). Amsterdam: Elsevier, 1982.
18. Hayes B, Czeisler CA. Chronobiology of human sleep and sleep disorders. In: Haus E, ed. Biological Rhythms in Clinical and Laboratory Medicine. New York: Springer-Verlag, 1992:256–264.
19. Honma K, Kohsaka M, Fukuda N, Morita N, Honma S. Effects of vitamin B_{12} on plasma melatonin rhythm in humans: increased light sensitivity phase-advances the circadian clock? Experientia 1992; 48:716–720.
20. Horne JA, Ostberg O. A self-assessment questionnaire to determine morningness-eveningness in human circadian rhythms. Int J Chronobiol 1976; 4:97–110.
21. Kamgar-Parsi B, Wehr TA, Gillin JC. Successful treatment of human non-24-hour sleep-wake syndrome. Sleep 1983; 6:257–264.
22. Kim L, Choi Y, Suh K, Shin D, Pollak CP. Recovery sleep on weekends and daytime sleepiness [abstr]. Sleep 1998; 21(3 suppl):258.
23. Kokkoris CP, Weitzman ED, Pollak CP, Spielman AJ, Czeisler CA, Bradlow H. Long-term ambulatory temperature monitoring in a subject with a hypernycthermal sleep-wake cycle disturbance. Sleep 1978; 1:177–190.
24. Lewy AJ, Sack RL, Singer CM. Treating phase typed chronobiologic sleep and mood disorders using appropriately timed bright artificial light. Psychopharmacol Bull 1985; 21:368–372.
25. Lewy AJ, Ahmed S, Sack RL. Phase shifting the human circadian clock using melatonin. Behav Brain Res 1996; 73:131–134.
26. Lucas EA, Scheving LE, Halberg F. Circadian rhythmometry before and after relief of delayed sleep-onset insomnia following total caffeine withdrawal. Adv Biosciences 1982; 41:29–42.
27. Moldofsky H, Musisi S, Phillipson EA. Treatment of a case of advanced sleep phase syndrome by phase advance chronotherapy. Sleep 1986; 9:61–65.
28. Moore RY. The suprachiasmatic nucleus and the mammalian circadian system. Adv Biosci 1987; 73:97–105.
29. Ohta T. Circadian rhythm sleep disorders: a brief review with special reference to long-term follow-up. Nagoya J Med Sci 1995; 58:85–93.
30. Okawa M, Nanami T, Wada S, Shimizu T, Hishikawa Y, Sasaki H, Nagamine H, Takehashi K. Four congenitally blind children with circadian sleep-wake rhythm disorders. Sleep 1987; 10:101–110.
31. Okawa M, Mishima K, Nanami T, Shimizu T, Iijima S, Hishikawa Y, Takahashi K. Vitamin B12 treatment for sleep-wake rhythm disorders. Sleep 1990; 13:15–23.
32. Oren DA, Turner EH, Wehr TA. Abnormal circadian rhythms of plasma melatonin and body temperature in the delayed sleep phase syndrome [letter]. J Neurol Neurosurg Psychiatry 1995; 58:379.
33. Ozaki S, Uchiyama M, Shirakawa S, Okawa M. Prolonged interval from body temperature nadir to sleep offset in patients with delayed sleep phase syndrome. Sleep 1996; 19:36–40.
34. Patten SB, Lauderdale WM. Delayed sleep phase disorder after traumatic brain injury. J Am Acad Child Adolesc Psychiatry 1992; 31:100–102.
35. Pittendrigh CS, Daan S. A functional analysis of circadian pacemakers in nocturnal

rodents. IV. Entrainment: pacemaker as clock. J Compar Physiol 1976; 106:291–331.
36. Regestein QR, Pavlova M. Treatment of delayed sleep phase syndrome. Gen Hosp Psychiatry 1995; 17:335–345.
37. Regestein QR, Monk TH. Delayed sleep phase syndrome: a review of its clinical aspects. Am J Psychiatry 1995; 152:602–608.
38. Richardson GS, Malin HV. Circadian rhythm sleep disorders: pathophysiology and treatment. J Clin Neurophysiol 1996; 13:17–31.
39. Rosenthal NE, Joseph-Vanderpool JR, Levenkosky AA, Honston SH, Allen R, Kelly KA, Souetre E, Schultz PM, Starz KE. Phase-shifting effects of bright morning light as treatment for delayed sleep phase syndrome. Sleep 1990; 13:354–361.
40. Roth B. Narcolepsy and Hypersomnia. New York: S Karger, 1980.
41. Schrader H, Bovim G, Sand T. The prevalence of delayed and advanced sleep phase syndromes. J Sleep Res 1993; 2:51–55.
42. Schrader H, Bovim G, Sand T. Depression in the delayed sleep phase syndrome [letter]. Am J Psychiatry 1996; 153:9.
43. Terman M, Lewy AJ, Dijk DJ, Boulos Z, Eastman CI, Campbell SS. Light treatment for sleep disorders: consensus report. IV. Sleep phase and duration disturbances. J Biolog Rhythms 1995; 10:135–147.
44. Thorpy MJ, Korman E, Spielman AJ, Glovinsky PB. Delayed sleep phase syndrome in adolescents. J Adolesc Health Care 1988; 9:22–27.
45. Tzischinski O, Dagan Y, Lavie P. The effects of melatonin on the timing of sleep in patients with delayed sleep phase syndrome. In: Pevet P, ed. Melatonin and the Pineal Gland: From Basic Science to Clinical Application. Amsterdam: Elsevier Excerta Medica, 1993:351–354.
46. Wagner DR, Moline ML, Pollak CP, Czeisler CA. Entrained sleep and temperature rhythms in delayed sleep phase syndrome [abstr]. Sleep Res 1986; 15:179.
47. Wehr TA, Wirz-Justice A, Goodwin FK, Duncan W, Gillin JC. Phase advance of the circadian sleep-wake cycle as an antidepressant. Science 1979; 206:710–713.
48. Weitzman ED, Czeisler CA, Coleman RM, Spielman AJ, Zimmerman JC, Dement W, Richardson G, Pollak CP. Delayed sleep phase syndrome: a chronobiologic disorder associated with sleep onset insomnia. Arch Gen Psychiatry 1981; 38:737–746.
49. Weitzman ED, Czeisler CA, Coleman R, Dement W, Richardson G, Pollak C. Delayed sleep phase syndrome: a biological rhythm sleep disorder [abstr]. Sleep Res 1979; 8:221.
50. Weyerbrock A, Timmer J, Hohagen F, Berger M, Bauer J. Effects of light and chronotherapy on human circadian rhythms in delayed sleep phase syndrome: cytokines, cortisol, growth hormone, and the sleep-wake cycle. Biol Psychiatry 1996; 40:794–797.
51. Wirz-Justice A, Pringle C. The non-entrained life of a young gentleman at Oxford. Sleep 1987; 10:57–61.

8

Insomnia in Neurology

Elio Lugaresi, Federica Provini, and Giuseppe Plazzi
University of Bologna
Bologna, Italy

INTRODUCTION

Insomnia, defined as difficulty in initiating or maintaining sleep, is not a disease itself but mostly a clinical sign of an underlying disease. Between 10 and 20% of the population in the Western world are deemed to be chronic insomniacs (1,2). The number of chronic insomniacs rises with age from under 5% at age 20 to over 30% in those over 60; women complain of insomnia more often than men (2) (Figure 1).

Patients often link their insomnia to a wide variety of mental states, from anxiety or depression to difficulties in interpersonal relationships, family discord, problems at work, and financial troubles. In individual cases, it is not easy to establish which of these factors is responsible for sleep impairment. However, insomnia is not entirely the result of psychological events: a disordered lifestyle; alcohol and drug abuse; bone, joint, and muscle pain; bronchitis; gastritis; colitis; and prostate hypertrophy can all lead to insomnia. This is especially true in the elderly, whose sleep is lighter and more fragmented and who frequently suffer from aches and pains and resort to chronic sleep medication. Last but not least, insomnia tends to run in families, and patients often have other relatives who suffer from anxiety, depression, irritability, and insomnia. Hence, both a genetic predisposition and living with emotionally disturbed people can lead to chronic insomnia in the same family.

Neurological disorders entail sensory-motor deficits and behavioral problems and may thus favor the onset of insomnia as they are a source of serious

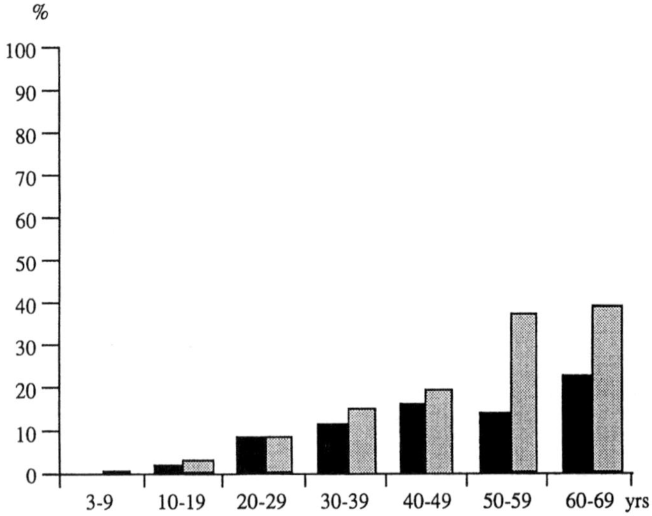

Figure 1 Prevalence of insomnia in a large sample of the San Marino population (2). Overall prevalence = 13.4%. Solid bars = male (9.9%); shaded bars = female (16.8%).

worry for the patient and his or her family. CNS diseases may, however, involve the nervous-system structures responsible for the physiological control of wake and sleep and therefore lead to sleep impairment.

INSOMNIA IN ELDERLY PATIENTS WITH DEMENTIA

Aging accompanied by mental deterioration caused by a degenerative (e.g., Alzheimer's) or vascular disease (multi-infarct dementia) can compromise the sleep–wake rhythm more than the physiological aging process. In patients with senile dementia of the Alzheimer's type and in those with multi-infarct dementia, nocturnal motor activity is more pronounced than in subjects of the same age without dementia (3,4).

The circadian fluctuations in body temperature and secretion of melatonin and cortisol are impaired in patients with dementia compared with an age-matched normal population. It remains unsettled whether insomnia in the elderly with dementia is due to an anatomical-functional impairment of the suprachiasmatic nucleus or to a more complex disruption of the circuits that control body homeostasis (5). *Sundowning* is the term used to define the tendency of many people with dementia, especially those in nursing homes, to present a nocturnal exacerbation of disruptive behavior and agitation. The concept of a "sundowning syndrome'' is useful for practical purposes, but it is more difficult to define in physiopathological terms. Isolated from their families and from society because of their dementia, patients often confuse day and night and present episodes of sleep alternating randomly with hours of agitation and confusion throughout the 24 hours. The nocturnal exacerbation characterized by confused oneiric episodes could be caused by disturbing dreams or REM behavior disorders (4–6). Transient delusions may persist during the daytime as a result of the nocturnal oneiric episodes.

To improve the nocturnal sleep of the elderly with dementia, it is advisable to try to re-establish a more normal sleep–wake rhythm by keeping patients in well-lit rooms during the day, whereas their sleeping quarters should be dark and quiet during the night. Benzodiazepine administration, especially drugs with a long half-life, should be avoided because, paradoxically, they can exacerbate nocturnal confusion and agitation. In some cases, phenothiazines or butyrophenones may be useful at low dosage (4–7).

When patients present a severe impairment of circadian rhythms of body temperature, morning sessions of hyperillumination, given for a few hours, or 3–5 mg melatonin administered 2 hours before bedtime may be of some benefit (5).

INSOMNIA IN DEGENERATIVE DISEASES OF THE CNS WITH MOTOR-SYSTEM INVOLVEMENT

This group of diseases includes Parkinson's disease and Parkinsonian syndromes, Huntington's chorea, hereditary ataxia, progressive dystonia, and Tourette's syndrome. Literature reports on insomnia in these diseases are fragmentary, controversial, and mainly anecdotal (8,9).

In idiopathic *Parkinson's disease*, both motor impairment and the depression that often accompanies the disease can give rise to insomnia, which may respond to administration of benzodiazepines or amitriptyline. Patients with Parkinson's disease have a marked reduction of spindling, fragmentation of sleep, and a shorter total sleep time. In diffuse Lewy body disease, characterized by dementia associated with parkinsonism, sleep is disrupted by hallucinatory episodes and REM-sleep behavior disorder, which are clinical features complicating the disorder (10,11).

Progressive supranuclear palsy (PSP) is characterized clinically by axial rigidity, impaired voluntary gaze, dysarthria, and subcortical dementia, and pathologically by extensive damage to the basal ganglia, median thalamus, and pontomesencephalic reticular formation. The involvement of the subcortical neurological structures responsible for sleep–wake regulation accounts for the sleep impairment commonly encountered. Polygraphic recordings in patients with PSP show a shortening of total sleep time, a drastic reduction of spindling, and a decreased percentage of REM sleep; slow-wave sleep is usually associated with atonia (12). Another characteristic feature of PSP seems to be daytime somnolence. In these patients, however, subjective findings of sleepiness may not coincide with objective measurement (multiple sleep latency test). In some cases, daytime somnolence was the most prominent clinical symptom for both the patients and their families.

In *multiple system atrophy* (MSA), which encompasses neurodegenerative diseases previously described as striatonigral degeneration, sporadic olivopontocerebellar atrophy, and Shy-Drager syndrome, sleep is often disturbed by motor (REM-sleep behavior disorders and periodic limb movements) and respiratory events (laryngeal stridor or snoring with apneas) that cause recurrent arousals, lightening and fragmenting sleep (13,14).

The circadian rhythms of temperature and melatonin secretion are also impaired in both propriospinal myoclonus and MSA and reflect a severe disruption of the mechanisms controlling homeostasis of the autonomic and endocrine systems that could contribute to sleep impairment (14,15; personal observation).

In *Huntington's chorea*, polysomnography shows reduced sleep efficiency with sleep fragmentation, decreased slow-wave and REM sleep, and a characteristic marked increase in amplitude and density of sleep spindling (8).

In *idiopathic torsion dystonia*, characterized by generalized dystonic posturing, the degree of sleep disruption is related to the severity of the disease (8). In *Tourette's syndrome*, characterized by multiple vocal and motor tics and compulsive behavior, sleep complaints are frequent. The degree of sleep disturbance is correlated with disease severity. In addition, around 40% of children with Tourette's syndrome have a history of somnambulism, night terrors, or enuresis and are prone to confusional arousal. Sleep analysis shows an increased number of awakenings and increased motor activity and body movements during sleep (16).

INSOMNIA LINKED WITH MOVEMENT DISORDERS

Some neurological disorders are characterized by abnormal movements that hinder sleep onset. These include the restless-legs syndrome, nocturnal myoclonus or periodic limb movements, and propriospinal myoclonus. In particularly severe cases of nocturnal frontal-lobe epilepsy and REM-sleep behavior disorders, sleep continuity may also be disrupted, leading to a complaint of chronic insomnia.

Restless-legs syndrome (RLS) is characterized by an undefinable feeling of discomfort typically localized deep in the tissues between the knee and the ankle. Paresthesias arise during rest, especially when the patient is about to fall asleep. Any movement of the limbs—such as rubbing the legs together, making bicycling movements, and pacing across the room—transiently relieves symptoms (17).

In milder forms of the syndrome, the disorder lengthens the time it takes to fall asleep and is not a true medical problem; in the most severe forms, however, the patient suffers severe and persistent insomnia that not only hinders falling asleep but triggers recurrent prolonged awakenings throughout the night. The most disturbing forms of RLS affect 1–2% of the population, whereas the mild forms were experienced by 5% of people interviewed (17,18).

A family history of the disorder is found in 90% of idiopathic cases, with an autosomal dominant pattern of inheritance in 2–10% of cases (19). The genetic impairment responsible for these hereditary forms has yet to be identified. The onset of hereditary-familial forms of RLS and severe sporadic cases occurs in the first and second decades and persists throughout life. In other cases, the disorder becomes clinically relevant after the fifth to sixth decades. The etiology and physiopathology of RLS remain unknown. Some symptomatic forms arise in cases of iron-deficiency anemia (20), familial amyloid neuropathy (21), and uremic (22) and diabetic polyneuropathies (23).

Over 80% of patients with RLS present *periodic limb movements during sleep* (PLMS) confined to the lower limbs. PLMS appear on falling asleep and continue in light sleep (Figure 2). In the most severe cases, PLMS may persist

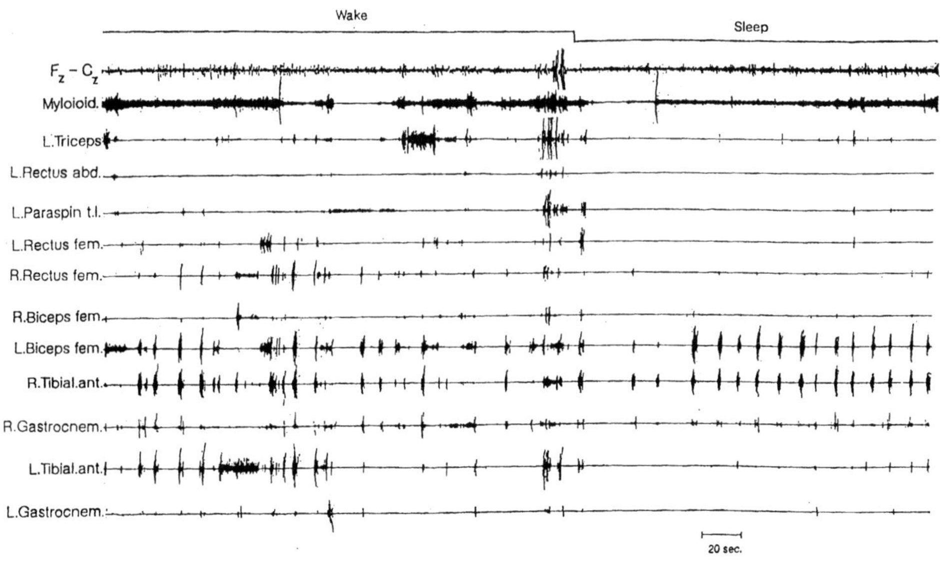

Figure 2 Restless-legs syndrome (RLS) and nocturnal myoclonus (NM). While asleep, the patient displays repetitive, quasi-rhythmic polyclonic jerks in the lower and upper limbs, intermingled with voluntary movements. As soon as the patient falls asleep, periodic movements (NM) persist in the lower limbs.

in deep (slow-wave) sleep and, more seldom, REM sleep. Since PLMS are associated with EEG signs of arousal, they make sleep lighter and more fragmented, and have been deemed an independent cause of insomnia, although this view remains a matter of debate (23,24).

Patients with iron deficiency (ferritin <45 μg/L) respond favorably to iron-replacement therapy (20). In other forms, either idiopathic or symptomatic, dopa-carbidopa therapy has proved to be the most effective, administered at doses of levodopa between 100 and 500 mg at bedtime. This dosage should not be exceeded because there is a risk that the RLS symptoms will recur during the night or the following day—exacerbation of symptoms may give rise to akathisia. Dopaminergic medication, especially pergolide at a dose of 0.15–0.50 mg twice daily (at lunch and 2 hours before retiring), may prove equally effective and has fewer side effects (25). Other forms of treatment include benzodiazepines, particularly clonazepam at a dose of 0.5–2 mg, gabapentin (26), and opiates, which should be administered only to patients with very severe resistant forms (27).

PLMS may occur independently of RLS in other neurological conditions such as narcolepsy, stiff-man syndrome, Isaacs' syndrome, chronic myelopathies, neuropathies, anemia, gastric surgery, uremia, pregnancy, and obstructive sleep apnea syndrome (23). These movements may also appear in healthy subjects, exceptionally under the age of 30 (5%) but in around a third of the population over 50. PLMS present in similar percentages in good and poor sleepers alike and therefore, unless they are associated with RLS, they are not a definite cause of insomnia. Nonetheless, the high frequency of periodic muscle jerks can fragment sleep, giving patients the impression of having slept little and badly. In these exceptional cases, PLMS may be a major cause of chronic insomnia (28,29).

Propriospinal myoclonus (PSM) is characterized by muscle jerks, usually very intense, that arise from an axial muscle (in the neck, chest, and abdomen) extending via the multisynaptic pathways both caudally and rostrally (for a clinical and electrophysiological description of PSM, see Ref. 30 and Chapter 9 of this volume).

PSM typically arises when patients are about to fall asleep, when the alpha rhythm spreads to the anterior regions or is replaced by low-amplitude theta activity (stage 1 of non-REM sleep). This triggers an arousal followed by another attempt at falling asleep, during which another myoclonic jerk occurs (Figure 3). The jerks may recur every 20 seconds to 1 minutes for 10s of minutes or hours at a time, preventing patients from falling asleep. Sensory activation (noise, lights, or other environmental stimuli) or mental tasks (speaking, thinking, mental arithmetic) temporarily impede the muscular jerks. The appearance of sleep spindling in stage 2 non-REM sleep (transition from stages 1 to 2) is immediately followed by a cessation of muscular jerks. Physiological sleep, when initiated, usually continues until the morning. Once the patient is awake, PSM seldom

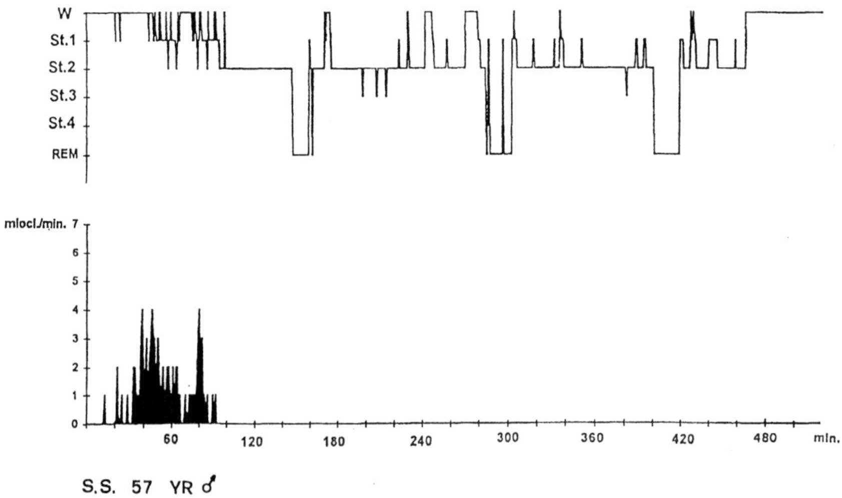

Figure 3 Propriospinal myoclonus hypnogram. The histogram (bottom) indicates the number of jerks per minute. Jerks persist over 90 minutes, increasing sleep latency; they disappear with sleep onset.

recurs and in any case is much milder. The insomnia caused by PSM is severe and often disrupts the family and social life of the patient.

Clonazepam (at a dose of 0.5–2 mg) can alleviate the disorder, making sleep more restful. However, a patient we saw at age 70 had had PSM since early adulthood. Since only opiates had proved beneficial, he had developed opiate drug dependence (30).

Nocturnal frontal-lobe epilepsy is a recently identified clinical entity (31) in which seizures are mainly or exclusively linked to non-REM sleep. Nocturnal frontal-lobe seizures (see Chapter 15) may consist of a sudden arousal (paroxysmal) accompanied by stereotyped abnormal movements (32), a dystonic attack lasting 1–2 minutes (nocturnal paroxysmal dystonia) (33), and agitated sleepwalking (episodic nocturnal wandering) (34,35). These three types of seizures often coexist in the same patient. The shortest seizures may recur several times every night, giving patients the feeling of having slept little and badly. Some patients with very frequent nocturnal seizures feel tired and weary on awakening in the morning and complain of daytime sleepiness. If seizures disappear or decline in frequency with antiepileptic drug treatment, this sense of tiredness and daytime somnolence may subside (36).

REM-sleep behavior disorders (RBDs) are basically linked to a dysfunction in the system blocking muscles during REM sleep (REM sleep without atonia).

This results in repeated episodes of motor agitation of varying intensity during REM sleep. The disorder may be idiopathic (40% of cases) or secondary to CNS disease (Ref. 37 and Chapter 9 of this volume).

When RBDs are intense and prolonged, as occurs in MSA, nocturnal sleep is disrupted and patients may feel tired and weary upon awakening.

NEUROLOGICAL DISORDERS CAUSING INABILITY TO SLEEP

Some rare neurological disorders are characterized by a virtually total loss of the ability to sleep, accompanied by episodes of confusion, agitation, and enacted dreams. The term *agrypnia excitata* (*agrypnia* = *agrein* or *agreiein*, ''to hunt''; *hypnos* = ''sleep'') can be used to distinguish this psychopathological condition from trivial insomnia. These disorders include: 1) fatal familial insomnia, a recently identified prion disease, 2) Morvan's syndrome, a rare disorder described for the first time more than a century ago, and 3) acute psychotic states induced by withdrawal of alcohol (delirium tremens) or drugs (barbiturates, benzodiazepines).

Fatal familial insomnia (FFI) is characterized clinically by apathy and an inability to sleep (agrypnia) accompanied by enacted dreams, sympathetic hyperactivity, and motor signs (ataxia, dysarthria, myoclonias), and pathologically by selective degeneration of the anteroventral and mediodorsal thalamic nuclei (38). FFI is a hereditary prion disease genetically linked to a point mutation at codon 178 of the prion protein at chromosome 20, in conjunction with methionine in the methionine/valine polymorphic position 129 of the mutant allele (39).

The sleep disorder comprises an early disappearance of spindling and increasing difficulties in initiating and maintaining sleep. Sleep disintegration leads to a persistent state of wakefulness or subwakefulness interspersed with episodes of more or less purposeful gesturing in which the patient enacts the content of a dream. These episodes occur when atypical episodes of REM sleep emerge directly from wakefulness.

Severe impairment of nocturnal sleep and daytime hypersomnolence characterize other disorders affecting the anteromedian thalamic nuclei, such as paramedian thalamic stroke syndrome (40).

Morvan's fibrillar chorea was first identified in 1890 and mainly reported by French researchers. The disorder consists of insomnia with subacute onset associated with anxiety and restlessness, hyperhydrosis, tachycardia, cramps, and fasciculations (41).

Fewer than 100 patients have been described to date. The disease course is usually benign with spontaneous remissions, but the disease progressively worsens, leading to death in about 10% of cases. One case with a malignant evolution was recorded polygraphically by Fischer-Perroudon et al. (42), who documented a virtually total inability to sleep in the 4 months preceding the patient's death. Autopsy failed to disclose gross macroscopic brain lesions.

In a similar case we followed until death, the clinical features were characterized by a typical aspect of neuromyotonia (Isaacs' syndrome) associated with an inability to sleep, dream enactment, and hallucinations. The PSG features showed continuous wakefulness or presleep behavior accompanied by an atypical EEG pattern characterized by alpha-theta activity (Figure 4). Plasma-exchange treatment led to a marked improvement of both central and peripheral signs. The patient died suddenly 2 years later. No major brain lesions were noted at autopsy, but the patient had a small-cell lung carcinoma.

Acute psychotic syndromes are due to withdrawal of alcohol (delirium tremens) or drugs (barbiturates, benzodiazepines). Studies by Tachibana et al. (43) and Kotorii et al. (44) have made a major contribution to the pathophysiology of acute psychotic conditions caused by sudden withdrawal of alcohol or drugs.

Delirium tremens, a typical example, is characterized by a confusional state with restlessness and dream enactment accompanied by signs of sympathetic activation (hyperhydrosis, tachycardia, hypertension, fever). Polysomnographic recording of a special case showed the disappearance of physiological sleep, replaced by continuous wakefulness from which atypical fragments of REM sleep emerged (Figure 5). Similar findings have been reported following sudden withdrawal of meprobamate, barbiturates, and benzodiazepines (45).

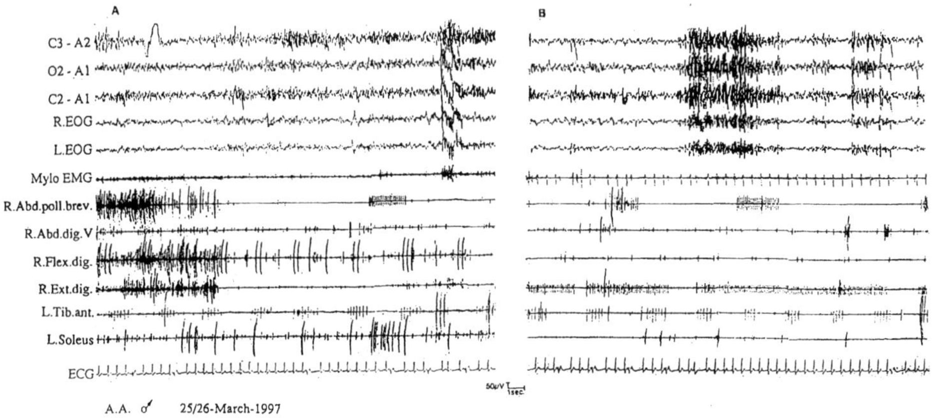

Figure 4 Morvan's syndrome. (A) The patient is agitated and presents dream-enacting behavior. The polysomnogram is characterized by wake-activity rhythms, muscle artifacts, and the characteristic continuous muscle-fiber activity on EMG. ECG shows multiple arrhythmic abnormalities. (B) Sleeplike behavior: the patient is quiet, but the EEG lacks any characteristic sleep pattern.

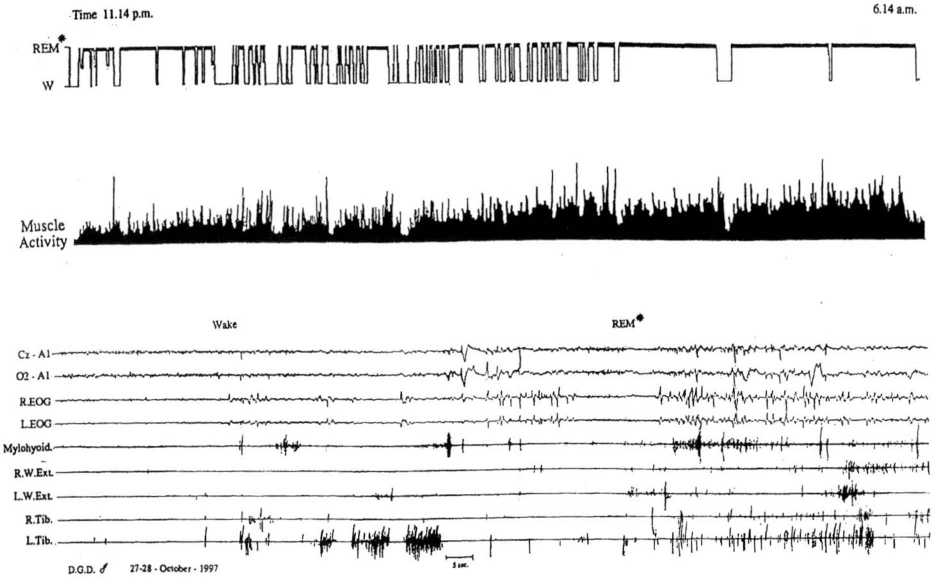

Figure 5 Delirium tremens. The hypnogram is characterized by continuous fluctuation from wakefulness to REM sleep without atonia (REM*). During REM* the patient displays complex oneiric hallucinatory behavior. ''Muscle activity'' recorded by the mylohyoid muscle shows a lack of atonia during REM sleep. Polysomnography documents an abrupt onset of REM* from wakefulness.

Pathogenetic mechanisms: FFI, Morvan's syndrome, and delirium tremens are three pathological conditions with a similar sleep disorder but different etiology. The clinical and polysomnographic similarities between them could be the result of a common underlying mechanism linked to the involvement of the same circuits responsible for sleep–wake regulation. The underlying mechanism responsible for these ''agitated agrypnias'' could be a functional imbalance characterized by the prevalence of activating (probably cholinergic) systems over deactivating (probably GABAergic) ones in the CNS. In FFI, this could result from atrophy of the mediodorsal thalamic nuclei, preventing GABAergic impulses originating in the reticular nucleus from reaching other cortical and subcortical structures involved in sleep regulation (46).

In delirium tremens, a similar outcome (inability to sleep and sympathetic activation) could ensue from downregulation of the GABA receptors caused by the chronic intake of GABAergic substances (alcohol, barbiturates, and benzodiazepines). The sudden withdrawal of alcohol or drugs acting on the GABAergic system could lead to the same functional imbalance between activating structures (promoting wakefulness) and deactivating structures (promoting sleep) observed in FFI.

In Morvan's syndrome, the mechanism responsible for such symptoms remains unclear, but the same circuits responsible for sleep–wake regulation could be implicated yet again as a consequence of an imbalance due to some channel-specific antibodies, leading to the functional prevalence of activating over deactivating systems. The beneficial effect of plasma exchange observed in our case is consistent with this tentative pathogenetic explanation of the inability observed in our patient to generate EEG sleep patterns.

REFERENCES

1. Mellinger GD, Balter MB, Uhlenhuth EH. Insomnia and its treatment: prevalence and correlates. Arch Gen Psychiatry 1985; 42:225–232.
2. Lugaresi E, Cirignotta F, Zucconi M, Mondini S, Lenzi PL, Coccagna G. Good and poor sleepers: Epidemiological Survey of the San Marino Population. In: Guilleminault C, Lugaresi E, eds. Sleep/Wake Disorders: Natural History, Epidemiology, and Long-Term Evolution. New York: Raven Press, 1983:1–12.
3. Mishima K, Okawa M, Satoh K, Shimizu T, Hozumi S, Hishikawa Y. Different manifestations of circadian rhythms in senile dementia of Alzheimer's type and multi-infarct dementia. Neurobiol Aging 1997; 18:105–109.
4. Bliwise DL. Dementia. In: Kryger MH, Dement W, Roth T, eds. Principles and Practice of Sleep Medicine. 2nd ed. Philadelphia: WB Saunders, 1994:790–800.
5. Mishima K, Hishikawa Y. Chronotherapy for circadian rhythm disorders in elderly patients with dementia. In: Hayaishi O, Inoué S, eds. Sleep and Sleep Disorders: From Molecule to Behavior. Tokyo: Academic Press, 1997:177–191.
6. Lipowski ZJ. Delirium in the elderly patient. N Engl J Med 1989; 320:578–582.
7. Evans LK. Sundown syndrome in institutionalized elderly. J Am Geriatr Soc 1987; 35:101.
8. Aldrich MS. Sleep and degenerative neurological disorders involving the motor system. In: Thorpy MJ, ed. Handbook of Sleep Disorders. New York: Marcel Dekker, 1990:673–692.
9. Culebras A. Sleep disorders associated with psychiatric, medical, and neurologic disorders. In: Culebras A, ed. Clinical Handbook of Sleep Disorders. Boston: Butterworth-Heinemann, 1996:233–281.
10. Uchiyama M, Isse K, Tanaka K, Yokota N, Hamamoto M, Aida S, Ito Y, Yoshimura M, Okawa M. Incidental Lewy body disease in a patient with REM sleep behavior disorder. Neurology 1995; 45:709–712.
11. Turner RS, Chervin RD, Frey KA, Minoshima S, Kuhl DE. Probable diffuse Lewy body disease presenting as REM sleep behavior disorder. Neurology 1997; 49:523–527.
12. Montplaisir J, Petit D, Décary A, Masson H, Bédard MA, Panisset M, Rémillard G, Gauthier S. Sleep and quantitative EEG in patients with progressive supranuclear palsy. Neurology 1997; 49:999–1003.

13. Plazzi G, Corsini R, Provini F, Pierangeli G, Martinelli P, Montagna P, Lugaresi E, Cortelli P. REM sleep behavior disorders in multiple system atrophy. Neurology 1997; 48:1094–1097.
14. Chokroverty S. The assessment of sleep disturbance in autonomic failure. In: Bannister R, Mathias CJ, eds. Autonomic Failure: A Textbook of Clinical Disorders of the Nervous System. 3rd ed. London: Oxford University Press, 1992:442–461.
15. Cortelli P, Pierangeli G, Provini F, Plazzi G, Lugaresi E. Blood pressure rhythms in sleep disorders and dysautonomia. In: Portaluppi F, Smolensky MH, eds. Time-Dependent Structure and Control of Arterial Blood Pressure. New York: Annals of the New York Academy of Sciences, 1996:204–221.
16. Glaze DG, Frost JD, Zughbi HY, Percy AK. Rett syndrome: characterization of respiratory patterns and sleep. Ann Neurol 1987; 21:377–382.
17. Ekbom KA. Restless legs syndrome. Neurology 1960; 100:868–873.
18. Lavigne GJ, Montplaisir JY. Restless legs syndrome and sleep bruxism: prevalence and association among Canadians. Sleep 1994; 17:739–743.
19. Ondo W, Jankovic J. Restless legs syndrome: clinicoetiologic correlates. Neurology 1996; 47:1435–1441.
20. O'Keeffe ST, Gavin K, Lavan JN. Iron status and restless legs syndrome in the elderly. Age Ageing 1994; 23:200–203.
21. Salvi F, Montagna P, Plasmati R, Rubboli G, Cirignotta F, Veilleux M, Lugaresi E, Tassinari CA. Restless legs syndrome and nocturnal myoclonus: initial manifestation of familial amyloid polyneuropathy. J Neurol Neurosurg Psychiatry 1990; 53: 522–525.
22. Callaghan N. Restless legs syndrome in uremic neuropathy. Neurology (Minn) 1966; 16:359–361.
23. Lugaresi E, Cirignotta F, Coccagna G, Montagna P. Nocturnal myoclonus and restless legs Syndrome. In: Fahn S, et al., eds. Advances in Neurology. Vol 43. Myoclonus. New York: Raven Press, 1986:295–307.
24. Diagnostic Classification Steering Committee; Thorpy MJ, Chairman. International Classification of Sleep Disorders: Diagnostic and Coding Manual. Rochester, MN: American Sleep Disorders Association, 1990.
25. Earley CJ, Allen RP. Pergolide and carbidopa/levodopa treatment of the restless legs syndrome and periodic leg movements in sleep in a consecutive series of patients. Sleep 1996; 19:801–810.
26. Mellick GA, Mellick LB. Management of restless legs syndrome with GABApentin (Neurontin®). Sleep 1996; 3:224–226.
27. Hening WA, Walters A, Kavey N, Gidro-Frank S, Côté L, Fahn S. Dyskinesias while awake and periodic movements in sleep in restless legs syndrome: treatment with opioids. Neurology 1986; 36:1363–1366.
28. Bixler EO, Kales A, Vela-Bueno A, Jacoby JA, Scarone S, Soldatos CR. Nocturnal myoclonus and nocturnal myoclonic activity in a normal population. Res Commun Chem Pathol Pharmacol 1982; 36:129–140.
29. Coleman RM, Pollak CP, Weitzman ED. Periodic movements in sleep (nocturnal myoclonus): relation to sleep disorders. Ann Neurol 1980; 8:416–421.
30. Montagna P, Provini F, Plazzi G, Liguori R, Lugaresi E. Propriospinal myoclonus

upon relaxation and drowsiness: a cause of severe insomnia. Mov Disord 1997; 12: 66–72.

31. Montagna P. Nocturnal paroxysmal dystonia and nocturnal wanderings. Neurology 1992; 42(suppl 6):61–67.
32. Montagna P, Sforza E, Tinuper P, Cirignotta F, Lugaresi E. Paroxysmal arousals during sleep. Neurology 1990; 40:1063–1066.
33. Lugaresi E, Cirignotta F, Montagna P. Nocturnal paroxysmal dystonia. J Neurol Neurosurg Psychiatry 1986; 49:375–380.
34. Pedley TA, Guilleminault C. Episodic nocturnal wanderings responsive to anticonvulsant drug therapy. Ann Neurol 1977; 2:30–35.
35. Plazzi G, Tinuper P, Montagna P, Provini F, Lugaresi E. Epileptic nocturnal wanderings. Sleep 1995; 18:749–756.
36. Peled R, Lavie P. Paroxysmal awakenings from sleep associated with excessive daytime somnolence: a form of nocturnal epilepsy. Neurology 1986; 36:95–98.
37. Schenck CH, Bundlie SR, Ettinger MG, Mahowald MW. Chronic behavioral disorders of REM sleep: a new category of parasomnia. Sleep 1986; 9:293–308.
38. Lugaresi E, Medori R, Montagna P, Baruzzi A, Cortelli P, Lugaresi A, Tinuper P, Zucconi M, Gambetti P. Fatal familial insomnia and dysautonomia with selective degeneration of thalamic nuclei. N Engl J Med 1986; 315:997–1003.
39. Goldfarb LG, Petersen RB, Tabaton M, Brown P, LeBlanc AC, Montagna P, Cortelli P, Julien J, Vital C, Pendelbury WW, Haltia M, Wills PR, Hauw JJ; McKeever PE, Monari L, Schrank B, Swergold GD, Autilio-Gambetti L, Gajdusek DC, Lugaresi E, Gambetti P. Fatal familial insomnia and familial Creutzfeldt-Jakob disease: disease phenotype determined by a DNA polymorphism. Science 1992; 258:806–808.
40. Guilleminault C, Quera-Salva MA, Goldberg MP. Pseudo-hypersomnia and presleep behaviour with bilateral paramedian thalamic lesions. Brain 1993; 116:1549–1563.
41. Morvan A. De la chorée fibrillaire. Gaz Heb Méd Chirurg 1890; 27:173–200.
42. Fischer-Perroudon C, Trillet M, Mouret J, Tommasi M, Jouvet M, Schott B, Girard PF. Investigations polygraphiques et métaboliques d'une insomnie durable avec hallucinations. Rev Neurol (Paris) 1974; 130:111–125.
43. Tachibana M, Tanaka K, Hishikawa Y, Kaneko Z. A sleep study of acute psychotic states due to alcohol and meprobamate addiction. In: Weitzman ED, ed. Advances in Sleep Research. 2nd ed. New York: Spectrum, 1976:177–203.
44. Kotorii T, Nakazawa Y, Yokoyama T, Kurauchi H, Sakurada H, Ohkawa T, Nonaka K, Hasuzawa H, Dainoson K, Inanaga K. The sleep pattern of chronic alcoholics during the alcohol withdrawal period. Folia Psych Neurol Jap 1980; 34:89–95.
45. Mahowald MW, Schenck CH. REM sleep behavior disorder. In: Kryger MH, Dement W, Roth T, eds. Principles and Practice of Sleep Medicine. 2nd ed. Philadelphia: WB Saunders, 1994:574–588.
46. Lugaresi E, Tobler I, Gambetti P, Montagna P. The pathophysiology of fatal familial insomnia. Brain Pathol 1998; 8:521–526.

9

Motor Disorders of Sleep

Periodic, Aperiodic, and Rhythmic Motor Disorders and Parasomnias

Pasquale Montagna
University of Bologna
Bologna, Italy

INTRODUCTION

The motor disorders of sleep represent a frequent challenge in the practice of sleep medicine. They are not, however, a uniform nosological category, as exemplified by the current International Classification of Sleep Disorders (ICSD) (1), in which sleep-related motor disorders fall under different headings, from the intrinsic sleep disorders—which includes periodic limb movement disorder and the restless-legs syndrome—to the parasomnias. Others are as yet only proposed sleep disorders. This chapter gives an overview of the principal motor disorders of sleep, i.e., those in which abnormal motor patterns are the prominent sign. The ICSD (1) is followed here as far as possible. However, a preliminary survey of the physiological mechanisms underlying motor control and normal motor activity during sleep reveals that the boundaries between normal and pathological events are not always clear-cut and that the classification rarely provides even a glimpse at the actual pathogenic mechanisms of each disorder.

PHYSIOLOGY OF MOTOR CONTROL DURING SLEEP

Progressive loss of muscle tone develops at the transition from wakefulness to light sleep, reaching full atonia during REM sleep. Especially observed in the antigravitary muscles such as the mental and nuchal muscles routinely monitored during polysomnography (PSG), muscle atonia is attended by reduced motor unit firing because of postsynaptic inhibition and dysfacilitation of the spinal and brainstem alpha motoneurons. In the cat, the neuronal membrane hyperpolarizes, only slightly during quiet non-REM sleep, but to a much greater degree—2 to 10 mV—during active REM sleep (2), making the motoneuron less excitable. Spontaneous motoneuron activity ceases, recurrent motoneuron discharges are inhibited, and excitatory postsynaptic potentials (EPSPs) induced by Ia fiber stimulation are all reduced during REM sleep, further so during the bursts of REMs, by a mechanism of postsynaptic inhibition. Spontaneous inhibitory postsynaptic potentials (IPSPs) also increase in number during REM sleep, and large-amplitude IPSPs appear during this sleep stage (2). While the neurotransmitter(s) implicated in the origin of the sleep-related inhibition of the EPSPs is still unknown, glycine appears to mediate the IPSPs that develop during sleep.

Atonia, however, is not complete during REM sleep. On the background of a potent inhibition, motoneuron spike potentials—isolated or in short bursts—can still be recorded, usually accompanied by brief motor activity in the shape of myoclonic twitches and jerky movements, especially of the facial or distal limb muscles. These sudden excitatory drives characterize the so-called phasic REM-sleep stage, as opposed to the tonic REM sleep from which it arises. The concomitant depolarization of the motoneuron membrane during such volleys is thus due not to relenting inhibition but to strong excitatory activity descending from supraspinal centers—currently, however, unknown.

The inhibitory influences impinging on the alpha motoneurons during sleep can instead be reproduced in the experimental animal by electric stimulation of the inhibitory reticular formation. Motor inhibition can be obtained in particular by activation of the gigantocellularis reticular nucleus, and it is thought that this nucleus is in turn activated, during REM sleep, by neurons of the nucleus pontis oralis (3). Lesions of the latter, in fact, cause a loss of the physiological muscle atonia typical of REM sleep (4), and provoke peculiar behavior abnormalities whereupon animals display complex motor activities such as fighting, searching for food, and ambulatory patterns, in the absence of any contact with the environment. The complex neurophysiological mechanisms underlying this so-called "REM sleep without atonia" have been further dissected by Sanford and coworkers (5) and need not be detailed here. Suffice it to say that sleep-related motor inhibition is equally seen in humans, associated with loss of tendon jerks and inhibition of the electrically evoked monosynaptic H-reflex of the soleus muscle

(6). The H-reflex, an indirect measure of the excitability of the motoneuronal pool, is progressively lost, in association with muscle tone, beginning from the 10 minutes of non-REM sleep preceding the REM-sleep stage until it totally disappears during REM sleep. Thus, muscle atonia during non-REM sleep in humans seems to parallel the findings in the experimental animal. Likewise, atonia during REM sleep and REM sleep without atonia have been recognized in humans following their description in the cat.

PHYSIOLOGICAL MOTOR ACTIVITY DURING SLEEP

In normal humans, sleep is not a period of absolute motor quiescence, and some degree of motor activity must be expected during sleep. In its most elementary form it is represented by the so-called *partial hypnic myoclonias* (PHMs), described for the first time by De Lisi in 1932 in humans and animals (7). PHMs are short, jerky contractions of parts of a muscle, or of an entire small muscle, resembling fasciculations and occurring mostly in the distal muscles of the hands and the face. They may or may not cause small displacements of the fingers, lips, or eyelids, and occur isolated or in short bursts. PHMs usually last less than 1 second, are especially frequent during non-REM sleep stage 1 and REM sleep, when they reach a peak, and tend to decrease during deep sleep (8). They closely resemble the brief jerky motor activity observed in the cat during the phasic REM-sleep periods, and are therefore thought to derive from strong excitatory volleys descending from the reticular formation, except that they are not associated with REMs. PHMs could otherwise be relayed through the corticospinal tracts, since they disappear on the side of a pyramidal lesion (9).

Sleep starts (also known as ''hypnic jerks'') represent another normal accompaniment of sleep. Although they are classified among the sleep–wake transition disorders, a kind of parasomnia according to the ICSD (1), they frequently occur in normal people, and at any age. In some cases they are a cause for concern and occasionally enter the differential diagnosis of epileptic myoclonic seizures. When particularly frequent and severe, however, they have been reported as a cause for sleep-onset insomnia (see ''Excessive Sleep Starts'' later). Oswald (10) described them as sudden contractions of one or more limbs or the entire body, usually involving the axial muscles, lasting for up to 1 second and especially evident when falling asleep and during light sleep. They are associated with EEG signs of arousal such as the K-complexes, autonomic activation (tachycardia, tachypnea, and sudomotor activity), and a peculiar sensory feeling of ''shock'' or ''falling into the void.'' Although their origin is still unknown, sleep starts are hypothetically due to descending volleys within the pyramidal tracts at the transititon from wakefulness to sleep (11).

Benign neonatal sleep myoclonus (BNSM) is another condition in which physiological myoclonic activity during sleep may mimic an epileptic seizure. Described by Coulter and Allen (12), BNSM presents in the first weeks or months of life with repetitive myoclonic jerks, involving one part, one or more limbs or the whole body or migrating between muscle groups, often repeated in clusters and recurring for several minutes. BNSM is especially evident during non-REM sleep and least evident during REM sleep, is absent in wakefulness, and remains unassociated with any other neurological or developmental abnormality. EEG is normal. BNSM rarely persists into childhood, and its mechanisms, whether due to a transient immaturity of the serotonergic system or to changes in activity of the reticular centers at the transition to or during sleep as hypothesized, remain unknown.

Finally, the so-called *gross body movements*, another normal motor activity of sleep, consists of global movements and shifts that modify the body position. They occur at least three or four times an hour, in particular during the second part of the night, prior to awakening. They are more frequent at the beginning and end of REM episodes, but may also be seen during light and REM sleep, preceded by EEG signs of arousal. Particularly evident during infancy, their decrease with adulthood has been taken to reflect maturational events of the brain and of the sleep–wake cycle.

Mimic acts and such gestures as smiling, sighing, scratching, or grinding the teeth are also commonly seen during every sleep stage but especially during light sleep.

Periodic Limb Movements During Sleep (PLMS) and Nocturnal Myoclonus

Nocturnal myoclonus (NM) was the term that Symonds first applied to sudden jerks arising during light sleep or when falling asleep (13). In the absence of neurophysiological studies, he thought the jerks were epileptic in nature. Retrospectively, it is apparent that he lumped together benign conditions such as the sleep starts, and also the periodic motor activity of periodic limb movements during sleep (PLMS). Later polysomnographic studies documented the motor activity and the EEG correlates of these jerks, and the term nocturnal myoclonus was applied to peculiar repetitive dorsiflexion movements of the toes, ankles, and knees, occurring either as an isolated phenomenon or in the setting of the restless-legs syndrome (RLS). Later still came the recognition that such movements were not truly myoclonic in aspect, and therefore the introduction of the term periodic limb movements of sleep, and the periodic limb movement disorder encompassed within the intrinsic sleep disorders, a subheading of the dyssomnias according to the ICSD (1).

In their simplest form, PLMS consist of repetitive dorsiflexion movements of the toes and ankle, often spreading to the knee and hip (Figure 1), and some-

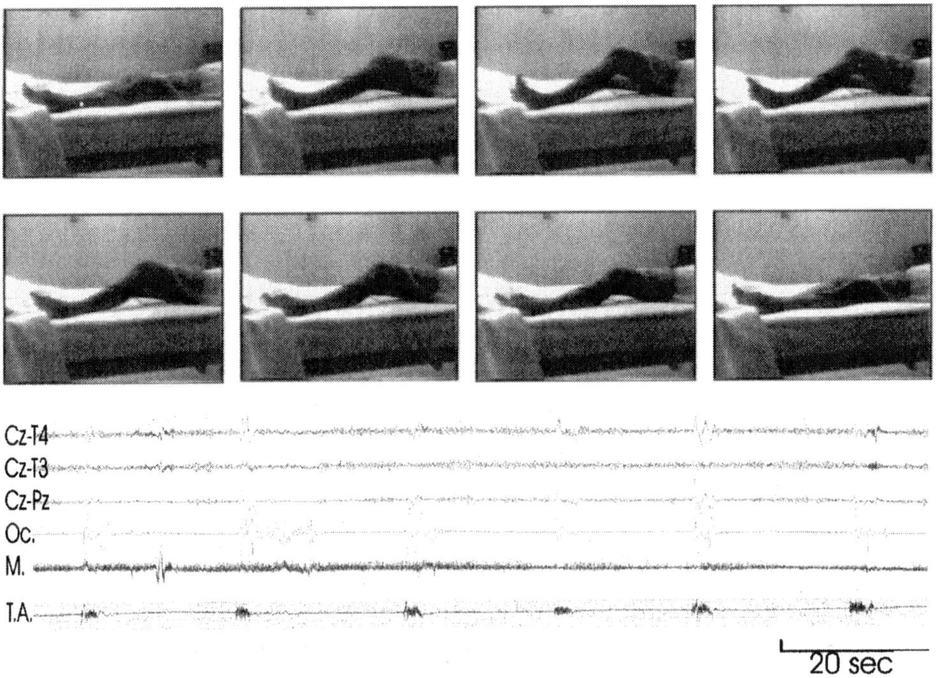

Figure 1 Videorecordings (selected frames) of a single jerk in a patient with PLMS and RLS. The initial movement is a dorsal flexion at the left ankle and knee. In the lower panel, polygraphic EEG (C_z–T_4, C_z–T_3, C_z–P_z), oculographic (Oc), and EMG (M: mylohyoideus; T.A.: tibialis anterior muscles) findings in the same patients show the EMG bursts in the TA lasting 2–3 s and repeated at intervals of 20–25 s.

times even involving the wrist and elbow. The movements occur during light-sleep stages 1 and 2, progressively diminish during deep-sleep stages 3 and 4, and nearly always disappear during REM sleep. In extreme cases, however, PLMS may persist into REM sleep or occur during drowsiness, when the patient is not yet fully asleep. In such cases, the patient finds PLMS annoying and an impediment to falling asleep.

On polygraphic recordings, the EMG activity during the jerks may take different forms: a tonic activity lasting several hundreds of milliseconds, which may or may not be followed by myoclonic activity, or an initial myoclonic jerk followed by tonic activity or several myoclonic jerks in clusters (polymyoclonus), which may or may not be followed by tonic activity (14). The duration of the EMG activity measured on the tibialis anterior muscle ranges between 0.5 and 5 seconds, with a peak at 2 seconds (15), and the jerks may or may not arise synchronously between the two legs. Sometimes they may be seen to occur only in one leg or on one side of the body, or to alternate between the two sides. The periodic jerks may be interspersed with a more continuous EMG activity, in the shape of an irregular tonic discharge of motor units. At least four repeated jerks are required for a diagnosis of PLMS, but usually PLMS recur hundreds of times for long stretches of the night, since their most characteristic feature is the quasi-periodic repetition at intervals of 20–40 seconds as a mean (range 4–90 seconds) (15) throughout light sleep. The PLMS may have no EEG correlate, but usually they are loosely associated with K-complexes on the EEG and other manifestations of arousal (tachycardia, tachypnea, an increase in systemic blood pressure). They have therefore been viewed as merely the motor counterpart of the periodic arousals that typify light sleep, since these sleep stages are characterized by intrinsic periodic fluctuations in excitability of the nervous system that affect the motor, autonomic, and vigilance systems at the same time (14). The EEG physiological fluctuations in excitability recurring every 20–40 seconds during light sleep were termed the cyclic alternating pattern by Terzano et al. (16). Epidemiological studies support the notion that PLMS, when isolated, should be considered a quasi-physiological phenomenon. In the normal population, in fact, PLMS are nearly absent in those under the age of 30 years, but progressively increase—especially after age 50, when about 29% of people are found to experience PLMS (17,18). Moreover, PLMS may be recorded in the absence of any sleep disturbance, and their prevalence is comparable between good and poor sleepers (19). It thus remains doubtful whether PLMS should be considered an intrinsic sleep disorder or merely a phenomenon of aging. When an accidental polysomnographic finding is unassociated with EEG signs of arousal, PLMS are probably best regarded as paraphysiological.

PLMS have been associated in anecdotal reports with several other pathological conditions, from ALS to the stiff-person and Isaacs' syndrome, peripheral neuropathies and myelopathies, narcolepsy, and sleep apnea, but in the absence of controlled studies and given their high prevalence in the adult and elderly normal population, it is difficult to judge whether any such association is significant.

The mechanisms underlying the PLMS are also unclear. They are known to occur in patients distally to a complete spinal cord transection, and are observed during the induction of spinal anesthesia. Back-averaging techniques exclude a cortical origin because of the absence of any premovement *bereitschaftpotential* (14,20), and detailed EMG analysis of the jerks (21) has shown that the motor activity originates first in such muscles as the quadriceps femoris, spreading thereafter to other leg and axial muscles, according to a pattern of propagation typical of the propriospinal pathways. All these observations imply that the PLMS are actually generated within the spinal cord, probably at a lumbosacral level (21). On the other hand, PLMS closely resemble a Babinski sign and, when more evident, a triple flexion reflex, and studies of mono- and polysynaptic reflexes demonstrate increased spinal segmental excitability (22), suggesting a role for supraspinal, possibly pyramidal, influences. PLMS may be induced in affected individuals and their characteristic periodicity entrained by exteroceptive stimulations, such as by electrical stimuli applied to the peroneal nerve at the fibular head (14). These features and the peculiar rhythmicity of the jerks, inscribed within the spectrum of more general fluctuations in excitability during sleep, have been taken to indicate that PLMS are modulated in their periodicity by descending supraspinal, probably reticular, influences. This hypothesis received some support from functional MRI studies implicating the red nucleus and other brainstem regions in the generation of the PLMS (23). The hypothesized role of an overactive sympathetic nervous system also fits well with an integrated view of the brainstem as the generator of PLMS.

Several medications have been reported to influence the PLMS, and have been advocated to curtail the phenomenon. However, since it is doubtful whether PLMS, when isolated, are of any clinical significance, it may be wise to reserve medications for patients with PLMS who also suffer from the RLS.

The Restless-Legs Syndrome

RLS is another disorder of sleep classified among the dyssomnias as an intrinsic sleep disorder (1). Described for the first time by Willis in 1672 and called *anxietas tibiarum* (''anxiety of the legs'') by Wittmaack in 1861, it was extensively studied by Ekbom (24). RLS is characterized by paresthesia in the legs, especially between the knee and the ankle but sometimes spreading to the thighs and the forearms, and described as a deep aching, gnawing, burning, or crawling sensation. It typically occurs at rest, especially when trying to fall asleep, dozing, or reclining in an armchair, and is relieved by such motor activity as rubbing, stretching, kicking, or, more generally, by walking. The diagnostic criteria for RLS set by the International RLS Study Group (25) include a desire to move the extremities, motor restlessness, worsening with rest and relief by motor activity, and worsening in the evening and at night. The importance of RLS as a motor disturbance of sleep lies in its nearly obligate association with the PLMS: at least 80% of patients with RLS are found to display PLMS upon PSG. Moreover, RLS patients, while awake, also display additional characteristic fidgeting movements of the legs, sometimes with dyskinetic features that have been termed ''resting dyskinesia while awake'' and that may represent, at least in part, voluntary attempts at motor relief.

RLS is quite common (2–5% of the population) and may occur as either a primary disease or secondary to other pathological conditions. Primary RLS is an independent nosological entity, hereditary in 50–92% of cases and transmitted as an autosomal dominant trait (26,27). Symptoms arise in the second decade of life, and persist with an oscillating course for a lifetime (28). Except for the

PLMS, primary RLS is not associated with neurological disturbances. PLMS have been reported as an isolated sign in siblings of families with RLS (26). The origin of the RLS is unknown—linkage studies in RLS families have been so far inconclusive, and widely different pathogenic theories rely mainly on pharmacological and neurophysiological data. Thus, defects in the endogenous opioid system (27) and abnormalities in iron metabolism with ferritin deficiency (29) have been hypothesized. Brain SPECT studies with IBZM have been reported as showing defects in striatal dopamine D_2 receptors (30), while Iannaccone et al. (31) found neurophysiological and sural nerve biopsy evidence for loss of peripheral sensory nerve fibers, indicating that RLS is a peripheral neuropathy.

RLS may also occur secondary to other pathological conditions, especially peripheral neuropathies. It is particularly frequent and troubling in the setting of uremia, and occurs in vitamin B_{12} deficiency and before or at the onset of familial amyloid neuropathy (32). RLS has also been reported to occur more frequently in Parkinson's disease, Huntington's chorea, and Tourette's syndrome, and is exacerbated or sets in more frequently during pregnancy.

For many years treatment of RLS has been based on anecdotal reports. Among the benzodiazepines, clonazepam at single doses of 0.5–2 mg at bedtime is effective without major side effects except for occasional drowsiness the morning after. Its long-term (more than 6 months) efficacy has been confirmed. Alternatively, levodopa plus decarboxylase inhibitors, 100–500 mg at bedtime, may be used with success. With levodopa, however, there is the problem that symptoms may rebound during the night or the morning after, and if doses are escalated to control the symptoms, RLS may worsen and spread to the daytime. Increasing levodopa dosages should therefore be discouraged to avoid this "augmentation effect." Other therapies effective in RLS include bromocriptine, carbamazepine, baclofen, clonidine, and opioids (methadone, oxycodone, codeine, and propoxyphene) (33); the latter should be reserved for treatment of severe cases only.

PARASOMNIAS

According to the ICSD (1), parasomnias are "clinical disorders with undesirable physical phenomena that occur predominantly during sleep." Parasomnias comprise several subcategories: arousal disorders, sleep–wake transition disorders, parasomnias associated with REM sleep, and others. Motor features that constitute a true motor disorder during sleep are prominent in only some parasomnias, especially the arousal disorders, the sleep–wake transition disorders, and some other parasomnias. Nightmares, a parasomnia occurring during REM sleep, are not associated with relevant motor phenomena and, as such, shall not be dealt with here. Other sleep-related motor disorders categorized among the parasomnias, such as sleep starts and the benign neonatal sleep myoclonus, have already been described in the section "Physiological Motor Activity During Sleep."

Arousal Disorders

Arousal disorders are attributed to disordered-arousal mechanisms, and occur typically during non-REM sleep. Foremost among them are the so-called ''sleep terrors'' (pavor nocturnus) and ''sleepwalking'' (somnambulism). In contrast, the ''confusional arousals''—in which automatic behaviors associated to mental confusion, impaired contact with the environment, and amnesia occur after awakening by definition—have no prominent motor features, in particular, no motor agitation or ambulation.

Pavor Nocturnus

Pavor nocturnus, also colloquially called ''sleep terror'' (and ''incubus'' when it occurs in an adult) is a paroxysmal event occurring during deep-sleep stages 3 and 4 in children, and characterized by sudden arousal and disordered motor agitation, screaming, and features of intense panic and autonomic activation, such as tachycardia, tachypnea, diaphoresis, and flushing. Patients do not usually leave the bed, although in severe cases they have jumped from windows, injuring themselves, and remained unresponsive or only dimly responsive to the environment throughout the episode. Attacks usually last between 1 and 20 minutes, occur mainly in the first half of the night, and almost never recur the same night. Patients may not even recall them the morning after, or may report a feeling of suffocation, as a weight on the chest (hence *incubus*, ''which sits upon''), or a number of frightening but imprecise panic sensations. Polygraphic recordings during the episodes, although usually masked by gross motor artefacts, do not show epileptic activity but rather high-voltage synchronized delta activity prior to the episode (34). Episodes of pavor nocturnus may be induced in predisposed individuals by external stimuli, and psychological stress and sleep deprivation are favoring factors.

Pavor nocturnus is quite prevalent: 1–6% of children are affected, with a peak between 5 and 7 years of age (35). Episodes spontaneously wane in frequency after puberty, but 1% of adults are reported as still suffering from sleep terrors. Pavor nocturnus shows a strong familial clustering, and indeed in some families it has been considered to recur as an autosomal dominant trait (36). Patients with pavor also share some predisposition to other parasomnias, such as somnambulism.

Disordered-arousal mechanisms are hypothesized to account for the origin of pavor (37): patients would undergo a partial awakening during deep sleep, with marked behavioral, emotional, and autonomic activation but without full consciousness during the episode. Developmental factors may explain the disappearance of pavor by late adolescence.

Pavor nocturnus should be considered a benign condition, usually outgrown in adulthood, but in severe cases, especially those with disordered ambulation and potential self-injuries, benzodiazepines or imipramine at bedtime may be employed.

The differential diagnosis of pavor nocturnus is sometimes difficult, especially with the sleep-related epileptic seizures. The recognition that attacks of nocturnal frontal-lobe epilepsy (NFLE), such as the paroxysmal arousals and nocturnal paroxysmal dystonia, commonly occur without scalp EEG epileptic activity and that they show a predilection for non-REM sleep should prompt in-depth studies of any paroxysmal motor event during non-REM sleep associated with bizarre motor patterns and ambulation. A high rate of same-night recurrence, the presence of dystonic motor features during the attacks, their stereotypical repetition, their response to antiepileptic medication, and persistence into adulthood are all features favoring the diagnosis of NFLE rather than parasomnia (see below).

Somnambulism (Sleepwalking)

Somnambulism is a disorder of arousal that may show overlapping features with pavor nocturnus. It is characterized by ambulation, which may occur in a quiet, ordered way with the patient calmly wandering around displaying normal-appearing motor patterns and gestures (Figure 2), or instead be associated, especially in grown children, with frantic running around, jumping, kicking, and sometimes injurious behavior, particularly when patients are physically restrained. Ambulation may follow a confusional arousal, in which case somnambulism overlaps with pavor nocturnus. Patients are poorly in contact, if at all, and amnesia is associated with the episodes. Recall of the episodes is therefore imperfect, especially in younger children.

Somnambulism is seen during non-REM deep sleep in children aged 5 to 16, with a peak at 10 years of age: 15% of all children 5–12 years of age have at least one episode of somnambulism (35). Just like pavor nocturnus, somnambulism has a strong familial influence. Its pathogenic mechanisms and pharmacological management overlap with those of pavor nocturnus. Differential diagnosis of somnambulism likewise includes the sleep-related epileptic seizures arising during non-REM sleep and characterized by ambulation. Epileptic nocturnal wanderings (38,39) may be especially difficult to distinguish from agitated somnambulism, and the difficulty is sometimes compounded by the presence of forensic issues due to injurious, even homicidal, behavior during the episode.

Wake–Sleep Transition Disorders

Jactatio Capitis Nocturna

A rhythmic motor disorder at the transition from wakefulness to sleep (rhythmic movement disorder according to the ICSD) (1), jactatio capitis nocturna (JCN), also called "head-banging" or "head-rolling," consists of repetitive movements of the head and neck that occur at sleep onset or during short arousals in light sleep. The head is thus rolled side to side, or may be forcibly banged into the pillow and mattress. The whole body or parts of it, such as hands, arms, or legs,

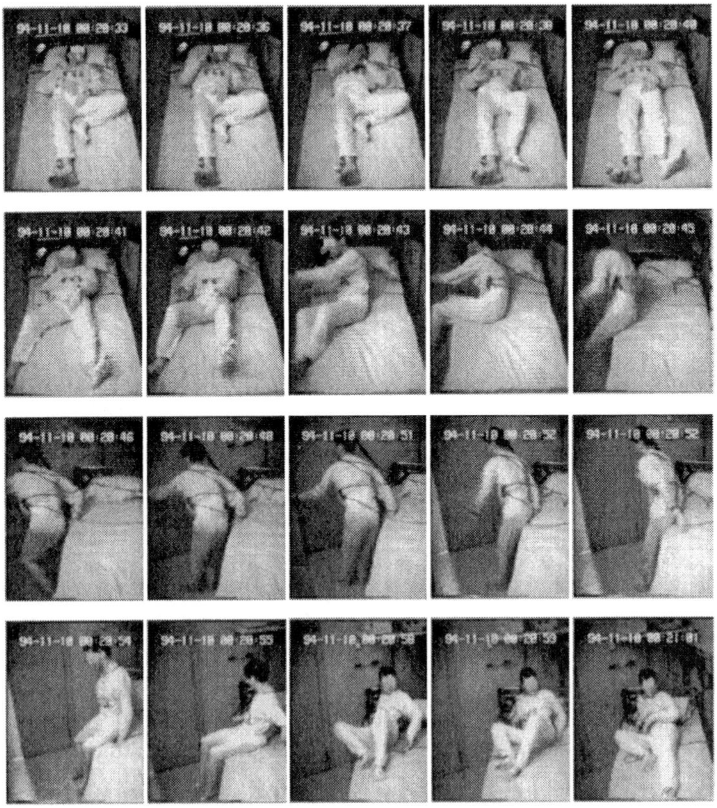

Figure 2 Sleepwalking episode in a 21-year-old boy. The boy arises from the bed and quietly walks to the door of the laboratory, tries the handle, and then returns to bed. Total duration of the episode: 40 seconds.

may also be rolled and rocked repetitively (''body-rocking''). These stereotypical movements may last a few or several minutes, repeated at a frequency of 0.5 to 2 per second. JCN is seen in otherwise normal children, but it has also been reported in mentally retarded and autistic patients. It usually disappears after the age of 3–4 years, and does not require any medication, although benzodiazepines may be useful in selected severe cases.

Excessive Sleep Starts

''Sleep starts,'' or ''hypnic jerks,'' although listed as a wake–sleep transition disorder (1), represent a physiological and universal accompaniment of sleep, especially light sleep (see above). In some patients, however, they may be so severe and frequent as to represent a cause of sleep-onset insomnia. This condition has been termed ''excessive sleep starts'' by Broughton et al. (11), and may respond to clonazepam. Its relationship to the polysomnographic readings observed at the transition from wakefulness to sleep (see above) needs clarification.

Somniloquy (Sleep Talking)

Another wake–sleep transition disorder according to the ICSD (1)—somniloquy, or sleep talking—is characterized by the utterance of single words or even complex and intelligible speech during sleep. Somniloquy is especially observed during light non-REM or REM sleep, and may be induced by conversation with the affected sleeping individual. It is found most often in children 3 to 10 years of age, but also in adults, in times of psychological stress or sleep deprivation. Somniloquy is a benign condition and does not require treatment. It shares some familial predisposition with other parasomnias, such as somnambulism.

Nocturnal Leg Cramps

Nocturnal leg cramps consist of painful, involuntary contractions of the leg, especially the triceps surae, or foot muscles, that arise suddenly during sleep or in the transition from wakefulness to sleep. Lasting several seconds, they are associated with palpable contraction of the muscles involved and subside either spontaneously or after lengthening of the contracting muscles. They may be a cause of insomnia. Nocturnal muscle cramps are especially frequent during non-REM sleep, and may recur aperiodically for long stretches of time. In some patients, cramps may also be present during wakefulness.

Whereas the usual cramping conditions during the day are often related to electrolyte disturbances or to muscle and endocrine disorders such as myotonic syndromes, muscle glycogenosis, or hypothyroidism, the exact mechanism underlying the nocturnal leg cramps is still unclear. Pregnancy, Parkinson's disease, and diabetes mellitus are known factors associated with them. Jacobsen et al. (40) described a familiar condition of nocturnal leg cramps, associated with myoclonic jerks and also involving trunk, limb, and face muscles, transmitted as an autosomal dominant trait. The pathogenesis remained unclear, but in their cases the cramps responded favorably to clonazepam. Carbamazepine, quinine, vitamin E, and verapamil are other medications described in anecdotal reports as being useful.

REM-Sleep Behavior Disorders

REM-sleep behavior disorders (RSBDs) are parasomnias occurring during REM sleep (41). They therefore most often arise in the second half of the night, when REM sleep is more abundant, and are characterized by loss of the physiological muscular atonia that typifies this sleep stage (REM sleep without atonia), and by sudden paroxysmal motor activities, sometimes in the form of simple or massive, irregular muscle jerks only, or instead of more complex and seemingly purposeful motor activities, including yelling, speaking, raising the head and trunk from the bed, swinging the arms, and punching or even getting out of bed (veritable REM-sleep behaviors). All the while, patients are not in contact with the environment and, if awakened, usually report that they are dreaming, and the motor behavior may then be seen to correspond to the dream content (dream enactment). The motor behavior is often quite violent, and may be injurious to the patient or the bed partner, sometimes with serious forensic consequences. Patients return to sleep after the episodes, which last only a few minutes, and are usually oblivious of them—the morning after, the only complaint is often only of insomnia. Eighty to 90% of RSBDs are seen in males.

RSBDs usually begin in the adult and elderly age range, and may recur from once every few months to several times each night. The reasons for the strikingly lower prevalence among women, who also display distinctly less violent behaviors during the episodes, remain unknown. On PSG, RSBDs are seen to correspond to an abnormal REM sleep characterized by the persistence of muscle tone in antigravitary muscles, and by the development of phasic motor activities in the limbs (42). Autonomic activation is typically absent during the episodes. RSBDs are often not easy to diagnose on purely clinical grounds; therefore, PSG, by documenting the onset of the episodes during REM sleep, is required for differentiation from the other non-REM parasomnias. RSBDs are known to occur without other associated clinical abnormalities (so-called idiopathic RSBDs). In about 60% of the cases, however, they may be associated with, or even be the harbinger of, neurodegenerative diseases such as Parkinson's disease, multiple-system atrophy (MSA), and Shy-Drager syndrome, Lewy body disease, olivopontocerebellar atrophy (43), or cerebrovascular—especially pontine—lesions (44). In particular, RSBDs are found in 90% of MSA patients, and they precede the onset of the parkinsonian and autonomic signs characteristic of this disease by more than 1 year in 44% of the cases (45). RSBDs instead remain absent in pure autonomic failure (46), a disease unassociated with CNS involvement. Therefore, the importance of the RSBD as an early sign of these neurodegenerative diseases has been emphasized, and patients with "idiopathic" RSBD need be followed up for an adequate length of time in order to exclude their being really symptomatic cases.

RSBDs, lasting a few nights only, may also present acutely upon administration of drugs (such as tricyclic, MAOI, and SSRI antidepressants) or sudden withdrawal of alcohol, barbiturates, or benzodiazepines (47). Such cases of acute RSBD are self-limiting, and resemble the confusional oneiric states of delirium tremens.

Clonazepam, 0.5 to 2 mg given nightly, is the most effective medication in both idiopathic and symptomatic RSBD cases (48). Alprazolam may also have comparable efficacy (49). From a pathophysiological point of view, it is interesting that REM sleep without atonia was first produced in the experimental animal by Jouvet and Delorme (4), by lesioning the pontine tegmentum. As we have already seen, the abolition of the peri–locus coeruleus neural structures responsible for the tonic suppression of muscle tone is thought to permit the emergence of the complex motor patterns during REM sleep (oneiric behavior). Accordingly, lesioned cats display complex behaviors such as fighting, sniffing, and walking during REM sleep, reminiscent of RSBD in humans. Lesions in different parts of the pons produce different patterns of motor behavior (5). Abnormalities in the pontine reticular substance in neurodegenerative diseases may likewise be thought to originate the RSBD in humans. However, the mechanisms underlying the so-called idiopathic RSBD remain unclear. It is worth mentioning here that the dissociation between the motor and the other—mental and EEG—aspects of REM sleep characteristic of the RSBD is just an example of the so-called status dissociatus, a concept recently developed by Mahowald and Schenck (50) that can be usefully employed in the explanation of the pathophysiology of the parasomnias.

Sleep Bruxism

Sleep bruxism, or teeth-grinding, is a kind of parasomnia that consists of grinding and clenching movements of the jaws during sleep, which produce a loud, annoying noise and, when long-lasting, is a remarkable cause of tooth wear. Sleep bruxism should be differentiated from bruxism during wakefulness, which is silent and characterized by clenching only, and not grinding movements.

Sleep bruxism occurs most commonly in children aged 3–12 years, but also in adults, without any sex prevalence (51). Patients are unaware of the jaw movements, and may come to medical observation only because of unexplained dental problems. Polysomnographic recordings demonstrate that bruxism occurs during non-REM—especially stage 2—sleep, in particular during arousals, and is due to forceful short rhythmic or prolonged tonic contractions of the masticatory muscles (51).

Sleep bruxism has been variously ascribed to craniomandibular—such as malocclusion—disorders, hyperthyroidism, psychological factors, or even encephalopathies with basal ganglia disorders or cerebral palsy. It may be exacerbated by the use of drugs such as levodopa, alcohol, amphetamines, and serotonin-reuptake inhibitors. In most cases, however, sleep bruxism remains an isolated condition. Treatment is warranted in patients in whom bruxism causes severe damage to the teeth and even to the mouth and tongue. Bite splints, benzodiazepines, and biofeedback therapy may be of help.

Nocturnal Paroxysmal Dystonia

Nocturnal paroxysmal dystonia (NPD) was reported for the first time by Lugaresi and Cirignotta in 1981 (52), who used the term hypnogenic paroxysmal dystonia.

They described cases of recurrent attacks during non-REM sleep characterized by sudden arousal; motor agitation associated with extrapyramidal features such as tremor, chorea, and dystonic posturing; and ballism of the limbs, in the absence of clear-cut epileptic figures on the ictal EEG. Their patients responded to antiepileptic medications such as carbamazepine, but the normal EEG precluded their being considered definite cases of epilepsy arising during sleep (morpheic epilepsy) or instances of sleep-related motor disorders. Since patients with NPD often complain of disturbed sleep, NPD was included within the sleep disorders as a category of parasomnia (1). NPD attacks of different duration were reported, and short- and long-lasting ones (> 2–3 minutes) were later recognized as having different features.

Later studies, however, documented that patients with otherwise typical short-lasting NPD had epileptic EEG activity detected over the frontal regions by means of sphenoidal electrodes (53), and NPD was thus included within the spectrum of nocturnal frontal-lobe epilepsy (NFLE). These observations were corroborated by Meierkord et al. (54), who demonstrated that NPD attacks with and without ictal epileptic discharges were indistinguishable, and by concomitant studies of frontal-lobe epileptic seizures showing that, when arising from the mesial and orbital frontal regions, epileptic seizures are characterized by complex and bizarre motor patterns involving axial muscles and bipedal or bimanual activity with rocking movements and sometimes ambulation, very similar to those observed during short-lasting NPD attacks.The origin of the discharges from deep-seated foci explains why EEG often remains normal even during the attacks.

NPD attacks have been further characterized according to their duration and the motor patterns observed during the videopolysomnographic recordings. Thus, paroxysmal arousals (PAs) represent attacks, often recurring several—up to 20—times during the night, several nights in a row, of stereotypical motor activity, such as abruptly raising the head from the pillow, staring, moving the arms in a dystonic posture and crying aloud as if in distress. These episodes, which last about 20 seconds or less, are associated with autonomic activation (Figure 3) (55). PAs are sometimes accompanied by frank epileptic activity and respond to carbamazepine, sometimes at very low dosages. PAs may recur quasi-periodically during non-REM—especially light—sleep stages, showing a periodicity (every 20 to 40 seconds) reminiscent of that found in the PLMS. That PA and NPD belong to the same spectrum of sleep-related frontal-lobe seizures is shown by the facts that in many patients they recur during the same night and that PA can be seen on videorecordings to initiate a typical NPD attack. Still more elaborate and complex motor patterns may be seen in the so-called episodic nocturnal wanderings (ENWs) first described by Pedley and Guilleminault (38). Patients with ENW display peculiar attacks of violent motor activity, with screaming, yelling, flailing of limbs, associated with frantic ambulation such as running about, jumping, and kicking. They may injure themselves or their bed partner, especially when restrained, but they are not in full contact with the envi-

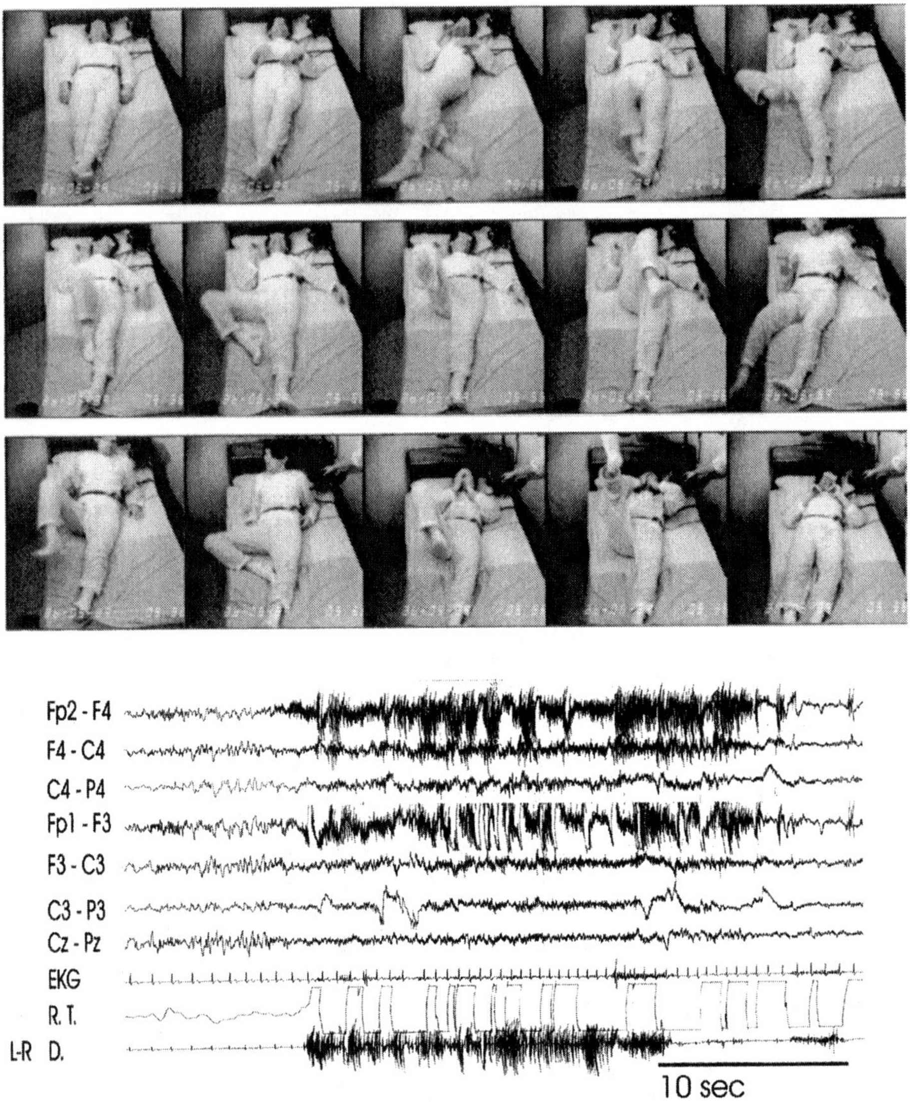

Figure 3 Attack of paroxysmal arousal in a 19-year-old man. The attack starts with sudden flexion of the right arm and leg; the left limbs are later stiffened and the right leg kicked about. The lower panels show excerpts from the polygraphic recordings of the same episode. The EMG movement artefacts are preceded by EEG signs of arousal from stage 2 sleep with tachycardia (R.T.: thoracic respiration; L-R D: left–right deltoid).

ronment. The attacks, always arising from non-REM sleep, sometimes respond to antiepileptic medications, which led Pedley and Guilleminault to suppose their epileptic nature. This view, refuted by others, was confirmed in three cases in which epileptic activity over the frontal regions was recorded during the ambulatory episode (39). ENWs are therefore thought to represent another example of sleep-related seizures, encompassed within the spectrum of NFLE.

PA, NPD, and ENW pose particular problems in their differential diagnosis, as they may be easily mistaken for non-REM parasomnias such as sleep terrors or somnambulism. The diagnostic problem is worsened by the fact that even ictal EEGs are often unrevealing and by the presence of a familial predisposition for both parasomnias and NFLE. The latter may, in fact, be inherited in an autosomal dominant fashion (56). Useful diagnostic markers for NFLE are: 1) the lifetime persistence of the attacks—usually well into adulthood—while parasomnias disappear after adolescence, 2) the high rate—up to 20–30—of same-night repetition of the episodes, clearly unusual for a parasomnia, and 3) their stereotypical features, that is, their recurrence with the same motor pattern over several nights. Moreover, parasomnias do not display dystonic or choreic motor patterns, and do not respond consistently to antiepileptic drugs. A high degree of suspicion, repeated polysomnographies, and the use of tentative trials with antiepileptic medications are warranted in cases that cannot be easily classified. Even after thorough neurophysiological studies, there remain cases with motor agitation during non-REM sleep that cannot in any way be ascribed to epileptic discharges. The symptoms of patients with NPD of long duration, with episodes lasting up to half an hour or more, and of children having puppet-like dystonic-dyskinetic attacks of long duration both during both non-REM sleep and after prolonged exercise in wakefulness (57) are thought to represent true movement disorders occurring during sleep, and should be differentiated from those of the more common short-lasting NPD epileptic attacks.

OTHER MOTOR DISORDERS OF SLEEP

Excessive Fragmentary Myoclonus During Non-REM Sleep

Excessive fragmentary myoclonus during non-REM sleep (EFMNS) was identified by Broughton et al. (11) as a pathological motor activity of small myoclonic twitches and fasciculation potentials, isolated or organized into repetitive discharges lasting less than 150 ms, throughout all non-REM sleep stages and usually apparent in the muscles of the legs.

The authors found that such activity was particularly prominent in patients with sleep apnea or excessive daytime sleepiness, and attributed its origin to hypoxia during sleep. The exact nosological status of this syndrome, however, is still under scrutiny, and EFMNS is listed in the ICSD (1) as a proposed sleep disorder.

Propriospinal Myoclonus at the Transition from Wakefulness to Sleep

Propriospinal myoclonus (PSM) was characterized by Brown and coworkers (58) as a form of myoclonus arising within the spinal cord (spinal myoclonus), usually in axial thoracolumbar segments and then propagated at low speed to other spinally innervated muscles presumably along propriospinal multisynaptic pathways intrinsic to the cord. Therefore, PSM—in contrast to the spinal myoclonus, which persists in the same segmentally innervated muscles—is a multisegmental propagated phenomenon, in which the myoclonic jerks travel in a progressive manner to more rostral and caudal segments in a descending and ascending pattern. The myoclonic jerks are usually irregular, last from 150 to 300 ms, and only in occasional patients may be evoked by external stimuli. Their propagation velocity along the spinal cord is low, calculated to around 3–11 m/s. PSM must surely originate in subcortical areas, as shown by the fact that the jerks lack any cortical premovement potential (*bereitschaftspotential*) upon back-averaging studies, and probably in the spinal cord as indicated by the few patients in whom a spinal lesion is found. It shows an effect of posture, being sometimes worsened by sitting or lying down.

Some cases of otherwise typical PSM, however, show a striking relationship of the myoclonic jerks with the state of vigilance of the patient. In these cases, PSM occurs only during the relaxed wakefulness state, when patients are trying to fall asleep lying down on a couch or in bed, and when the EEG alpha activity has spread to involve the anterior brain regions (59). In such a situation, the jerks can recur quasi-rhythmically every 10–20 seconds and are of such intensity as to propel the patient out of bed or in any case severely impede his falling asleep (Figure 4). Yet whenever the patients undergo sensory or mental stimulation or are asked to perform a mental task, the jerks, together with the EEG alpha activity, disappear. PSM again disappears as soon as the patient finally achieves sleep, and remains conspicuously absent thoughout all sleep stages. Occasionally, the jerks can also show up for a short time upon awakening in the morning. Only partial improvement is afforded in these patients by the use of clonazepam.

The peculiar relation of the PSM with the relaxed wakefulness prior to sleep is attributed to supraspinal modulatory influences acting on the spinal cord where the jerks are thought to originate (59). It also shows that wakefulness prior to sleep represents a peculiar vigilance state with intrinsic mental and neurophysiological characteristics—the predormitum, as defined by Critchley (60)—and that PSM should be considered a cause of sleep-onset insomnia and categorized as a parasomnia within the sleep–wake transition disorders.

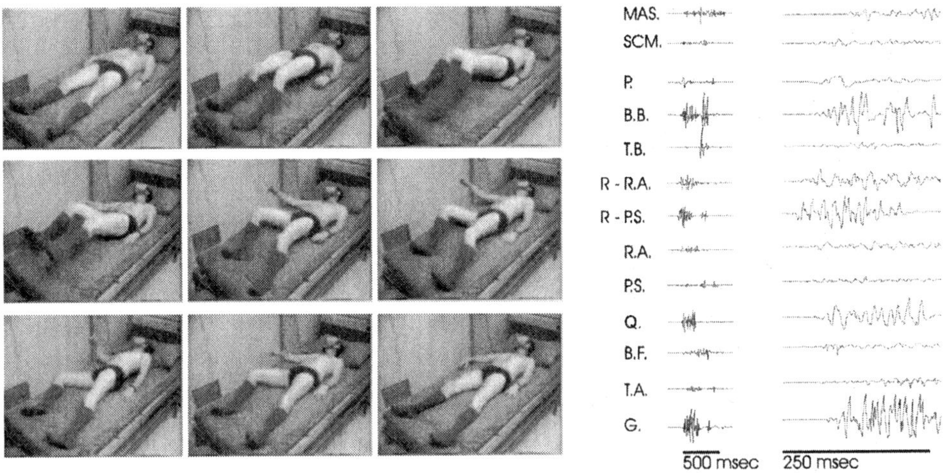

Figure 4 Videorecordings of a jerk of PSM in a 41-year-old man. Total duration of the jerk: 0.5 s. The panels on the right show the EMG recordings of the same jerk, at low and high speed, respectively. The EMG activity originates in the right paraspinal muscles (R-PS), thereafter propagating to more rostral (RA: rectus abdominis; TB: triceps brachii; BB: biceps brachii; P: pectoralis; SCM: sternocleidomastoideus; MAS: masseter, all on the left) and caudal (RA; PS; Q: quadriceps femoris; BF: biceps femoris; TA: tibialis anterior; G: gastrocnemius) muscles.

CONCLUSION

The nosography of the motor disorders that arise during sleep has gained much in the last few decades by the widespread use of videopolysomnographic recordings, which enable audiovisual monitoring of the different motor episodes concomitantly with the relevant neurophysiological EEG, EMG, and autonomic features. While permitting the recording and a detailed analysis of the motor episodes, videopolysomnography seldom discloses the pathophysiological mechanisms underlying the motor events. In other words, it is a purely descriptive means, and lacks etiological power. Thus, this field is still far from being completely characterized, and even the boundaries between the physiological and the pathological are not always completely clear. The increasing application of molecular biology and modern imaging techniques such as functional MRI or PET imaging will doubtless offer further insight into the pathogenic mechanisms behind many sleep-related motor disorders, with important implications for our knowledge of the sleep mechanisms involved in their origin.

ACKNOWLEDGMENTS

I wish to thank Ms. A. Laffi for typing the manuscript, Ms. A. Collins for reviewing the English text, and Mr. C. Grassi for help with the figures. Dr. F. Provini, Dr. G. Plazzi, and Professor E. Lugaresi gave invaluable advice.

REFERENCES

1. Diagnostic Classification Steering Committee; Thorpy MJ, Chairman. International Classification of Sleep Disorders: Diagnostic and Coding Manual. Rochester, MN: American Sleep Disorders Association, 1997.
2. Chase MH, Morales FR. The control of motoneurons during sleep. In: Kryger MH, Roth T, Dement WC, eds. Principles and Practice of Sleep Medicine. Philadelphia: WB Saunders, 1989:74–85.
3. Moruzzi G. The sleep-waking cycle. Ergeb Physiol 1972; 64:1–165.
4. Jouvet M, Delorme F. Locus coeruleus et sommeil paradoxal. C Roy Soc Biol 1965; 159:895–899.
5. Sanford LD, Morrison AR, Mann GL, Harris JS, Yoo L, Ross RJ. Sleep patterning and behaviour in cats with pontine lesions creating Rem without atonia. Sleep Res 1994; 3:233–240.
6. Hodes R, Dement WC. Depression of electrically induced reflexes (''H-reflexes'') in man during low voltage EEG ''sleep.'' Electroenceph Clin Neurophysiol 1964; 17:617–629.
7. De Lisi L. Su di un fenomeno motorio costante del sonno normale: le mioclonie ipniche fisiologiche. Riv Pat Ment 1932; 39:481–496.
8. Montagna P, Liguori R, Zucconi M, Sforza E, Lugaresi A, Cirignotta F, Lugaresi E. Physiological hypnic myoclonus. Electroenceph Clin Neurophysiol 1988; 70: 172–176.
9. Dagnino N, Loeb C, Massazza G, Sacco G. Hypnic physiological myoclonias in man: an EEG-EMG study in normal and neurological patients. Eur Neurol 1969; 2: 47–58.
10. Oswald I. Sudden bodily jerks on falling asleep. Brain 1959; 82:92–102.
11. Broughton R, Tolentino MA, Krelina M. Excessive fragmentary myoclonus in NREM sleep: a report of 38 cases. Electroenceph Clin Neurophysiol 1985; 61:123–133.
12. Coulter DL, Allen RJ. Benign neonatal sleep myoclonus. Arch Neurol 1982; 39: 191–192.
13. Symonds CP. Nocturnal myoclonus. J Neurol Neurosurg Psychiatry 1953; 16:166–171.
14. Lugaresi E, Cirignotta F, Coccagna G, Montagna P. Nocturnal myoclonus and restless legs syndrome. In: Fahn S, et al, eds. Advances in Neurology. Vol 43. Myoclonus. New York: Raven Press, 1986:295–307.
15. Coleman RM. Periodic movements in sleep (nocturnal myoclonus) and the restless legs syndrome. In: Guilleminault C, ed. Sleeping and Waking Disorders: Indications and Techniques. Menlo Park, CA: Addison-Wesley, 1982:265–295.

16. Terzano MG, Mancia D, Salati MR, Costani G, Decembrino A, Parrino L. The cyclic alternating pattern as a physiological component of normal NREM sleep. Sleep 1985; 8:137–145.
17. Bixler EO, Kales A, Vela Bueno A, Jacoby JA, Scarone S, Soldatos CR. Nocturnal myoclonus and nocturnal myoclonic activity in a normal population. Res Commun Chem Pathol Pharmacol 1982; 36:129–140.
18. Coleman RM, Bliwise DL, Sajben N, De Bruyn L, Boomkamp A, Menn ME, Dement WC. Epidemiology of periodic movements during sleep. In: Guilleminault C, Lugaresi E, eds. Sleep/Wake Disorders: Natural History, Epidemiology, and Long-Term Evolution. New York: Raven Press, 1983:217–229.
19. Kales A, Bixler EO, Soldatos CR, Vela-Bueno A, Caldwell AB, Cadieux RJ. Biopsychobehavioral correlates of insomnia. Part 1. Role of sleep apnea and nocturnal myoclonus. Psychosomatics 1982; 23:1–5.
20. Trenkwalder C, Bucher SF, Oertel WH, Proeckl D, Plendl H, Paulus W. Bereitschaftspotential in idiopathic and symptomatic restless legs syndrome. Electroenceph Clin Neurophysiol 1993; 89:95–103.
21. Trenkwalder C, Bucher SF, Oertel WH. Electrophysiological pattern of involuntary limb movements in the restless legs syndrome. Muscle Nerve 1996; 19:155–162.
22. Wechslar LR, Stakes JW, Shahani BT, Busis NA. Periodic leg movements of sleep (nocturnal myoclonus): an electrophysiological study. Ann Neurol 1986; 19:168–173.
23. Bucher SF, Seeleos KC, Oertel WH, Reiser M, Trenkwalder T. Cerebral generators involved in the pathogenesis of the restless legs syndrome. Ann Neurol 1997; 5: 639–645.
24. Ekbom KA. Restless legs. Acta Med Scand 1945; 185:5–123.
25. Walters AS. The International Restless Legs Syndrome Study Group. Towards a better definition of the restless legs syndrome. Mov Disord 1995; 10:634–642.
26. Boghen D, Peyronnard JM. Myoclonus in familial restless legs syndrome. Arch Neurol 1976; 33:368–370.
27. Walters A, Hening W, Côté L, Fahn S. Dominantly inherited restless legs with myoclonus and periodic movements of sleep: a syndrome related to the endogenous opiates? In: Fahn S, et al, eds. Advances in Neurology. Vol 43. Myoclonus. New York: Raven Press, 1986:309–319.
28. Montagna P, Coccagna G, Cirignotta F, Lugaresi E. Familial restless legs syndrome: long-term follow-up. In: Guilleminault C, Lugaresi E, eds. Sleep/Wake Disorders: Natural History, Epidemiology, and Long-Term Evolution. New York: Raven Press, 1983:231–235.
29. O'Keeffe ST, Gavin K, Lavan JN. Iron status and restless legs syndrome in the elderly. Age Ageing 1994; 23:200–203.
30. Staedt J, Stoppe G, Kogler A, Munz D, Riemann H, Einrich D, Ruther E. Dopamine D_2 receptor alteration in patients with periodic movements in sleep (nocturnal myoclonus). J Neural Transm Gen Sect 1993; 93:71–74.
31. Iannaccone S, Zucconi M, Marchettini P, Ferini-Strambi L, Nemni R, Quattrini A, Palazzi S, Lacerenza M, Formaglio F, Smirne S. Evidence of peripheral axonal neuropathy in primary restless legs syndrome. Mov Disord 1995; 10:2–9.

32. Salvi F, Montagna P, Plasmati R, Rubboli G, Cirignotta F, Veilleux M, Lugaresi E, Tassinari CA. Restless legs syndrome and nocturnal myoclonus: initial clinical manifestation of familial amyloid polyneuropathy. J Neurol Neurosurg Psychiatry 1990; 53(6):522–525.
33. Hening WA, Walters A, Kavey N, Gideo-Frank S, Côté L, Fahn S. Dyskinesias while awake and periodic movements in sleep in restless legs syndrome: treatment with opioids. Neurology 1986; 36:1363–1366.
34. Fisher C, Kahn E, Edwards A, Davis DM, Fine J. A psycho-physiological study of nightmares and night terrors. J Nerv Ment Dis 1974; 158:174–188.
35. Kales JD, Kales A, Soldatos CR, Caldwell AB, Charney DS, Martin ED. Night terrors: clinical characteristics and personality patterns. Arch Gen Psychiatry 1980; 37:1413–1417.
36. Hallstrom T. Night terror in adults through three generations. Acta Psychiatr Scand 1972; 48:350–352.
37. Broughton RJ. Sleep disorders: disorders of arousal? Science 1968; 159:1070–1078.
38. Pedley TA, Guilleminault C. Episodic nocturnal wanderings responsive to anticonvulsant drug therapy. Ann Neurol 1977; 2:30–35.
39. Plazzi G, Tinuper P, Montagna P, Provini F, Lugaresi E. Epileptic nocturnal wanderings. Sleep 1995; 18:749–756.
40. Jacobsen JH, Rosenberg RS, Huttenlocher PR, Spire JP. Familial nocturnal cramping. Sleep 1986; 9:54–60.
41. Schenck CH, Bundlie SR, Ettinger MG, Mahowald MW. Chronic behavioral disorders of human REM sleep: a new category of parasomnia. Sleep 1986; 9:293–308.
42. Lapierre O, Montplaisir J. Polysomnographic features of REM sleep behavior disorder: development of a scoring method. Neurology 1992; 42:1371–1374.
43. Schenck CH, Bundlie SR, Mahowald M. Delayed emergence of a parkinsonian disorder in 38% of 29 older men initially diagnosed with idiopathic rapid eye movement sleep behavior disorder. Neurology 1996; 46:388–393.
44. Culebras A, Moore JT. Magnetic resonance findings in REM sleep behavior disorder. Neurology 1989; 39:1519–1523.
45. Plazzi G, Corsini R, Provini F, Pierangeli G, Martinelli P, Montagna P, Lugaresi E, Cortelli P. REM sleep behavior disorders in multiple system atrophy. Neurology 1997; 48:1094–1097.
46. Plazzi G, Cortelli P, Montagna P, De Monte A, Corsini R, Contin M, Provini F, Pierangeli G, Lugaresi E. REM sleep behaviour disorder differentiates pure autonomic failure from multiple system atrophy with autonomic failure. J Neurol Neurosurg Psychiatry 1998; 64:683–685.
47. Silber MH. REM sleep behavior disorder associated with barbiturate withdrawal. Sleep Res 1996; 25:371.
48. Schenck CH, Mahowald MW. Polysomnographic, neurologic and psychiatric and clinical outcome report on 70 consecutive cases with REM sleep behavior disorder (RBD): sustained clonazepam efficacy in 89.5% of 57 treated patients. Cleve Clin J Med 1990; 57:10–24.
49. Schenck CH, Mahowald MW. Long-term, nightly benzodiazepine treatment of injurious parasomnias and other disorders of disrupted nocturnal sleep in 170 adults. Am J Med 1996; 100:333–337.

50. Mahowald MW, Schenck CH. Status dissociatus—a perspective on states of being. Sleep 1991; 14:69–79.
51. Rugh JD, Harlan J. Nocturnal bruxism and temporo-mandibular disorders. Adv Neurol 1988; 49:329–341.
52. Lugaresi E, Cirignotta F. Hypnogenic paroxysmal dystonia; epileptic seizures or a new syndrome? Sleep 1981; 4:129–138.
53. Tinuper P, Cerullo A, Cirignotta F, Cortelli P, Lugaresi E, Montagna P. Nocturnal paroxysmal dystonia with short-lasting attacks: three cases with evidence for an epileptic frontal lobe origin of seizures. Epilepsia 1990; 31:549–556.
54. Meierkord H, Fish DR, Smith SJM, Scott CA, Shorvon SD, Marsden CD. Is nocturnal paroxysmal dystonia a form of frontal lobe epilepsy? Mov Disord 1992; 7:38–42.
55. Montagna P, Sforza E, Tinuper P, Cirignotta F, Lugaresi E. Paroxysmal arousals during sleep. Neurology 1990; 40:1063–1066.
56. Scheffer IE, Bathia KP, Lopes-Cendes I, Fish DR, Marsden CD, Andermann E, Andermann F, Desbiens R, Keen D, Cendes F, et al. Autosomal dominant nocturnal frontal lobe epilepsy: a distinctive clinical disorder. Brain 1995; 118:61–73.
57. Montagna P, Cirignotta F, Giovanardi Rossi P, Lugaresi E. Dystonic attacks related to sleep and exercise. Eur Neurol 1992; 32:185–189.
58. Brown P, Thompson PD, Rothwell JC, Day BL, Marsden CD. Axial myoclonus of propriospinal origin. Brain 1991; 114:197–214.
59. Montagna P, Provini F, Plazzi G, Liguori R, Lugaresi E. Propriospinal myoclonus upon relaxation and drowsiness: a cause of severe insomnia. Mov Disord 1997; 12: 66–72.
60. Critchley M. The pre-dormitum. Rev Neurol (Paris) 1955; 93:101–106.

10

Sleep in Neurodegenerative Diseases

Sudhansu Chokroverty
Saint Vincents Hospital and
New York Medical College
New York, New York

INTRODUCTION

The scientific understanding of the molecular mechanism responsible for degeneration of nerve cells is beginning to change the concept of neurodegenerative diseases. The DNA analytical techniques are rapidly expanding the disorders resulting from the DNA mutation; hence, many neurodegenerative diseases may be determined by the DNA mutation and gene location. For example, DNA analytical techniques identified the gene location in Huntington's chorea (1) and familial Parkinson's disease (2), and spinocerebellar ataxias (3) have been classified into several types based on molecular analysis. Great strides have also been made in understanding the nature of the neurodegenerative diseases based on neuroimaging (MRI, fMRI, PET), neurochemical, and immunohistochemical methods. However, until further clarification and refinement of the molecular DNA analysis of various neurodegenerative diseases, we will continue to use the traditional definition of neurodegenerative diseases as a group of heterogeneous diseases of the central nervous system for which no causal agent can be identified by the currently available diagnostic techniques. The disorders generally affect one or more systems symmetrically and run an inexorably progressive course.

Many of the sleep–wake-promoting neurons are involved in the process of diffuse degeneration in various neurodegenerative diseases. Furthermore, in many of these degeneration disorders, central respiratory and autonomic neurons are also degenerated. All these factors are responsible for a variety of sleep disorders in neurodegenerative diseases.

The neurodegeneration of the somatic neurons can be predominantly:

Cortical: e.g., Alzheimer's disease
Basal ganglia or basal ganglia plus syndromes: e.g., Parkinson's disease, progressive supranuclear palsy, Huntington's chorea, torsion dystonia, or Tourette's syndrome
Cerebellar or cerebellar plus syndromes: e.g., spinocerebellar ataxias, including olivopontocerebellar atrophy
Motor neurons of the cerebral cortex, brainstem, and spinal cord: e.g., amyotrophic lateral sclerosis or motor neuron disease

Neurodegeneration of the autonomic neurons will cause multiple-system atrophy (MSA) or the Shy-Drager syndrome.

GENERAL SLEEP COMPLAINTS IN NEURODEGENERATIVE DISEASES

Sleep complaints in neurodegenerative diseases include insomnia, hypersomnia, complaints related to circadian rhythm disorders, abnormal movements, and behavior during sleep (4). Many of these patients are at risk for additional sleep disturbances, such as sleep apnea or periodic limb movements in sleep (PLMS). It should also be noted that generally these are elderly individuals and that sleep quality declines even in the relatively healthy elderly. However, sleep will improve once effective therapy—e.g., dopaminergic treatment for Parkinson's disease (PD)—is instituted for the underlying condition (5).

Insomnia complaints may include difficulty in initiating sleep; repeated awakenings, including early-morning awakenings; and insufficient amounts of sleep (6). Other complaints accompanying poor sleep may include excessive daytime sleepiness (EDS), fatigue, anxiety, irritability, lack of concentration, muscle aches and pains, and sometimes depression. EDS may be a major problem in many of these patients, resulting from inadequate sleep, sleep apnea, sleep fragmentation, or circadian rhythm disturbances. The problem may be compounded by medications prescribed for specific neurodegenerative disease. Patients with hypersomnia complaining of EDS (6) may fall asleep at inappropriate places and under inappropriate circumstances. They may also have additional complaints of daytime fatigue, lack of concentration, impaired motor skills and cognition, and lack of relief of symptoms following additional sleep at night.

Some patients may have additional risk of sleep-related respiratory dysrhythmias and loud snoring during sleep, as well as PLMS (4). Especially vulnerable are patients with PD, olivopontocerebellar degeneration, and MSA resulting from alterations of the sleep–wake regulatory neurons and central respiratory neurons.

Circadian rhythm disturbances are seen particularly in the degenerative conditions (4). Many patients are elderly and severely incapacitated, and all these features may weaken the circadian regulation of activity. Other factors that may impair the circadian rhythm are medications prescribed for these patients that cause nocturnal confusion, or "sundowning."

PREDOMINANTLY CEREBELLAR OR CEREBELLAR PLUS SYNDROMES

The role of the cerebellum in the regulation of sleep and wakefulness in humans is uncertain but has been demonstrated in animal studies (7). Sleep disturbances occur in many patients with olivopontocerebellar degeneration or atrophy and other types of SCAs (8–11). The term olivopontocerebellar atrophy (OPCA) was introduced by Dejerine and Thomas (12) in 1900 to describe a chronic progressive, sporadic late-onset, predominantly cerebellar degeneration, often accompanied by parkinsonism and associated with atrophy of the pontine nuclei and cerebellar cortex, and degeneration of the pontocerebellar region. Earlier, Menzel (13) had described this dominant form of cerebellar degeneration, also known as olivopontocerebellar degeneration (OPCD). Before the SCAs were defined on the basis of DNA analytical technique, the classification of OPCA was based on the clinical phenomenology and pathological features, but there was chaos and confusion in the various classification systems. Later, several genes, SCA1, SCA2, SCA3, or Machado-Joseph disease, SCA6, and SCA7, as well as dentatorubral-pallidoluysian atrophy (DRPLA) with expanded CAG repeats responsible for autosomal dominant cerebellar ataxia, were described (3,14). However, about 40% of the dominant ataxias cannot yet be identified at a genotypical level (14). Cases of recessive or sporadic OPCA will now be classified under MSA (15). In many patients with OPCA, central, obstructive, or mixed apneas have been described (16,17), but the apneas are less frequent and less intense in this condition than in the Shy-Drager syndrome. Obstructive sleep apnea may be related partly to bulbar muscle involvement in OPCA, and in some patients nocturnal stridor occurs. Typical features of REM-sleep behavior disorder (RSBD) have been described in several cases of OPCA (18,19). OPCA has also been associated with hyposomnia.

Sleep disturbances in other neurodegenerative and heredodegenerative disorders have been described elsewhere in his book.

PATHOGENESIS IN NEURODEGENERATIVE DISEASES

Pathogenesis of Sleep Disturbance in Alzheimer's Disease

Both direct and indirect mechanisms are responsible for sleep disturbances in Alzheimer's disease (AD) (4,20). Direct mechanisms include degeneration of the neurons of the suprachiasmatic nucleus that may be responsible for the circadian dysrhythmia causing inversion of sleep rhythm, sundowning, and other sleep–wake-schedule disturbances in AD (20,21). Degeneration of the cholinergic neurons in the nucleus basalis of Meynert, the pedunculopontine tegmental and laterodorsal tegmental nuclei, and noradrenergic neurons of the brainstem may be responsible for decreased REM sleep in AD patients (20).

Indirect mechanisms consist of degeneration of the brainstem respiratory neurons and other degenerative changes in the supramedullary respiratory pathways causing sleep apnea-hypopnea and other respiratory dysrhythmias in sleep in AD (20). Other indirect mechanisms include medication effects, associated depression, increasing incidence of PLMS in elderly AD patients, and age-related alterations in sleep. Additionally, associated general medical diseases affecting the cardiovascular or respiratory systems, or environmental factors such as the artificial environment of the sleep laboratory and placement of AD patients in nursing homes or other long-term-care institutions, may also contribute to sleep disturbances.

Pathogenesis of Sleep Disorders in Parkinson's Disease

Both direct and indirect mechanisms are responsible for sleep disturbances in PD patients (4). Degenerative loss of dopaminergic, noradrenergic, serotonergic, and cholinergic neurons in the brainstem may be responsible for a variety of sleep disturbances in PD (4). Degeneration of the pedunculopontine tegmental nucleus, which is known to be affected in PD, may be responsible for RSBD in these patients (22).

Degeneration of the brainstem respiratory neurons as well as alterations of the neurochemical environment of the respiratory neurons and degenerative changes in the supramedullary respiratory pathways in PD patients may be responsible for sleep-related breathing disorders causing sleep–wake disturbances (20,23). Other indirect mechanisms in PD include increasing prevalence of PLMS, age-related alterations in sleep, associated conditions of depression, and associated general medical diseases affecting the cardiovascular or respiratory system.

Factors that may be responsible for sleep disturbances in PD also include the following (24): persistence of tremor, dystonia, rigidity, or dyskinesias during sleep, RSBD, PLMS (particularly in the elderly), REM-sleep-onset blinking, and repeated awakenings with reactivation of symptoms such as difficulty in changing position or inability to initiate movements. Depression, which occurs in many PD patients, and medication effects (e.g., levodopa-induced dyskinesia, psychosis, and nightmares) may also contribute to sleep abnormalities. In many patients, increased awakenings, frequent stage shifts, and repeated arousals along with immobility and abnormal movements may be responsible for increased time spent in wakefulness and decreased slow-wave and REM sleep. Rigidity, dystonia, and postural difficulties in PD may contribute to insomnia.

Pathogenetic Mechanisms of Sleep Disturbances in Other Somatic Neurodegenerative Diseases

The most severe sleep abnormalities in progressive supranuclear palsy (PSP) compared with PD may be due to the greater brainstem pathology, especially that in the pedunculopontine tegmental area, a region linked to control of REM sleep (25). Rigidity, dystonia, and postural difficulties in PSP may contribute to insomnia.

Pathogenetic mechanisms for sleep disturbances in Huntington's chorea (HC) may include one or more of the following (4): degenerative changes affecting structures regulating sleep–wakefulness, presence of chorea and dystonia, medication effects, and prominent psychological symptoms including depression and psychosis in many patients with HC.

Pathogenetic factors responsible for sleep disturbances in torsion dystonia may be related in part to reduced amounts of serotonin in the dorsal raphe nucleus and norepinephrine in the locus coeruleus, which are found in some patients with dystonia musculorum deformans, in addition to other mechanisms related to motor abnormalities as described above. In dystonia, there is no involvement of the descending inhibitory pathways of REM sleep as demonstrated by decreased amplitude and prolonged latency of motor-evoked potentials following magnetic brain stimulation in patients with dystonia.

The pathogenetic mechanisms for sleep disturbances in Tourette's syndrome may be related partly to an alteration of dopamine, serotonin, or norepinephrine metabolism noted in these patients (7).

In the Shy-Drager syndrome (multiple-system atrophy), as in other neurodegenerative diseases, both direct and indirect mechanisms are responsible for sleep disturbances (4). Some of these mechanisms are listed below.

In MSA, there is degeneration of the pontine tegmentum, nucleus tractus solitarius, nucleus ambiguous, hypoglossal nucleus, reticular formation of the brainstem, and, in some patients, the cervical and thoracic spinal cord. Respiratory dysrhythmias resulting from direct involvement of the region of the brainstem containing the respiratory neurons have been described by Lockwood (26) and Chokroverty et al. (27) correlating physiological and clinical findings. Impairment of respiratory control in the Shy-Drager syndrome, as manifested by impaired hypercapnic and hypoxic ventilatory and mouth occlusion pressure responses, has been described by McNicholas et al. (28) and Chokroverty (20). In some patients, apneustic or dysrhythmic breathing may have resulted from interference with the forebrain, midbrain, and pontine inputs to the medullary respiratory neurons. Other mechanisms for respiratory dysrhythmia may include direct involvement of the projections from the hypothalamus and central nucleus of amygdala to the respiratory neurons in the nucleus tractus solitarius and nucleus ambiguous. In addition, affection of the vagal input from the respiratory receptors to the central respiratory neurons and sympathetic denervation of the nasal mucosa may cause respiratory dysrhythmias. Alterations of the neurochemical environment may also be responsible for sleep-wake and respiratory dysrhythmias in MSA. Low levels of dopamine and noradrenaline in the limbic-hypothalamic region including the septal nuclei, basal ganglia, and the locus coeruleus have been described in patients with MSA (29). In addition, MSA patients may have specific catecholamine enzyme deficits in the brain and the sympathetic ganglia (30).

DIAGNOSTIC APPROACHES IN NEURODEGENERATIVE DISORDERS

Clinical Assessment

The first step in the diagnosis is a detailed history of sleep complaints, which should include present and past sleep history, family history, and drug/alcohol and medical/psychiatric histories. The history should also be specifically directed at possible respiratory dysrhythmias during sleep. It is important to perform physical examination for the diagnosis of the primary condition or associated medical, including neurological disorders that may be responsible for the sleep disturbances in MSA.

Laboratory Assessment

Laboratory investigations should be undertaken to diagnose the nature of the sleep disturbance and the primary neurological disorder. It is beyond the scope of this chapter to discuss all the laboratory tests to uncover the underlying neurological disorders. This section is limited to the pertinent laboratory tests to understand the nature of the sleep disturbances. Overnight polysomnographic (PSG) study and the multiple sleep latency test (MSLT) are the two most important laboratory tests for the diagnosis of sleep disturbances. In addition, pulmonary-function tests are important to address the question of sleep-related respiratory disturbances.

Overnight Polysomnographic Study

PSG study must be performed in patients suspected of sleep-related respiratory disorders or those complaining of daytime hypersomnia (6,20). However, the diagnosis and treatment of sleep disturbances may be problematic in neurodegenerative diseases with severe functional impairment. All-night PSG is important to assess the severity of the sleep-disordered breathing and to document sleep architecture. It should be noted that sleep may adversely affect respiration and the primary neurological disorder, and respiratory dysrhythmia or the primary neurological disorder may adversely affect sleep. Thus, sleep and breathing disturbances may alter the natural course of the illness and it is therefore important to study the sleep architecture. Overnight PSG should include simultaneous recordings of multiple channels of EEG, EMG, electro-oculogram, electrocardiogram, respiratory monitoring (to detect both effort and flow), and continuous recording of O_2 saturation by finger oxymetry. In suspected cases of upper-airway resistance syndrome (33) in extrapyramidal disorders, measurement of the intrathoracic pressure is important and is accomplished by inserting an intraesophageal balloon.

It is also important to record multiple channels of EEG to accurately identify different sleep stages as well as reveal any focal or diffuse cerebral lesions and epileptiform discharges that may be associated with sleep disturbance and sleep-related respiratory dysrhythmias in neurodegenerative disorders.

The overnight PSG findings in various neurodegenerative disorders are listed under the description of each entity in other chapters of this volume.

Multiple Sleep Latency Test

MSLT may document the presence of pathological sleepiness and any associated primary sleep disorder such as narcolepsy in some of these neurodegenerative diseases. MSLT has been standardized and consists of four or five daytime recordings of EEG, EMG, and electro-oculogram at 2-hour intervals, each recording lasting for a maximum of 20 minutes (34). MSLT measures the average sleep-onset latency (time to the first epoch of any sleep stage for the clinical purpose) as well as the presence of REM sleep and the measurement of REM latency (time from sleep onset to the first REM sleep). A mean sleep latency of less than 5 minutes is consistent with excessive sleepiness. Sleep-onset REM in two or more of the four or five recordings during MSLT is suggestive of narcolepsy. Abnormalities of REM-sleep regulatory mechanisms and circadian rhythm sleep disturbances may also lead to REM-sleep abnormalities during MSLT.

Other Laboratory Tests

In order to diagnose parasomnias such as RSBD that may be noted in patients with MSA, OPCA, PD, and AD, a video-PSG recording may be needed.

Actigraphy

Actigraphy is a recently developed technique that uses a motion detector to record activities during sleep and waking (35). Actigraphy is very useful in the diagnosis of circadian rhythm sleep disorders in patients with neurodegenerative diseases.

Pulmonary Function Tests

In order to exclude intrinsic bronchopulmonary disease, which may affect sleep-related breathing disorders, pulmonary-function tests may be needed. These tests will assess lung volumes, gas distribution and transfer, arterial blood gases, and chemical control of breathing.

MANAGEMENT OF SLEEP DISTURBANCES IN NEURODEGENERATIVE DISEASES

Management of the primary neurological condition is beyond the scope of this chapter and the reader is referred to the general neurological texts. It is important to emphasize, however, that treatment of the primary condition is important as it may improve the sleep disturbance. In this section, some general principles and specific treatment directed at sleep disturbances are discussed. The management can be discussed under the following four headings: 1) general measures, 2) pharmacotherapy, 3) phototherapy, and 4) treatment of sleep-related breathing disorders.

General Measures, Including Sleep Hygiene

The goal of treatment is to improve quality of life, and the general measures are directed at reducing or eliminating risk factors that may enhance the sleep-related respiratory disturbances. Certain general principles of treatment are helpful (4,20,24,36). An attempt should be made to reduce the dose or change the medications that could have an adverse effect on sleep and breathing. Associated conditions such as depression, anxiety, or pain due to arthritis should be treated with appropriate medications. The patients should be encouraged to develop good sleep habits and discouraged from taking daytime naps. They should not drink caffeine before bedtime or in the evening and should be encouraged to exercise—for example, by walking—during the day.

Pharmacotherapy

Sleep has not been consistently benefited by treating PD patients (4). Contradictory reports (24) have appeared, with some reporting parallel benefit (37) to sleep and movements and others showing persistent abnormalities in sleep (38). However, adjustment of timing and choice of medications may help patients with PD who experience reactivation of symptoms during the night. Patients who are taking medications early in the day may benefit from evening or bedtime doses. Longer-acting preparations of levodopa (Sinemet CR) may help when taken near bedtime. Administration of tolcapone (Tasmar) (39,40), a catachol-o-methyl transferase (COMT) inhibitor that has recently become available, can be useful for these patients by prolonging the action of levodopa. Dopamine agonists such as bromocriptine or pergolide, with their sustained action, may benefit sleep in some patients.

Two recently approved dopamine agonists, pramipexole (mirapex) and ropinirole (Requip), have not undergone adequate trial but may be useful (40,41). Antihistamines such as diphenhydramine may promote sleep in addition to its modest antiparkinsonian effect. It is important to remember that dopaminergic drugs have biphasic action (36): low doses may promote sleep by improving nocturnal mobility while high doses in the evening may disrupt sleep by inducing arousals and movements, especially during the first half of the night. In PD patients complaining of insomnia, a small dose of levodopa (Sinemet 25/100) with a second dose later at night if the patient awakens may sometimes be helpful (36). In PD patients with restless-legs syndrome, evening and late-night doses of levodopa may be helpful. Selegiline (Eldepryl) may improve sleep in some patients. Specific motor disorders of sleep in PD patients may be treated with appropriate medications such as clonazepam for RSBD or PLMS and clozapine, an atypical neuroleptic with D4 receptor antagonist, for nocturnal hallucination and psychosis. During clozapine treatment, however, usual precautions for monitoring blood count and testing liver function should be taken.

Patients with dopa-responsive dystonia or Segawa variant show circadian variability with significant symptomatic relief from sleep (42). Small doses of levodopa (Sinemet 25/100) may be effective for both the diurnal dystonia and the nighttime sleep abnormalities of dopa-responsive dystonia.

Pharmacotherapy for sleep disturbances in other neurodegenerative diseases has not been found to be very efective, but the general measures as outlined above with medications for selected patients with insomnia may be useful. In patients with insomnia, a trial with intermediate-acting benzodiazepines (e.g., Temazepam) or zolpidem (Ambien) should be tried for a short period. For nocturnal wanderings or agitation and sundowning, a trial with small doses (0.5–1 mg) of haloperidol should be instituted.

Phototherapy

Time exposure to bright light in the morning may be helpful in some patients. Satlin (43) and Okawa (44) and colleagues reported improvement in nighttime sleep and a decrease in daytime sleepiness following bright-light exposure in the evening in limited studies involving patients with AD. However, further studies are needed to confirm these encouraging results.

Treatment of Sleep-Related Breathing Disorders

The objectives of treatment of sleep-related breathing disturbances in neurodegenerative diseases are to improve the quality of life and prevent life-threatening cardiac arrhythmias and congestive cardiac failure. The quality of life may be improved by preventing repeated arousals, sleep fragmentation, nocturnal episodes of hypoxemia associated with sleep apnea, and daytime hypersomnolence. The treatment of sleep-related breathing disturbances in neurodegenerative diseases may be divided into four approaches: general, pharmacological, mechanical, and surgical measures (4,20).

General Measures

These should follow the general principles as outlined in the beginning of this section. Patients undergoing such treatment should avoid alcohol and sedative-hypnotic drugs, which may depress breathing during sleep, causing further deterioration in sleep-disordered breathing.

Pharmacological Therapy

Pharmacological treatment for sleep-disordered breathing has not been very successful. Three agents that have been tried in patients with mild to moderate sleep apnea with partial success are protriptyline, medroxyprogesterone acetate, and acetazolamide. Acetazolamide has had some good results in patients with central sleep apnea but may cause obstructive apnea or aggravate orthostatic hypotension owing to its diuretic and natriuretic effects.

Mechanical Measures

Nasal continuous positive airway pressure (CPAP) is an important measure for treatment of obstructive sleep apnea in patients with neurodegenerative diseases. Such treatment often improves the quality of sleep and reduces daytime symptoms by eliminating or reducing sleep-related obstructive or mixed apneas and O_2 desaturation. Instead of CPAP, some patients will require bilevel positive airway pressure (BiPAP); the latter delivers different pressures during inspiration and expiration, and some patients may find it comfortable with reduced expiratory pressure. It should be noted, however, that CPAP or BiPAP treatment has not been very useful in patients with neurodegenerative diseases with a natural history of progression of the disorder. An adequate study in a sufficient number of patients using such treatment has not been conducted.

Ventilatory support may be needed for sleep apnea and hypoventilation in patients with amyotrophic lateral sclerosis (ALS). Two types of ventilatory support are available for patients with sleep-related apnea or hypoventilation: negative-pressure and positive-pressure ventilators. Some patients with ALS may need negative-pressure ventilation by cuirass, which alleviates respiratory problems and quality of sleep, but the current standard of care for chronic ventilatory failure is mainly nasal intermittent positive pressure ventilation (NIPPV) using a nasal mask or prongs. Long-term NIPPV is not suitable, however, for those with diffuse oropharyngeal muscle weakness who cannot ventilate on their own. Some patients with sleep apnea or hypoventilation due to diaphragmatic or bulbar muscle weakness may require initial treatment with cuirass, CPAP, and later NIPPV at night with symptomatic relief.

Surgical Treatment

Other than tracheostomy, no surgical measure is practical in patients with neurodegenerative diseases with an unrelenting course. Tracheostomy is the only effective measure for emergency treatment of severe respiratory dysfunction and hypoxia in patients with marked laryngeal stridor due to laryngeal abductor paralysis in patients with MSA. Tracheostomy has also been performed in patients with sudden respiratory arrest after resuscitation by intubation. In patients with neurodegenerative diseases with a relentlessly progressive and unfavorable course, a decision for tracheostomy must be weighed carefully.

REFERENCES

1. The Huntington's Disease Collaborative Research Group. A novel gene containing a trinucleotide repeat that is expanded and unstable on Huntington's disease chromosome. Cell 1993; 72:971.
2. Polymeropoulos MH, Higgins JJ, Golbe LI, et al. Mapping of a gene for Parkinson's disease to chromosome 4q21–q23. Science 1996; 274:1197–1199.
3. Conner KE, Rosenberg RN. The genetic basis of ataxia. In: Rosenberg RN, Prusiner SB, DiMauro S, Barchi RL, eds. The Molecular and Genetic Basis of Neurological Disease. Boston: Butterworth-Heinemann, 1997:503–544.
4. Chokroverty S. Sleep and degenerative neurologic disorders. Neurolog Clin 1996; 14:807–826.
5. Askenasy JJM, Yahr MD. Reversal of sleep disturbance in Parkinson's disease by antiparkinsonian therapy: a preliminary study. Neurology 1985; 35:527.
6. Chokroverty S. An approach to a patient with sleep complaints. In: Chokroverty S, ed. Sleep Disorders Medicine: Basic Science, Technical Considerations, and Clinical Aspects. 2nd ed. Boston: Butterworth-Heinemann, 1999:277.
7. Cunchillos JD, DeAndres I. Participation of the cerebellum in the regulation of the sleep-wakefulness cycle: results in the cerebellectomized cats. Electroencephalogr Clin Neurophysiol 1982; 53:549–558.
8. Katayama S, Yokoyama S, Hirano Y, et al. TRH and sleep abnormalities in spinocerebellar degeneration (SCD). In: Sobue I, ed. TRH and Spinocerebellar Degeneration. Amsterdam: Elsevier, 1986:227.
9. Neil JF, Holzer BC, Spiker DG, et al. EEG sleep alterations in olivopontocerebellar degeneration. Neurology 1980; 390:660–662.
10. Osorio J, Daroff RB. Absence of REM and altered NREM sleep in patients with spinocerebellar degeneration and slow saccades. Ann Neurol 1980; 7:277–280.
11. Shimizu T, Sugita Y, Injima S, et al. Sleep study in Shy-Drager syndrome. Clin Neurol (Japan) 1981; 21:218–227.

12. Dejerine J, Thomas A. L'atrophic olivo-ponto-cerebellum. Nouv Icon de la Salpet 1900; 13:330.
13. Menzel P. Beitrag zur Kenntnis der hereditaren ataxie und Kleinhirnatrophie. Archiv fur Psychiatrie 1891; 22:160–190.
14. Subramony SH. Inherited ataxias. In: Gilchrist JM, ed. Prognosis in Neurology. Boston: Butterworth-Heinemann, 1998:147–155.
15. Consensus statement on the definition of orthostatic hypotension, pure autonomic failure and multiple system atrophy. Neurology 1996; 46:1470.
16. Chokroverty S, Sachdeo R, Masdeu J. Autonomic dysfunction and sleep apnea in olivopontocerebellar degeneration. Arch Neurol 1984; 41:926–931.
17. Salazar-Grueso EF, Rosenberg RS, Roos RP. Sleep apnea in olivopontocerebellar degeneration: treatment with trazodone. Ann Neurol 1988; 23:399–401.
18. Quera-Salva MA, Guilleminault C. Olivopontocerebellar degeneration, abnormal sleep and REM sleep without atonia. Neurology 1986; 36:576–577.
19. Shimizu T, Sugita Y Iijima S, et al. Sleep study in Shy-Drager syndrome. Clin Neurol (Japan) 1981; 21:218–227.
20. Chokroverty S. Sleep, breathing and neurological disorders. In: Chokroverty S, ed. Sleep Disorders Medicine: Basic Science, Technical Considerations and Clinical Aspects. 2nd ed. Boston: Butterworth-Heinemann, 1999:509.
21. Bliwise DL. Dementia. In: Kryger MH, Roth T, Dement WC, eds. Principles and Practice of Sleep Medicine. Philadelphia, WB Saunders, 1994:790.
22. Schenck CH, Bundie SR, Mahowald MW. Delayed emergence of a parkinsonian disorder in 38% of 29 older men initially diagnosed with idiopathic rapid eye movement sleep behavior disorder. Neurology 1996; 46:388. (Erratum appears in Neurology 1996; 46:1787.)
23. Chokroverty S. The spectrum of ventilatory disturbances in movement disorders. In: Chokroverty S, ed. Movement Disorders. Costa Mesa, CA: PMA, 1990:365.
24. Hening WA, Walters AS, Chokroverty S. Motor function and dysfunction of sleep. In: Chokroverty S, ed. Sleep Disorders Medicine: Basic Science, Technical Considerations and Clinical Aspects. 2nd ed. Boston: Butterworth-Heinemann, 1999:441.
25. Montplasir J, Petit D, Decary A, et al. Sleep and quantitative EEG in patients with progressive supranuclear palsy. Neurology 1997; 49:999.
26. Lockwood AH. Shy-Drager syndrome with abnormal respirations and antidiuretic hormone release. Arch Neurol 1976; 33:292–295.
27. Chokroverty S, Sharp JT, Barron KD. Periodic respiration in erect posture in Shy-Drager syndrome. J Neurol Neurosurg Psychiatry 1978; 41:980–986.
28. McNicholas WT, Rutherford R, Grossman R, et al. Abnormal respiratory pattern generation during sleep in patients with autonomic dysfunction. Am Rev Respir Dis 1983; 128:429–433.
29. Spokes EG, Bannister R, Oppenheimer DR. Multiple system atrophy with autonomic failure: clinical, histological and neurochemical observations on 4 cases. J Neurol Sci 1979; 43:59–82.
30. Black IB, Petio CK. Catecholamine enzymes in the degenerative neurological disease idiopathic orthostatic hypotension. Science 1976; 192:910–912.
31. Chokroverty S. An approach to a patient with sleep complaints. In: Chokroverty S,

ed. Sleep Disorders Medicine: Basic Science, Technical Considerations, and Clinical Aspects. Boston: Butterworth-Heinemann, 1994:181.
32. Chesson AL Jr, Ferber RA, Fry JM, et al. The indications for polysomnography and related procedures. Sleep 1997; 20(6).
33. Guilleminault C, Stoohs R, Clerk A, et al. From obstructive sleep apnea syndrome to upper airway resistance syndrome. Sleep 1992; 15:513–516.
34. Carskadon MA, Dement WC, Mitler M, et al. Guidelines for the multiple sleep latency test (MSLT): a standard measure of sleepiness. Sleep 1986; 9:519–524.
35. Saadeh A, Hauri PJ, Kripke DF, Lavie P. The role of actigraphy in the evaluation of sleep disorders. Sleep 1995; 18:288–302.
36. Aldrich MS. Parkinsonism. In: Kryger MH, Roth T, Dement WC, eds. Principles and Practice of Sleep Medicine. Philadelphia: WB Saunders, 1994:783.
37. Askenasy JJ. Sleep in Parkinson's disease. Acta Neurol Scand 1993; 87:167–170.
38. Apps MCP, Scheaff PC, Ingram DA, et al. Respiration and sleep in Parkinson's disease. J Neurol Neurosurg Psychiatry 1985; 48:1240–1245.
39. Rajput AH, Martin W, Saint-Hilaire MH, et al. Tolcapone improves motor function in parkinsonian patients with the "wearing off" phenomenon: a double-blind, placebo-controlled, multicenter trial. Neurology 1997; 49:1066.
40. LeWitt PA. New options for treatment of Parkinson's disease. Baillieres Clin Neurol 1997; 6:109.
41. Gottwald MD, Bainbridge JL, Dowling GA, et al. New pharmacotherapy for Parkinson's disease. Ann Pharmacother 1997; 31:1205.
42. Segawa M, Nomura Y. Hereditary progressive dystonia with marked diurnal fluctuations. In: Riederer P, Nagatsu T, Beckmann H, Carlsson A, Gershon S, Narabayashi H, Yoshida MC, eds. Parkinson's Disease: From Clinical Aspects to Molecular Basis. New York: Springer, 1992:167.
43. Satlin A, Volicer L, Ross V, et al. Bright light treatment of behavioral and sleep disturbance in Alzheimer's disease. MJ Psychiatry 1992; 114:1028–1032.
44. Okawa M, Mishima K, Shirakawa S, et al. Sleep disorders in elderly patients with dementia and attempts of bright light therapy: in senile dementia of Alzheimer's type and muti-infarct dementia. In: Hairoshige T, Honma K, eds. Evolution of Circadian Clock. Sapporo, Japan: Hokkaido University Press, 1994:313–322.

11

Parkinson's Disease and Extrapyramidal Disorders

Robert L. Rodnitzky
University of Iowa College of Medicine
Iowa City, Iowa

Disturbed sleep in patients with Parkinson's disease (PD) was noted by James Parkinson in his original description of the disorder in 1817 (1). Since then, considerable knowledge and experience have accumulated regarding the interaction of sleep with PD as well as with other extrapyramidal disorders. The steady growth in this body of knowledge has paralleled our evolving understanding of the physiology of sleep and the etiopathogenesis of clinical disorders of the extrapyramidal system. More is known about the relationship between sleep and PD than about the interaction between sleep and other extrapyramidal disorders because PD is the most prevalent and the most extensively studied condition of this class of clinical disorders.

MECHANISMS OF INTERFERENCE WITH SLEEP

There are a variety of mechanisms through which extrapyramidal disorders can interfere with sleep. In many instances, particularly in advanced stages of illness when there is severe motoric and cognitive dysfunction that requires more intense pharmacotherapy, sleep may be disrupted concurrently by several different mechanisms that are operative in a single patient.

One of the most basic ways that these conditions affect sleep is through disruption of sleep architecture. Abnormalities in the sequence or duration of sleep stages have been noted in PD and several other extrapyramidal disorders.

When a disturbance of sleep architecture occurs in an individual receiving drug therapy for an underlying extrapyramidal syndrome, it is often difficult to determine whether the abnormality represents a primary neurobiological effect of the neurological disorder or a medication effect. Two additional mechanisms by which sleep may be disturbed in extrapyramidal disorders are disruption of circadian rhythm and the appearance of one or more parasomnias. In the latter circumstance, the appearance of a parasomnia may antedate the onset of the typical neurological signs associated with the underlying basal ganglia disorder. Lastly, the motoric symptoms present in most extrapyramidal disorders have significant potential to interrupt sleep. In this regard, either hyperkinetic or hypokinetic abnormalities can interfere with sleep onset or maintenance. One final mechanism of sleep disturbance has to do not with extrapyramidal disorders but rather with the medications prescribed to treat them. These drugs may exert their influence either through a primary effect on sleep, by exacerbating a previously existent parasomnia, or by inducing nocturnal motoric or behavioral side effects.

To devise rational corrective therapy for sleep dysfunction appearing in the context of an extrapyramidal disorder, it is critical to recognize which of these mechanisms, singly or in combination, is contributing to disturbed sleep. At the same time, it is important to avoid choosing a therapy that may exacerbate the underlying neurological illness. With these considerations in mind, understanding the spectrum of sleep abnormalities that can occur in each of the common extrapyramidal disorders is the next step in planning effective therapy.

PARKINSON'S DISEASE

The Effect of Parkinson's Disease on Sleep

It is widely accepted that sleep abnormalities are common in PD (2–6). In two large surveys, prominent complaints of sleep disturbance were noted in 74% (3) and 93% (4) of PD patients. In these studies, and most others, it is often difficult to ascertain whether the reported sleep disturbance is related to PD itself or the medications used to treat it. In patients in whom the sleep disturbance is clearly related to PD alone, it may be difficult to discern which of the many ways that PD can affect sleep is at play. Specifically, it may be difficult to determine whether sleep disruption unrelated to drugs is caused by nocturnal akinesia, nocturnal rigidity and pain, re-emergence of tremor, associated parasomnias, disruption of the circadian rhythm, or a primary alteration of sleep architecture. Some studies have suggested that there are no sleep abnormalities inherent to PD and have found that sleep parameters in untreated PD patients are not different from those of a normal, age-matched population (7). It should be noted, however, that most PD patients who are untreated are those in whom motoric abnormalities such as rigidity, tremor, and akinesia are very mild and nondisabling. To the extent that nocturnal re-emergence of these symptoms contributes to disrupted sleep, untreated patients with mild PD would be expected to suffer from fewer sleep disturbances. Virtually all the other mechanisms by which PD can affect sleep also become more prominent as the illness progresses, again explaining why studies of mild PD patients may not uncover the full spectrum of sleep disturbances in Parkinson's disease.

Sleep Fragmentation

Parkinson's disease patients suffer from an increase in nocturnal arousals (2), and the degree of this abnormality appears to correlate with the severity of the underlying neurological disorder (8). This propensity to frequent arousals may stem in part from abnormalities in sleep architecture that are present in PD, including reduction in total slow-wave and REM sleep (2,8,9) and a decrease in sleep spindle density (9). The cardinal motor signs of PD—tremor, rigidity, and bradykinesia—also play a role in sleep fragmentation (5,10), and such complaints as immobility in bed and pain related to nocturnal rigidity correlate with abnormalities of sleep. What is not clear is the exact sequence of events that lead to awakening in patients with nocturnal symptoms. Polysomnographic studies suggest that tremor (11) usually occurs in stage 1 or 2 sleep, after arousals, and during sleep-stage transitions, but occasionally with no relationship to any of these events (11–13). When tremor does appear during sleep, it is often in an attenuated form consisting of lower-amplitude movements and repetitive but nonalternating muscle activity of the previously tremorous muscles (14,15). The mild tremor that occurs during sleep stage 1 or 2 may not result in an awakening, but more severe tremor can appear shortly after an awakening that occurs for whatever cause (16), and is often reported by patients to be associated with sleep disturbance. By the same token, severe tremor may prevent patients from initiating sleep at bedtime. Bradykinesia can also contribute to disturbed sleep. In some patients, especially those with advanced disease in whom the effect of dopaminergic medication wears off as the night progresses, sleep disturbance is caused by severe immobility and inability to shift to a comfortable position (10). Lees et al. (4) found this to be present in 65% of PD patients surveyed and to be the most troublesome sleep complaint in 39%. As another indication of the impact of nocturnal bradykinesia, 79% had the need to void at night, yet 35% were unable to get out of bed unaided. Similarly, patients in whom significant rigidity appears during an awakening may complain of associated pain that prevents the resumption of sleep.

The potential for the re-emergence of motoric parkinsonian symptoms to disrupt sleep suggests that nighttime dosages of antiparkinson medications might improve sleep. There is some controversy, however, about whether a bedtime dose of levodopa or a dopamine agonist improves sleep in PD (5). One large survey (4) indicated that sleep complaints in PD are not related to the timing of the last daily dosage of antiparkinson medication, but this study did not separately analyze this relationship in advanced patients, whose sleep is more likely to be interrupted by immobility, rigidity, or tremor. In many moderately severe to advanced PD patients, nocturnal amelioration of significant motoric signs of PD is often an important therapeutic goal in attempting to normalize sleep (17,18). The most useful strategy to achieve this goal is the use of a bedtime dose of a dopaminergic agent with a relatively long efficacy half-life. Long-acting dopamine agonists are useful for this purpose, and perhaps even more useful are the sustained-release levodopa preparations (19,20). The use of a COMT inhibiting agent along with levodopa at bedtime might further prolong the dopaminergic effect during the night. Bedtime dosing in PD patients with nocturnal disabilities results in less tremor, reduced rigidity, improved mobility, and fewer awakenings, at least during the early part of the night and often through the entire night (17,18,20). Some patients may require additional dosing of a sustained-release or standard levodopa preparation after early awakening to allow uninterrupted sleep for the remainder of the night.

The question remains as to whether bedtime dopaminergic agents are useful in PD patients with milder disease and less potential for sleep-disrupting motoric symptoms. Low dosages of levodopa can promote sleep in some PD patients with insomnia unrelated to nocturnal emergence of tremor or immobility (21). However, higher bedtime dosages in such patients can be counterproductive and may actually prolong sleep latency (16). Van Hilten et al. (5), for example, found that in less severe PD patients, sleep disruption was positively correlated with the total daily dosage of levodopa or dopamine agonist. A caveat is that a bedtime dose of a dopaminergic medication, irrespective of its purpose, has the potential to induce vivid dreaming and nocturnal hallucinosis, both of which are often associated with reduced sleep efficiency, less total sleep time, and a reduction in REM sleep (22). This side effect, should it occur, can be dealt with by reducing or eliminating the bedtime dose of the offending dopaminergic drug or by appropriate pharmacotherapy as discussed below.

Many PD patients, or their physicians, initiate bedtime dosing of levodopa or a dopamine agonist in the absence of nocturnal motoric symptoms or PD-related sleep disturbance, in the belief that antiparkinson medication is required around the clock. This practice should be discouraged because it unnecessarily raises the dosages of medication and because in some patients dopaminergic drugs can actually interfere with sleep by inducing dyskinesias (see below) or through the aforementioned tendency for high dosages to induce insomnia. Bedtime dosing with dopaminergic medications can either improve or interfere with sleep, and a clinical judgment in individual patients needs to be made to determine which effect is likely to prevail. In general, advanced PD patients who experience nocturnal emergence of motoric symptoms are more likely to benefit from bedtime dosing, and patients with milder PD symptoms stand a greater chance of experiencing medication-related sleep disturbance.

In addition to pharmacological treatment of the sleep-disrupting motoric features of PD, several nonpharmacological strategies are also useful. To minimize the effect of nocturanl immobility, the use of stain bedsheets can be recommended as a means of reducing friction between the body and the sheets, allowing easier mobility in bed. Ambient stimuli (noises, drafts, a restless bed partner) that might lead to brief arousals followed by a major emergence of tremor of rigidity and pain should be avoided to the extent possible.

Depression

Depression occurs in over 40% of PD patients (23). Depressed PD patients have a higher incidence of sleep complaints than those who are not depressed (24,25). The typical clinical and polygraphically defined sleep changes of depression, including shortened REM-sleep latency, increased arousals, and early awakening occur more frequently in depressed PD patients than in nondepressed ones (26).

The relative contributions of depression and the underlying features of PD to disturbed sleep can be difficult to separate. Menza and Rosen (25), while noting poorer overall sleep in depressed PD patients, found that compared to depression, age, illness-related variables, and levodopa dose were greater determinants of sleep disturbance in this population. Starkstein et al. (24), on the other hand, found that depression correlated with sleep disturbance more than any motoric or demographic variable. Furthermore, these investigators found a graded relationship between sleep dysfunction and depression, the greatest sleep disruption appearing in the most seriously depressed PD patients. Depression-related sleep disturbances in PD are treated in much the same manner as those in the non-PD population with only minor differences in choices of drug. The sedating antidepressants such as amitriptyline or doxepin administered at bedtime are very useful for this purpose (27). For some PD patients, especially those with dementia, agents with less anticholinergic effect such as nortriptyline are a better choice to avoid exacerbating their cognitive deficit. There is some controversy as to whether the selective serotonin-reuptake inhibitor (SSRI) drugs exacerbate PD in a small percentage of patients (28). Also, the use of either SSRI or tricyclic antidepressants in patients receiving selegiline for PD has been reported to cause a severe, potentially fatal interaction in a small number of patients (29). However, a recent survey of PD specialists revealed that these adverse interactions were quite rare and SSRI agents were the first choice of therapy for depression in PD for 51% of the respondents (30). In this same survey, the most common reason to choose tricyclic antidepressants instead was their potential to improve sleep.

Circadian Rhythm Disorders

Reversal of the sleep cycle is common in PD, especially in elderly patients with advanced disease. Typically, affected patients nap frequently during the day and are awake at night. The cause for this circadian abnormality is multifactorial. Many of the standard external markers of diurnal rhythmicity such as mealtime and scheduled activities are altered by PD and by the timing of medications used to treat the disease. For example, meals may be scheduled at unusual times to coincide with peak drug effect or to avoid an adverse drug interaction at scheduled medication dosing times. Also, periodic immobility can occur during the day as a result of fluctuations in response to dopaminergic medications. Similarly, a natural circadian pattern of worsening and improvement in dopamine-dependent functions (31,32) may dictate certain periods of the waking day when the patient is ambulatory and active (typically the early morning) and other times when there is relative immobility and a tendency to nap (typically late afternoon). Factor et al. (33) found that circadian changes in symptom severity were most common in more advanced PD patients. Lastly, the sedative effect of antiparkinson medications experienced by some patients leads to daytime somnolence and napping, with resultant nighttime wakefulness. To reverse the sleep cycle toward normalcy, attempts should be made to restore mealtime to a typical morning, noon, and early-evening pattern and to plan scheduled activities during times of predicted somnolence, whether drug-induced or related to the patient's spontaneous diurnal cycle.

The sedating effects of antiparkinson medication can be countered to some extent by administration of a daytime dosage of selegiline (34,35). This drug, which is metabolized to amphetamine derivatives, has potential alerting properties. Stimulant agents such as pemoline, methylphenidate, or dextroamphetamine are sometimes used (27), but tachyphylaxis and the occasional induction of hallucinosis in the elderly or cognitively impaired PD patient limit their use. The potential for PD patients to develop hallucinosis when using wake-promoting drugs might be avoided through the use of alerting drugs such as modafinil, which have little or no dopaminergic activity (36).

The advanced-sleep-phase syndrome, although relatively common in the general elderly population, is even more prominent in PD. In some patients, the final daily dosage of antiparkinson medication is so early in the day that there is wearing off of its motoric benefit well before bedtime, leaving the patient relatively immobile and unstimulated in the early evening. The advanced sleep phase may coincide with this period of evening immobility, leaving the PD patient at risk for falling asleep for the night. In this circumstance, an additional evening dosage of levodopa or dopamine agonist 2 to 3 hours before the desired bedtime may ameliorate the problem. In refractory cases, the use of nighttime phototherapy as a zeitgeber can be considered to shift the endogenous clock governing sleep toward a more normal time of night (37). Of interest is the recent discovery that this endogenous clock can be entrained by light application to extraretinal sites on the body, such as the popliteal space, where photoreceptors in intravascular hemoglobin are stimulated (38).

Respiratory Disorders

Significant respiratory dysfunction is not seen in mild PD (39), but in more advanced patients there may be an increased frequency of obstructive and central apneas and arterial oxygen desaturations during sleep (40). In at least one study, sleep apnea was not observed in any PD patients irrespective of the severity of the underlying illness, although tachypnea during REM sleep was commonly observed (41). Although there is little exact clinical data, it is common clinical experience that obstructive sleep apnea is much more common in multiple-system atrophy than in idiopathic PD. Nonetheless, advanced PD patients may be at risk for sleep-related respiratory dysfunction that has the potential to contribute to sleep fragmentation.

The Effect of Antiparkinson Drugs on Sleep

Although, as mentioned, antiparkinson drugs can improve sleep by lessening the nocturnal motor symptoms of PD, they also have the potential to impact sleep adversely in three ways: 1) by inducing unwanted sleep, 2) by inhibiting normal sleep, or 3) by resulting in motoric or behavioral side effects that interrupt sleep.

Daytime Somnolence Related to Antiparkinson Drugs

Most of the commonly used antiparkinson medications, including levodopa, amantadine, dopamine agonists, COMT inhibitors, and anticholinergic agents, have some potential to induce excessive daytime somnolence. Selegiline, on the other hand, is virtually never associated with excessive daytime sleepiness. Among the antiparkinson drugs, levodopa is the most common cause of medication-related somnolence. Typically, patients complain of an irresistible desire to sleep within 30 minutes of a dosage of standard or sustained-release carbidopa/levodopa. Nausieda et al. (3) found that polysomnographic study in such patients demonstrated a transition into stage 1–2 sleep within 30 to 60 minutes of a dosage of levodopa, but multiple sleep latency tests in these patients were normal if evaluated while they were not under treatment with levodopa. The pathogenesis of this phenomenon is unclear since levodopa infusion, at least at high levels, suppresses REM sleep (42). It is likely that in some PD patients exhibiting this apparent relationship the appearance of daytime somnolence simply reflects the high incidence of this problem in a normal aged population, a problem that occurs independently of levodopa administration. In these patients, a cause–effect relationship between levodopa and somnolence can be mistakenly assumed by the patient or the physician. In one study comparing PD patients with age-matched healthy individuals, the incidence of daytime somnolence was identical in both groups (43). While some excessive daytime somnolence in PD undoubtedly occurs independently of medications being administered, the striking temporal relationship between somnolence and the administration of the last dosage of levodopa in some patients suggests that—at least in these circumstances—a true cause–effect relationship exists.

The treatment of this problem can be difficult. One simple strategy to control medication-related somnolence is to alter environmental stimuli and activity schedules in the immediate postdose period when somnolence is most likely to occur. During this at-risk period, dark, quiet, poorly ventilated rooms should be avoided and vigorous activities such as a morning or afternoon walk can be scheduled. Fortunately, from a motoric point of view, many PD patients are best able to engage in such physically demanding activities immediately after a dosage of medication, when they are "on." If this strategy fails, an attempt can be made to change to another antiparkinson drug. Some patients may be less somnolent on standard carbidopa/levodopa than on the sustained-release preparation (27), and in a small percentage of patients the reverse is true. Similarly, each of the available dopamine agonists may have a different potential to induce somnolence in a given patient.

Stimulant drugs are occasionally indicated to combat this form of excessive daytime sleepiness in PD, but must by used with caution in this patient population, especially because of the risk of behavioral side effects (27). As mentioned previously, there is some reason to believe that stimulant drugs without dopaminergic properties may be better tolerated (36).

Insomnia Related to Antiparkinson Medications

Antiparkinson drugs can also result in insomnia. Selegiline, because of its potentially alerting metabolites, can result in insomnia, especially when administered after noon (27). Levodopa has the potential to alter sleep architecture, at least in the period immediately after the initiation of therapy (43,44) and possibly chronically (45). As discussed previously, in some patients dopaminergic agents administered at high dosages late in the evening have the potential to increase sleep latency and result in sleep fragmentation (42). Accordingly, for most patients, if a late-evening dosage of levodopa or dopamine agonist is not required to control nocturnal motoric symptoms, it should be eliminated, decreased, and/or distanced from bedtime.

Nocturnal Neuropsychiatric Disturbances Related to Medication

A variety of behavioral side effects are possible as a result of antiparkinson therapy, including memory loss, confusion, paranoia, psychosis, hallucinations, and vivid dreaming (27). Of these, nocturnal hallucinations and vivid dreaming have the greatest potential to interrupt sleep. With chronic dopaminergic therapy, some patients report that dreams become increasingly vivid, although dream content remains unchanged. In the survey by Lees et al. of 250 PD patients (4), 48% acknowledged experiencing vivid dreams or nightmares and 9% identified this as their major sleep complaint. Medication-induced vivid dreams not only have the potential to interrupt sleep, but may also be a premonitory sign of hallucinations and advanced psychosis (3,46), suggesting that they not be left untreated. This progression is most likely to occur in PD patients who are aged, cognitively impaired, and already have disturbed nocturnal sleep of any cause (47,48).

Comella et al. (22) have postulated that the initial event in the behavioral cascade leading from vivid dreaming to overt hallucinations is a reduction in REM sleep related to levodopa therapy. Therefore, when vivid dreams appear, it is advisable to reduce the bedtime dosage of antiparkinson medication and/or distance it from bedtime. Although levodopa and the dopamine agonists are the most common offenders, anticholinergic drugs, including the anticholinergic antidepressant agents and amantadine, can also result in this syndrome and should be adjusted before attempting to taper the more clinically effective primary dopaminergic agents. Ultimately, a strategy of downward titration of late-evening and bedtime antiparkinson medications is undertaken while being vigilant for the inevitable re-emergence of disabling motoric signs of PD. If downward titration of antiparkinson drugs cannot be successfully accomplished without seriously exacerbating parkinsonism, small dosages of low-potency neuroleptic agents such as molindone or thioridazine can be administered at bedtime, usually without fear of significantly worsening the underlying illness (27). Similarly, olanzapine (49) and risperidone (50), each with reduced potential for extrapyramidal side effects, can be used at bedtime. If these strategies fail, low dosages of the atypical neuroleptic clozapine (12.5–50 mg per day) can be administered (51). All these agents can cause daytime somnolence if taken other than at bedtime. Clozapine must be used with caution because of its potential to induce agranulocytosis in a small percentage of patients.

Medication-Induced Involuntary Movements and Restlessness

Dyskinesias related to dopaminergic therapy are usually choreiform or dystonic. In some patients, both patterns are found (52). Typically, choreiform dyskinesias occur when the dopaminergic agent is manifesting its greatest central effect (peak-dose dyskinesia); less commonly, they occur when the central effect is just beginning to be manifest and again when it is just beginning to wane (biphasic dyskinesia). Choreiform dyskinesias, irrespective of their temporal pattern of occurrence, tend not to persist to a major degree or emerge during sleep and are seldom the cause of self-reported sleep disturbance. Dystonic dyskinesias, on the other hand, are more likely to affect sleep. While dystonia can also occur de novo in PD, it is much more commonly related to the administration of dopaminergic medications. Dystonic dyskinesias, like the choreic form, can occur concurrently with the peak effect of dopaminergic agents or in a biphasic pattern. Even more commonly, these abnormal movements occur exclusively at the end of an interdose period when the central effects of medication have nearly or totally worn off. End-of-dose dystonia can be especially prominent upon awakening in the morning after a prolonged medication-free interval while asleep. In this pattern of occurrence, referred to as early-morning dystonia, the lower extremities are usually involved, with painful plantar flexion of the feet and curling of the toes. Less commonly, the facial and upper-extremity musculature are affected as well. One-third of PD patients surveyed by Lees et al. (4) experienced nocturnal dystonia and 20% experienced early-morning foot dystonia. Since nocturnal or early-morning dystonia is most commonly related to the waning central effect of levodopa as the night progresses, the most useful treatment is to institute bedtime therapy with a relatively long-acting dopaminergic agent, such as controlled-release carbidopa/levodopa, or a long-acting dopamine agonist. Pahwa et al. (18) noted resolution of early-morning dystonia in eight of 14 patients after changing from standard to controlled-release carbidopa/levodopa. In some patients, a bedtime dosage of baclofen will also ameliorate this symptom. An additional strategy employed by some patients to prevent early-morning dystonia is to set their alarm so that they can administer a dose of levodopa 30 to 45 minutes before their usual waking time and then return to sleep to awaken for the day after the medication has begun to take effect. Another form of dystonia, blepharospasm, occurs in PD patients at the beginning of the night, but is not clearly related to dopaminergic medications (53).

Levodopa-induced myoclonus occurs predominantly, but not exclusively, at night (54). It typically involves axial and proximal muscles and can appear during non-REM sleep as often as 30 times per night. These movements usually emerge only after chronic administration of levodopa. Surprisingly, they seldom interrupt the sleep of the PD patient, but can pose a problem for the bed partner. It has been postulated that levodopa-induced myoclonus is related to enhanced central serotonergic activity, since serotonin-blocking agents have been reported to be effective treatment (54).

Akathisia, an irresistible internal desire to move, is seen in some PD patients receiving levodopa and, very rarely, in the untreated patient. It can be distinguished from the restless-legs syndrome by its lack of relationship to recumbency, by the absence of associated sensory phenomena, and by its involvement of the entire body, not just the legs. Although not totally confined to bedtime, it is commonly nocturnal and can inhibit sleep initiation (55). In individual patients, akathisia has a variable relationship to the timing of levodopa administration and can occur in either the "on" or "off" state (56). Accordingly, in treating PD patients with severe nocturnal akathisia it is sometimes necessary to experiment by first increasing and then decreasing the evening dosage of dopaminergic medication. Should both approaches fail, a bedtime dosage of the atypical neuroleptic clozapine is very effective in treating this symptom, keeping in mind its potentially severe side effects (55).

Parasomnias in Parkinson's Disease

PD patients can experience abnormal movements and behaviors during sleep (parasomnias), including somnambulism, somniloquy, nightmares, night terrors, REM-sleep behavior disorder (RSBD), and periodic limb movements of sleep (PLMS) (57,58). Since all of these sleep-related phenomena can also occur in an ostensibly healthy population, the question remains as to whether their incidence is greater in PD patients. The exact frequency of their occurrence in PD is not totally certain, but the two parasomnias most frequently reported in PD patients are RSBD and PLMS.

In RSBD there is a failure of the normal suppression of EMG activity during REM sleep and an absence of atonia (57). Affected individuals physically act out their dreams, often incurring serious injury as they move, run, or dive from bed in the course of a dream. That RSBD appears in PD is well established, but there are surprisingly few well-documented cases in the literature (22,59). The paucity of reported cases may simply reflect a relatively low threshold for recognition of this syndrome. In support of this notion is the report by Comella et al. (22), who unexpectedly discovered RSBD in 50% of 10 PD patients undergoing screening polysomnography as part of a research protocol. A single case has been reported in which there were no parkinsonian features in life, but Lewy bodies were found at postmortem in the locus coeruleus and substantia nigra (60). Another report detailed three PD patients in whom clinically apparent RSBD emerged only after beginning selegiline therapy (61).

The notion that there is an interrelationship between PD and RSBD has been strengthened by several reports demonstrating that patients with RSBD often develop PD later in life (62,63). Schenck et al. (63) followed 29 older men with RSBD and found that 38% developed PD at a mean interval of 13 years after the diagnosis of their parasomnia. The relationship of RSBD to Lewy body pathology was also demonstrated by a patient who developed diffuse Lewy body disease 17 years after onset of RSBD (64). Most hypotheses explaining the co-occurrence of RSBD and PD have centered on the fact that in both conditions there is involvement of the pedunculopontine nucleus, a structure that plays a major role in REM atonia and is reciprocally connected to the substantia nigra (62,63). The finding of pontine pathology on magnetic resonance imaging in RSBD patients supports this notion (65).

Because of the potential for serious injury to the patient and for disruption of both the patient's and bed partner's sleep, serious attention should be given to treating this disorder in PD. The potential for injury while acting out a dream by rising from bed is even greater than average in PD because these patients may be especially prone to fall in the middle of the night when antiparkinson medications have worn off. For PD patients with RSBD, the treatment is much the same as in non-PD patients, namely, clonazepam at bedtime. Because of the long efficacy half-life of clonazepam, a bedtime dosage can result in daytime somnolence. Accordingly, it is often useful to experiment with dosage times as far in advance of bedtime as possible to avoid this potential complication. PD patients who are not yet on levodopa therapy may find that this preparation ameliorates the symptoms of both PD and RSBD (62).

The syndrome of periodic limb movements of sleep (PLMS) is commonly encountered in PD patients although there is little documentation in the literature of its exact incidence in this population (66). In one study, the incidence of PLMS in PD patients increased in proportion to the severity of the parkinsonian symptoms (67). This syndrome, often erroneously referred to as nocturnal myoclonus, consists of stereotypical movements of the lower extremities characterized by extension of the great toe and ankle and flexion at the knee and sometimes the hip. Rarely, the upper extremities are involved. The patient may or may not be aware of these movements. Occasionally, only the bed partner is disturbed by them. PLMS is especially common in patients suffering from the restless-legs syndrome (RLS). Almost all patients with RLS also experience PLMS, but not all patients suffering from PLMS have RLS. As with RSBD, the treatment of PLMS in PD is similar to that in the non-PD population (68), with one exception. Levodopa is the drug of choice for PLMS in the non-PD population, but PD patients may already be receiving this medication. In this case, a bedtime dosage of sustained-release levodopa should be added if it is not already a part of the patient's regimen. Dopamine agonists administered at bedtime are also a useful therapy for this condition. Clonazepam is the next most effective therapy, followed by opioids such as oxycodone or propoxyphene. Benzodiazepines other than clonazepam, such as triazolam, are useful, especially for reducing PLMS-related arousals (69). Combination therapy with two agents is sometimes required in these patients (68).

Another parasomnia, somnambulism, has been reported to appear with increased frequency in PD. Merello et al. (70) reported a 5% incidence of sleepwalking among 312 PD patients studied, which is twice the frequency observed in a study of a large non-PD population (71).

Effect of Sleep on Parkinson's Disease

Sleep typically has a salutary effect on the symptoms of PD. The most common diurnal pattern of symptom severity in PD is that of improvement in motoric function just after arising in the morning. This is paralleled by improvement in nonmotoric dopamine-dependent functions at the same time of day (31). In a recent study, 25% of PD patients reported a greater than 40% improvement in PD symptoms following nocturnal sleep, with a duration of benefit ranging from 30 minutes to 3 hours (72). This effect was most prominent in younger patients and those with milder symptoms; however, two subsequent studies found sleep benefit of this type to be most common in patients with longer disease duration (70,73). In these two surveys, the incidence of sleep benefit was still higher, ranging between 33 and 55% of PD patients.

The beneficial effect of sleep on the symptoms of PD can be so prominent in some patients as to eliminate the need for antiparkinson medications for the first half of the day. The mechanisms underlying this phenomenon are not yet fully understood. Comella et al. (72) hypothesized that sleep benefit may result from the effect of sleep on residual dopamine storage, while Currie et al. (73) suggested that patients taking higher dosages of levodopa have higher residual tissue levodopa levels in the morning. Merello and colleagues' results (70) argue against both of these theories. Their findings indicated that sleep benefit does not correlate with the use of controlled-release levodopa, which would be expected to enhance residual tissue levodopa in the morning. They also noted that PD patients with the least restful sleep and the most nocturnal awakenings appear to have the greatest sleep benefit, arguing against the hypothesis that the restorative properties of sleep improve dopamine storage.

MULTIPLE-SYSTEM ATROPHY

Multiple-system atrophy (MSA) is a degenerative extrapyramidal disorder characterized by parkinsonism, symptoms of cerebellar dysfunction, and autonomic failure, each to various degrees of severity in individual patients. The condition is thought to represent the combined clinical and histological result of its component disorders: striatonigral degeneration (resulting in parkinsonism), olivopontocerebellar atrophy (resulting in cerebellar signs), and Shy-Drager syndrome (resulting in prominent autonomic symptoms) (74). Although these component symptoms can occur in any combination, parkinsonism is present in the great majority of patients, followed in frequency by autonomic failure and cerebellar dysfunction.

Disrupted sleep patterns are common in MSA. Manni et al. (75), studying patients with MSA and autonomic failure, found their sleep to be characterized by reduced total sleep time, less REM-sleep time, and prolonged REM latency. They also noted either obstructive, central, or mixed sleep apnea in approximately half of this patient population. Patients with the most severe autonomic dysfunction were at greatest risk for developing abnormal breathing during sleep.

A serious and potentially fatal sleep-related breathing disorder in MSA is nocturnal vocal-cord abductor paralysis (76–78). In the early stages of this dysfunction, vocal-cord movement may be normal during wakefulness and exhibit paradoxical movements only during sleep. At this stage, suspected vocal-cord paralysis can be confirmed reliably only by laryngoscopy performed during sleep (78). With further progression, there may be both daytime and nighttime inspiratory stridor. Also, at this time there may be the onset of peculiar snoring that is different in pitch from ordinary soft-palate snoring owing to its origin from the vibrating glottis (77,78). Sudden nocturnal death has occurred in several MSA patients with this vocal-cord syndrome, presumably due to respiratory arrest (77,79). Because of the potential seriousness of this syndrome, careful investigation, possibly including sleep laryngoscopy, is indicated in the MSA patient exhibiting loud, high-pitched snoring. If vocal-cord abductor paralysis is demonstrated, there should be consideration of early tracheostomy (76,77,79).

Another sleep-related disorder that has become increasingly recognized in MSA is RSBD. As in the case in Parkinson's disease, RSBD can occasionally be the presenting symptom of MSA (80). In addition, its overall prevalence in clinically established MSA is probably much higher than previously suspected. Plazzi et al. (81) reported the results of polysomnography in 39 consecutive patients with MSA. Of these patients, 69% reported nocturnal paradoxical episodes related to dreams, suggesting RSBD. By polysomnographic evaluation 90% of these patients were felt to have RSBD. Twelve of the patients reported symptoms of RSBD for at least 1 year preceding the clinical onset of MSA, again confirming the notion that RSBD not infrequently antedates the extrapyramidal disorders with which it is associated. Other forms of sleep disturbance were documented in this study. Six patients demonstrated obstructive sleep apnea, eight had laryngeal stridor, and 10 had PLMS. Based on these results, the authors suggested that RSBD may be the most common sleep disorder in MSA rather than sleep breathing disorders. The finding of absent REM atonia in a high percentage of MSA patients without sleep complaints supports this notion (82).

Another potential sleep-related problem in MSA is nocturnal hypertension. Patients with Shy-Drager syndrome frequently require medications such as fludrocortisone or midodrine to counteract orthostatic hypotension occurring during the day. These agents may result in significant hypertension while the patient is asleep and recumbent. It is usually advised that patients requiring these agents not take a large dosage close to bedtime. In addition, elevation of the head of the bed is often required to reduce the potential for nocturnal recumbent hypertension.

PROGRESSIVE SUPRANUCLEAR PALSY

Progressive supranuclear palsy (PSP) is a degenerative central nervous system disorder characterized by supranuclear gaze palsy, parkinsonism, axial dystonia and rigidity, and early gait disturbance (83). The most consistent sleep abnormality reported in PSP is an absence or severe reduction of REM sleep (84,85). This reduction in REM sleep results from REM periods that are both fewer in number and shorter in duration. Additionally, PSP patients have been found to have shorter total sleep time, reduced sleep efficiency, a marked reduction in sleep spindles, and atonic slow-wave sleep (85). REM-sleep atonia is preserved—a surprising finding in light of the fact that the frequent absence of REM atonia in PD has been attributed to dysfunction of the pedunculopontine nucleus, a structure that is typically abnormal in PSP (85). Frequent nocturnal awakenings are common in PSP (84–87), and several studies have concluded that the number of awakenings and reduction of sleep time in PSP is proportional to the severity of the underlying neurological symptoms (84,86). Sleep-related respiratory disorders are typically not a source of major disability in PSP. Aldrich et al. (84) found only mild central, obstructive, or mixed apneas in PSP and noted that they did not constitute a major source of sleep disability. Other investigators were unable to detect evidence of even mild nocturnal respiratory dysfunction in PSP patients, including those with severe underlying neurological dysfunction and those with a significant daytime disturbance of voluntary respiration (86).

OTHER PARKINSONIAN SYNDROMES

A variety of other neurological conditions may be associated with parkinsonian symptoms. Conditions such as corticobasal degeneration, Hallervorden-Spatz syndrome, and X-linked dystonia parkinsonism (Lubag) are relatively uncommon, and their potential interaction with sleep has not been well documented or studied. To the extent that patients with these disorders manifest nocturnal rigidity and akinesia, they are susceptible to the same types of sleep disruption caused by these motor symptoms as those experienced by PD patients. Another parkinsonian syndrome, diffuse Lewy body disease, is characterized by parkinsonian features and early dementia. These patients are even more susceptible to drug-induced nocturnal hallucinosis and vivid dreaming than PD patients are. In this syndrome, as in PD, RSBD can appear years before typical motor or cognitive symptoms (64).

DYSTONIA

Dystonia is an abnormal involuntary movement characterized by sustained and twisting postures. The pattern of body parts involved may be focal or generalized. One of the most common generalized dystonias is idiopathic torsion dystonia, and the most common focal dystonias are spasmodic torticollis and writer's cramp. Considerable investigation has centered on the degree to which dystonia persists or is altered during sleep. Most observers have suggested that in both generalized and focal dystonias the abnormal movement seen in the waking state is improved during sleep, and in some cases totally abolished (11,87–89). Fish et al. (11)

noted that dystonic movements, although greatly attenuated during sleep, were still present in stage 1 and 2 sleep, as well as during awakenings and lightening of sleep. In a parallel study, the same investigators demonstrated that dystonia disappears during REM sleep, and normal REM sleep atonia is maintained. This was further documented by the demonstration of reduced motor responses to scalp magnetic stimulation during REM sleep (90). Similarly, in two studies, oromandibular focal dystonia improved, especially in deeper sleep, but never totally disappeared (87,88).

The sleep benefit in spasmodic torticollis may be considerably more striking. In this condition, Lobbezzoo et al. (89) demonstrated that patients experienced a significant decrease in abnormal cervical-muscle activity immediately upon lying down, with subsequent disappearance of all abnormal muscle activity during the transition to light non-REM sleep. In this form of dystonia, which exclusively involves axial postural muscles, the beneficial effects of recumbency appeared to considerably enhance the primary benefit derived from sleep.

Although dystonic movements are typically improved at night, patients with this condition still suffer from a variety of sleep disturbances, including increased sleep latency (89,91), reduced sleep efficiency (88,91), and reduced slow-wave and REM sleep (88). Treatment of the underlying dystonic disorder may influence these sleep abnormalities. Jankel et al. (92) noted that unilateral stereotactic thalamotomy for idiopathic torsion dystonia not only improved the abnormal involuntary movements but also normalized previously experienced sleep abnormalities such as reduced REM sleep. Whether improvement in sleep parameters in this circumstance reflects a primary physiological effect of the thalamic lesion or simply corresponds to the benefit of less severe nocturnal dystonia after treatment remains uncertain.

Two forms of dystonia deserve special mention because of their unique relationship to sleep. Nocturnal paroxysmal dystonia (NPD) is a symptom complex occurring during non-REM sleep. It is characterized by sudden onset of axial and appendicular dystonic posturing, often associated with a variety of seemingly purposeful movements or vocalizations (93). Occasionally, similar episodes occur during the day while awake. Despite the fact that the electroencephalogram is often normal during these attacks, their clinical resemblance to frontal-lobe epilepsy, their excellent response to carbamazepine, and the appearance of typical seizures in the same patient at other times suggest that NPD is epileptic in origin and not truly a primary movement disorder (94,95). A preferred name for this syndrome is nocturnal frontal lobe epilepsy (NFLE), although for many patients in this category, nocturnal paroxysmal dystonia is an appropriate descriptive term, if physiologically imprecise. In a study of 40 patients with an autosomal dominant form of NFLE, over 42% were found to manifest dystonic or dyskinetic movements during the typical nocturnal episodes (96). In many instances, these patients had previously been diagnosed as having a parasomnia based on their abnormal nocturnal movements and behavior.

Dopa-responsive dystonia (DRD) is an autosomal dominant, heritable condition characterized by a marked diurnal variation in severity of symptoms. In this condition, dystonia is typically least severe in the morning and then worsens as the day progresses, only to be relieved by sleep. DRD is known to be remarkably responsive to small dosages of levodopa. The recent discovery of the genetic basis for this condition explains the marked benefit derived from levodopa. The responsible gene for DRD encodes GTP cyclohydrolase I, which is the rate-limiting enzyme in the synthesis of tetrahydrobiopterin, an important cofactor in the metabolic pathway for dopamine (97). Levodopa not only has the potential to completely reverse dystonia in DRD but may also improve the insomnia that sometimes accompanies this disorder.

HUNTINGTON'S DISEASE AND CHOREA

The great majority of sleep investigations in choreic disorders have been performed in patients with the relatively common adult condition Huntington's disease (HD). Polysomnographic evaluations in HD have revealed a variety of sleep disturbances, including reduced sleep efficiency (98–100), prolonged sleep latency (99), reduced slow-wave sleep (98–100), frequent awakenings (99), and increased sleep-spindle density (99–101). Chorea improves during sleep, but never completely disappears (11,100), often appearing after awakenings, during lightening of sleep, or in stage 1 sleep (11). One group of investigators (98,99) found that sleep abnormalities in HD correlated with the duration and severity of clinical symptoms of the disorder as well as with the degree of caudate atrophy demonstrated by neuroimaging. Respiration during sleep in HD is normal (102), although daytime respiratory dyskinesias are common.

Although other forms of chorea are somewhat rarer and may have a different pathophysiological basis, sleep abnormalities in these conditions may be very similar to those found in HD. Sleep evaluation in a patient with vascular hemichorea revealed reduced total sleep time, prolonged sleep latency, and reduced slow-wave and REM sleep (103). After treatment with haloperidol, all these sleep parameters improved. These observations suggest that a bedtime dose of antichorea medication such as haloperidol, and perhaps reserpine, can improve disturbed sleep in the choreic patient. This may be particularly true in vascular hemichorea-hemiballism, in which the involuntary movement itself may be so violent as to inhibit initiation or continuation of sleep.

TOURETTE'S SYNDROME

Tourette's syndrome (TS) typically presents in childhood with a succession of motor and phonic tics, often associated with obsessive-compulsive behaviors and attention-deficit hyperactivity disorder (ADHD). It is most common in boys, and in many cases improves as the patient passes into adulthood (104). Tics in this disorder are characterized as being either simple or complex. Simple motor tics are meaningless motions, such as a shoulder shrug; complex motor tics are more purposeful and integrated movements, such as jumping. Simple phonic tics are sounds or articulations without meaning, such as throat-clearing, while complex vocal tics are understandable utterances, such as a word or phrase. Perhaps most disabling are vocal tics known as coprolalia, in which the vocal utterance contains socially unacceptable obscene words.

To a certain extent, motor and phonic tics are suppressible in the waking state. Both kinds continue to occur during sleep, especially stages 1 and 2, but their frequency is decreased (105). Just as in the waking state, phonic tics may take the form of coprolalia during sleep as well (106). A variety of sleep disturbances have been documented in TS, including night terrors (107), somnambulism (107,108), PLMS (109), and reduced sleep time (109). In one study, the existence of sleep disturbances in patients manifesting both TS and ADHD was especially high (41%) compared to those with TS alone (26%) (110). Sleep apnea can appear in TS, and it has been suggested that the TS gene confers a lifelong susceptibility to disorders of ventilatory control during sleep, resulting in a higher incidence of such conditions as infantile apnea and sudden infant death syndrome early in life and sleep apnea in adults (111).

MYOCLONUS

Myoclonus can originate at several different levels within the central nervous system, including the cortex, the brainstem, and the spinal cord (see also Chapter 9). It is difficult to make a global statement about sleep and the myoclonic disorders because they are of such diverse etiology and anatomical origin and each interacts with sleep somewhat differently. The myoclonus of Creutzfeldt-Jakob disease is of cortical origin and continues to appear during sleep, just as in wakefulness (112). Reticular reflex myoclonus, a form of brainstem myoclonus, was documented to persist during sleep in a patient with levodopa-resistant parkinsonism (113). While it is relatively easy to discern the effect of sleep on myoclonus, this case illustrates the difficulty of determining the effect of myoclonus on sleep. In this patient with parkinsonism, sleep architecture was markedly abnormal, but assigning causality to myoclonus is not possible since it represented only one symptom appearing within a syndrome with much broader neurological dysfunction.

The relationship of myoclonus and sleep is much easier to understand in patients with palatal myoclonus since this is a monosymptomatic syndrome. There are two basic categories of palatal myoclonus: essential palatal myoclonus (EPT), in which no structural pathology of the central nervous system is apparent, and symptomatic palatal myoclonus (SPT), which arises from a lesion in the Guillain Mollaret triangle of the brainstem. The clinical syndromes of EPT and

SPT are only slightly different but their interaction with sleep is dissimilar. During sleep, EPT ceases while SPT continues, with only a slight change in frequency of the repetitive movements (114,115). Neither appears to have very much effect on sleep; in fact, many patients are unaware of the syndrome except for an audible ear click which usually accompanies each palatal movement in EPT.

Spinal myoclonus is affected variably during sleep, depending on the precise etiology and location of the causative lesion. Although the generator for this form of myoclonus is within the spinal cord, it is almost always subject to supraspinal influences, which may in turn be modified by sleep. In essential spinal myoclonus, in which there is no apparent structural spinal-cord pathology, the abnormal movement may disappear entirely during sleep and reappear only during arousals (115). Supraspinal influence is very apparent in propriospinal myoclonus, a syndrome characterized by abnormal activity spreading both rostrally and caudally within the spinal cord. In three patients with this condition, myoclonus appeared only during mental relaxation and mild drowsiness, but then disappeared entirely during sleep (116). The myoclonus appearing during drowsiness was a major cause of insomnia in these patients. As would be expected, spinal myoclonus originating in segments below a complete spinal-cord transection is deprived of supraspinal control and is not influenced by sleep (117).

PRINCIPLES OF TREATMENT

Each of the specific sleep disorders appearing in the movement disorders discussed here merit individual analysis and appropriately tailored treatment strategies. There are, however, some general principles of therapy that are useful in approaching sleep dysfunction appearing in the context of an extrapyramidal disorder. The simplest and one of the most useful principles is based on the observation that hyperkinetic or hypokinetic movements that persist into the night can themselves disrupt sleep. Accordingly, the first goal of therapy should be to ameliorate nocturnal symptoms such as severe tremor, dystonia, rigidity, chorea, ballism, and hypokinetic immobility. The same pharmacological treatment strategy used to control these symptoms during the waking day can be applied at bedtime. Having done this, the second principle of therapy is to weigh the potential that any medication being used for this purpose at bedtime has for producing a direct adverse effect on sleep. For example, as discussed previously, levodopa given at bedtime may ameliorate nocturnal rigidity, tremor, and hypokinesia on the one hand—but can also prolong sleep latency, induce vivid dreaming, or result in nocturnal hallucinosis, all of which are counterproductive.

A second principle of treatment is that the therapy required for parasomnias associated with extrapyramidal disorders is usually similar to that used for the same parasomnias in the general population. Thus, clonazepam is useful in RSBD associated with extrapyramidal disorders and levodopa, dopamine agonists, and opioids are useful for RLS, provided they do not adversely interact with the predominant underlying neurological condition.

A final principle of therapy has to do with the adjustment of medications that are required for control of the waking movement disorder but may have adverse effects on sleep. In this circumstance, it is critical to attempt to distance the last medication dosage of the day as far away from bedtime as is feasible. Parkinson's patients with insomnia, for instance, should take their last required dosage of selegiline no later than noon. Similarly, Shy-Drager patients requiring therapy for hypotension should have their last daily dosage of medication administered as early in the evening as possible to avoid nocturnal hypertension. Adherence to these general guidelines will often enable the clinician to make significant strides in improving the sleep of patients with extrapyramidal disorders.

REFERENCES

1. Parkinson J. An Essay on the Shaking Palsy. London: Sherwood, Neely, and Jones, 1817.
2. Askenasy JJM. Sleep patterns in extrapyramidal disorders. Int J Neurol 1981; 15: 62–76.
3. Nausieda PA, Weiner WJ, Kaplan LR, Weber S, Klawans HL. Sleep disruption in the course of chronic levodopa therapy: an early feature of the levodopa psychosis. Clin Neuropharmacol 1982; 5:183–194.
4. Lees AJ, Blackburn NA, Campbell VL. The nighttime problems of Parkinson's disease. Clin Neuropharmacol 1988; 11:512–519.
5. Van Hilten B, Hoff JI, Huub AM, Middelkoop AM, van der Velde E, Kerkhof GA, Wauquier A, Kamphulsen HA, Roos RA. Sleep disruption in Parkinson's disease. Arch Neurol 1995; 51:922–928.
6. Smith MC, Ellgring H, Oertel WH. Sleep disturbances in Parkinson's disease patients and spouses. J Am Geriatr Soc 1997; 45:194–199.
7. Carter J, Carroll S, Cannon MC. Sleep disruption in untreated Parkinson's disease. Neurology 1990; 40(suppl 1):220.
8. Friedman A. Sleep pattern in Parkinson's disease. Acta Med Pol 1980; 21:193–199.
9. Emser W, Brenner M, Stober T. Changes in nocturnal sleep in Huntington's and Parkinson's disease. J Neurol 1988; 235:177–179.
10. Laihinen A, Alihanka J, Raitasuo S, Rinne UK. Sleep movements and associated autonomic nervous activities in patients with Parkinson's disease. ACTA Neurol Scand 1987; 76:64–68.
11. Fish DR, Sawyers D, Allen PJ, Blackie JD, Lees AJ, Marsden CD. The effect of sleep on the dyskinetic movement of Parkinson's disease, Giles de la Tourette syndrome, Huntington's disease and torsion dystonia. Arch Neurol 1991; 48:210–214.
12. Tassinari CA, Broughton R, Poire R. An electro-clinical study of nocturnal sleep

in patients presenting abnormal movements. Electroencephalogr Clin Neurophysiol 1965; 18:95.
13. April RS. Observations on parkinsonian tremor in all-night sleep. Neurology 1977; 16:720–724.
14. Stein M, Roffwarg H, Duvoisin R. The parkinsonian tremor in sleep. J Nerv Ment Dis 1968; 147:202–210.
15. Askenasy JJM, Yahr MD. Parkinsonian tremor loses its alternating aspect during non-REM sleep. J Neurol Neurosurg Psychiatry 1990; 52:749–753.
16. Askenasy JJM, Yahr MD. Suppression of REM rebound by pergolide. J Neurol Trans 1984; 59:151–159.
17. Lees AJ. Sustained release of l-dopa (Madopar HBS) in the treatment of nocturnal and early morning disabilities in Parkinson's disease. Eur Neurol 1987; 27(suppl 1):126–134.
18. Pahwa R, Busenbark K, Huber SJ, Michalek D, Hubble JP, Koller WC. Clinical experience with controlled-release carbidopa/levodopa in Parkinson's disease. Neurology 1993; 43:677–681.
19. Rodnitzky RL, Dickens QS, Dobson JK. Long-term clinical efficacy of Sinemet CR in patients with Parkinson's disease. Neurology 1989; 39(suppl):92–95.
20. Jansen EN, Meerwaldtt JD. Madopar HBS in nocturnal symptoms of Parkinson's disease. Adv Neurol 1990; 53:527–531.
21. Leeman AL, Oneil CJ, Nicholson PW, Deshmuch AA, Denham MJ, Royston JP, Dobbs RJ, Dobbs SM. Parkinson's disease in the elderly: response to and optimal spacing of night time dosing with levodopa. Br J Clin Pharmacol 1987; 24:637–643.
22. Comella CL, Tanner CM, Ristanovic RL. Polysomnographic sleep measures in Parkinson's disease patients with treatment induced hallucinations. Ann Neurol 1993; 34:710–714.
23. Dooneief G, Mirabello E, Bell K, Marder K, Stern Y, Mayeux R. An estimate of the incidence of depression in idiopathic Parkinson's disease. Arch Neurol 1992; 49:305–307.
24. Starkstein SE, Preziosi TJ, Robinson RG. Sleep disorders, pain and depression in Parkinson's disease. Eur Neurol 1991; 31:352–355.
25. Menza MA, Rosen RC. Sleep in Parkinson's disease: the role of depression and anxiety. Psychosomatics 1995; 3G:262–266.
26. Kostic VS, Susic V, Przdborski S, Sternic N. Sleep EEG in depressed and nondepressed patients with Parkinson's disease. J Neuropsychiatr Clin Neurosci 1991; 3:176–179.
27. Koller WC, Silver DE, Lieberman A, eds. An algorithm for the management of Parkinson's disease. Neurology 1994;44(suppl 10):S1–52.
28. Jansen Steur ENH. Increase of Parkinson disability after fluoxetine medication. Neurology 1993; 43:211–213.
29. Suchowersky O, deVries JD. Interaction of fluoxetine and selegiline. Can J Psychiatry 1990; 35:571–572.
30. Richard IH, Kurlan R. A survey of antidepressant drug use in Parkinson's disease. Neurology 1997; 49:1168–1170.

31. Struck LK, Rodnitzky RL, Dobson JK. Circadian fluctuations of contrast sensitivity in Parkinson's disease. Neurology 1990; 40:467–470.
32. Rodnitzky RL, Dobson JK. Circadian variability of olfactory function in Parkinson's disease. Proceedings of the 10th International Symposium on Parkinson's disease. Tokyo, 1991:177.
33. Factor SA, McAlanarney T, Sanchez-Ramos JR, Weiner WJ. Sleep disorders and sleep effect in Parkinson's disease. Mov Disord 1990; 5:280–285.
34. Mayer G, Ewert Meier K, Klinik Hephata. Selegeline hydrochloride treatment in narcolepsy: a double-blind placebo-controlled study. Clin Neuropharmacol 1995; 18:306–319.
35. Reinish LW, MacFarlane JG, Sandor P, Shapiro CM. REM changes in narcolepsy with selegiline. Sleep 1995; 18:362–367.
36. U.S. Modafinil in Narcolepsy Multicenter Study Group. Randomized trial of Modafinil for the treatment of pathological somnolence in narcolepsy. Ann Neurol 1998; 43:88–97.
37. Lack L, Wright H. The effect of evening bright light in delaying the circadian rhythms and lengthening the sleep of early morning awakenings insomniacs. Sleep 1993; 16:436–443.
38. Campbell SS, Murphy PJ. Extraocular circadian phototransduction in humans. Science 1998; 279:396–399.
39. Ferini-Strambi L, Franceschi M, Pinto P, Zucconi M, Smirne S. Respiration and heart rate variability during sleep in untreated Parkinson's patients. Gerontology 1992; 38:92–98.
40. Hardie RJ, Efthimiou J, Stern GM. Respiration and sleep in Parkinson's disease. J Neurol Neurosurg Psychiatry 1986; 49:1326.
41. Apps MC, Sheaff PC, Ingram DA, Kennard C, Empey DW. Respiration and sleep in Parkinson's disease. J Neurol Neurosurg Psychiatry 1985; 48:1240–1245.
42. Gillin JC, Post RM, Wyatt RJ, Goodwin FK, Snyder F, Bunney WE. REM inhibitory effect of l-dopa infusion during human sleep. Electroencephalogr Clin Neurophysiol 1973; 35:181–186.
43. Van Hilten JJ, Weggeman M, van der Velde EA, Kerkhof GA, Van Dijk JG, Roos RA. Sleep, excessive daytime sleepiness and fatigue in Parkinson's disease. J Neurol Trans 1994; 5:235–244.
44. Kales A, Ansel R, Markham C, Scharf M, Tan T. Sleep in patients with Parkinson's disease and normal subsets prior to and following levodopa administration. Clin Pharmacol Ther 1971; 12:397–406.
45. Wyatt RJ, Chase TN, Scott J, Snyder S. Effect of l-dopa on the sleep of man. Nature 1970; 228:999–1001.
46. Factor SA, Molho ES, Podskalny GD, Brown O. Parkinson's disease: drug-induced psychiatric states. Adv Neurol 1995; 65:115–138.
47. Sanchez-Ramos J, Ortou R, Paulson GW. Visual hallucinations associated with Parkinson's disease. Arch Neurol 1996; 53:1265–1268.
48. Klein C, Kompf D, Pulkowski U, Moser A, Vieregge P. A study of visual hallucinations in patients with Parkinson's disease. J Neurol 1997; 244:371–377.
49. Wolters EC, Jansen EN, Tuynman-Qua HG, Bergmans PL. Olanzapine in the treat-

ment of dopaminergicpsychosis in patients with Parkinson's disease. Neurology 1996; 47:1085–1087.

50. Mecu G, Alessandri A, Gisutini P, Bonifati V. Risperidone in levodopa-induced psychosis in advanced Parkinson's disease: an open-label, long-term study. Mov Disord 1997; 12:610–612.
51. Friedman JH, Lannon MC. Clozapine in the treatment of psychosis in Parkinson's disease. Neurology 1989; 39:1219–1221.
52. Marconi R, Lefebure-Caparos D, Bonnet AM, Vidailhet M, Dubois B, Agid Y. Levodopa-induced dyskinesias in Parkinson's disease: phenomenology and pathophysiology. Mov Disord 1994; 9:2–12.
53. Mouret J. Differences in sleep in patients with Parkinson's disease. Electroencephalogr Clin Neurophysiol 1975; 38:653–65.
54. Klawans H, Goetz C, Bergen D. Levodopa-induced myoclonus. Arch Neurol 1975; 32:331–334.
55. Linazasoro, Marti Masso JF, Suarez JA. Nocturnal akathisia in Parkinson's disease, treatment with clozapine. Mov Disord 1993; 171–174.
56. Lang AE, Johnson K. Akathisia in idiopathic Parkinson's disease. Neurology 1987; 477–481.
57. Thorpy MJ, and the Diagnostic Classification Steering Committee. The International Classification of Sleep Disorders: Diagnostic and Coding Manual. Rochester, MN: American Sleep Disorders Association, 1990.
58. Dyken ME, Rodnitzky RL. Periodic, aperiodic, and rhythmic motor disorders of sleep. Neurology 1992; 42(suppl 6):68–74.
59. Silber MA, Ahlskog JE. REM sleep behavior disorder in parkinsonian syndromes. Sleep Res 1992; 21:313.
60. Uchiyama M, Isse K, Tanaka K, Yokota N, Hammamoto M, Aida S, Ito Y, Yoshimura M, Okawa M. Incidental Lewy body disease in a patient with REM sleep behavior disorder. Neurology 1995; 45:709–712.
61. Louden MB, Morehead MA, Schmidt HS. Activation by selegiline (Eldepryl) of REM sleep behavior disorder in parkinsonism. W Virginia Med J 1995; 91:101.
62. Tan A, Salgado M, Fahn S. Rapid eye movement sleep behavior disorder preceding Parkinson's disease with therapeutic response to levodopa. Mov Disord 1996; 11: 214–216.
63. Schenck CH, Bundlie SR, Mahowald MW. Delayed emergence of a Parkinsonian disorder in 38% of 29 older men initially diagnosed with idiopathic rapid eye movement sleep behavior disorder. Neurology 1996; 46:388–393.
64. Turner RS, Chervin RD, Minoshima S, Kuhl DE. Probable diffuse Lewy body disease presenting as REM sleep behavior disorder. Neurology 1997; 49:523–527.
65. Culebras A, Moore JT. Magnetic resonance findings in REM sleep behavior disorder. Neurology 1989; 9:1519–1523.
66. Askenasy JJ, Weitzman ED, Yahr MD. Are periodic movements in sleep a basal ganglia disorder? J Neural Trans 1987; 70:333–347.
67. Horiguchi J, Inami Y, Nishimatsu O, Innami T, Kakimoto Y. Sleep wake complaints in Parkinson's disease. Rinsho Shinkeigaku 1990; 30:214–216.
68. Henning WA, Walters AS, Chokroverty S. Treatment of the restless legs syndrome: current practices of sleep experts. Neurology 1995; 45(suppl 4):A285.

69. Bonnet MH, Arand DL. Chronic use of triazolam in patients with periodic leg movements, fragmented sleep and daytime sleepiness. Aging 1991; 3:313–324.
70. Merello M, Hughes A, Colosimo C, Hoffman M, Starkstein S, Leiguarda R. Sleep benefit in Parkinson's disease. Mov Disord 1997; 12:506–508.
71. Bixler EO, Kales A. Prevalence of sleep disorders in the Los Angeles metropolitan area. Am J Psychiatry 1979; 136:1257–1262.
72. Comella CL, Bohmer J, Stebbins GT. Sleep benefit in Parkinson's disease. Neurology 1995; 45(suppl 4):A286.
73. Currie LJ, Bennett JP, Harison MB, Trugman JM, Wooten GF. Clinical correlates of sleep benefit in Parkinson's disease. Neurology 1997; 1115–1117.
74. Wenning GK, Ben-Shlomo Y, Magalhaes M. Clinical features and natural history of multiple system atrophy: an analysis of 100 cases. Brain 1994; 117:835–845.
75. Manni R, Morini R, Martignoni E, Pacchetti C, Micieli G, Tartara A. Nocturnal sleep in multisystem atrophy with autonomic failure: polygraphic findings in ten patients. J Neurol 1993; 240:249–250
76. Isozaki E, Naito A, Heriguhi S, Kawamura R, Hayashida T, Tanabe H. Early diagnosis and stage classification of vocal cord abductor paralysis in patients with multiple system atrophy. J Neurol Neurosurg Psychiatry 1996; 60:399–402.
77. Sadaoka T, Kakitsuba N, Fujiwara Y, Kanai R, Takahashi H. Sleep-related breathing disorders in patients with multiple system atrophy and vocal fold palsy. Sleep 1996; 19:479–484.
78. Kakitsuba N, Sadaoka T, Kanai R, Fujiwara Y, Takahashi H. Peculiar snoring in patients with multiple system atrophy: Its sound source, acoustic characteristics, and diagnostic significance. Ann Otol Rhinol Laryngol 1997; 106:380–384.
79. Munschauer FE, Loh L, Bannister R, Newson-Davis J. Abnormal respiration and sudden death during sleep in multiple system atrophy with autonomic failure. Neurology 1990; 40:670–679.
80. Tison F, Wenning GK, Quinn NP, Smith SJ. REM sleep behavior disorder as the presenting symptom of multiple system atrophy. J Neurol Neurosurg Psychiatry 1995; 58:379–380.
81. Plazzi G, Corsini R, Provini F, Pierangeci G, Martinelli P, Montagna P, Lugaresi E, Cortelli P. REM sleep behavior disorders in multiple system atrophy. Neurology 1997; 48:1094–1097.
82. Tachibana N, Kimura K, Kitajima K, Nagamine T, Kimura J, Shibasaki H. REM sleep without atonia at early stage of sporadic olivopontocerebellar atrophy. J Neurolog Sci 1995; 132:28–34.
83. Golbe L, Davis PH, Schoenberg BS, Duvoisin RC. Prevalence and natural history of progressive supranuclear palsy. Neurology 1988; 38:1031–1034.
84. Aldrich MS, Foster NL, White RF, Bluemlein L, Prokopowicz G. Sleep abnormalities in progressive supranuclear palsy. Ann Neurol 1989; 25:577–581.
85. Montplasir J, Petit D, Deeary A, Masson H, Bedard MA, Panisset M, Remillard G, Gauthier S. Sleep and quantitative EEG in patients with progressive supranuclear palsy. Neurology 1997; 49:999–1003.
86. DeBruin VS, Machado C, Howard RS, Hirsch NP, Lees AJ. Nocturnal and respiratory disturbances in Steele-Richardson-Olszewski syndrome (progressive supranuclear palsy). Postgrad Med J 1996; 72:293–296.

87. Silvestri R, DeDomenico P, DiRosa AE, Bramanti P, Serra S, DiPerri R. The effects of nocturnal physiologic sleep on various movement disorders. Mov Disord 1990; 5:8–14.
88. Sforza E, Montagna P, Defazio G, Lugaresi E. Sleep and cranial dystonia. Electroencephalogr Clin Neurophysiol 1991; 79:166–169.
89. Lobbezzoo F, Thu Thon M, Remillard G, Montplaisir JY, Lavigne GJ. Relationship between sleep, neck muscle activity, and pain in cervical dystonia. Can J Neurol Sci 1996; 23:285–290.
90. Fish DR, Sawyers D, Smith SJ, Allen PJ, Murray NM, Marsden CD. Motor inhibition from the brainstem is normal in torsion dystonia during REM sleep. J Neurol Neurosurg Psychiatry 1991; 54:140–144.
91. Jankel WR, Allen RP, Niedermeyer E, Kalsher MJ. Polysomnographic findings in dystonia musculorum deformans. Sleep 1983; 6:281–285.
92. Jankel WR, Niedermeyer E, Graf M, Kalsher MJ. Case report: polysomnographic effects of thalamotomy for torsion dystonia. Neurosurgery 1984; 14:495–498.
93. Lugaresi E, Cirignotta F, Montagna P. Nocturnal paroxysmal dystonia. J Neurol Neurosurg Psychiatry 1986; 49:375–380.
94. Tinuper P, Cerullo A, Cirignotta F, Cortelli D, Lugaresi E, Montagna P. Nocturnal paroxysmal dystonia with short-lasting attacks: three cases with evidence for an epileptic frontal lobe origin of seizures. Epilepsia 1990; 31:549–556.
95. Hirsch E, Sellal F, Maton B, Rumbach L, Mareseaux C. Nocturnal paroxysmal dystonia: a clinical form of focal epilepsy. Neurophysiol Clin 1994; 24:207–217.
96. Oldani A, Zucconi M, Asselta R, Modugno M, Bonati MA, Dalpra L, Malcovati M, Tenchini ML, Smirne S, Ferini-Strambi L. Autosomal dominant nocturnal frontal lobe epilepsy. Brain 1998; 121:205–223.
97. Ichinose H, Ohye T, Takahashi E. Hereditary progressive dystonia with marked diurnal fluctuation caused by mutations in GTP cyclohydrolase I gene. Nature Genet 1994; 8:236–242.
98. Wiegand M, Moller AA, Schreiber W, Lauer C, Krier JC. Brain morphology and sleep in patients with Huntington's disease. Eur Arch Psychiatry Clin Neurosci 1991; 240:148–152.
99. Wiegand M, Moller AA, Lauer CJ, Stultz S, Schreiber W, Dose M, Krier JC. Nocturnal sleep in Huntington's disease. J Neurol 1991; 238:203–208.
100. Silvestri R, Raffaele M, DeDomenico P, Tisano A, Mento G, Casella C, Tripoli MC, Serra S, Diperri R. Sleep features in Tourette's syndrome, neuroacanthocytosis and Huntington's chorea. Neurophysiol Clin 1995; 25:66–77.
101. Emser W, Brenner M, Stuber T, Schimrick K. Changes in nocturnal sleep in Huntington's and Parkinson's disease. J Neurol 1998; 235:177–179.
102. Bollen EL, Den Heijer JC, Ponsioen C, Kramer C, Van der Velde EA, Van Dijk JG, Roos RA, Kamphuisen HA, Buruma OJ. Respiration during sleep in Huntington's chorea. J Neurolog Sci 1988; 84:63–68.
103. Pucca FM, Mineruini MG, Savarese M, Quarta F, DeMarzo C, Lanave C. Sleep in a case of hemiballism. Boll Soc Ital Biol Sper 1984; 60:981–987.
104. Kurlan R. Tourette's syndrome: current concepts. Neurology 1989; 39:1625–1630.
105. Glaze DG, Frost JD, Jankovic J. Sleep in Gilles de la Tourette syndrome: disorder of arousal. Neurology 1983; 33:586–592.

106. Burd L, Kerbeshian J. Nocturnal coprolalia and phonic tics. Am J Psychiatry 1988; 145:132.
107. Comings DE, Comings BG. A controlled study of Tourette syndrome. VI. Early development, sleep problems, allergies and handedness. Am J Hum Genet 1987; 41:822–838.
108. Barabas G, Matthews WS, Ferrari M. Somnambulism in children with Tourette's syndrome. Dev Med Child Neurol 1984; 26:457–460.
109. Voderholzer U, Muller N, Haag C, Riemann D, Straube A. Periodic limb movements during sleep are a frequent finding in patients with Gilles de la Tourette's Syndrome. J Neurol 1997; 244:521–526.
110. Allen RP, Singer HS, Brown JE, Salam MM. Sleep disorders in Tourette syndrome: a primary or unrelated problem? Pediatr Neurol 1992; 8:275–280.
111. Sverd J, Montero G. Is Tourette Syndrome a cause of sudden infant death syndrome and childhood obstructive sleep apnea? Am J Med Genet 1993; 46:494–496.
112. Callena J, Carpizo R, Berchiano J, Quintial C, Polo J. Serial waking-sleep EEGs and evaluation of somato-sensory potentials in Creutzfeldt-Jakob disease. Electroencephalogr Clin Neurophysiol 1985; 60:504–508.
113. Clouston PD, Lim CL, Fung V, Yiannikas C, Morris JG. Brainstem myoclonus in a patient with non-dopa-responsive parkinsonism. Mov Disord 1996; 11:404–410.
114. Deuschl G, Toro C, Valls-Sole J, Zeffiro T, Zee DS, Hallett M. Symptomatic and essential palatal tremor. I. Clinical, physiological and MRI analysis. Brain 1994; 117:775–788.
115. Bauleo S, DeMitri P, Coccagna G. Evolution of segmental myoclonus during sleep: polygraphic study of two cases. Ital J Neurolog Sci 1996; 17:227–232
116. Montagna P, Provini F, Plazzi G, Liguori R, Lugaresi E. Propiospinal myoclonus upon relaxation and drowsiness: a cause of severe insomnia. Mov Disord 1997; 12:66–72.
117. Yokota T, Hirose K, Tanabe H, Tsukagoshi H. Sleep-related periodic leg movements (nocturnal myoclonus) due to spinal cord lesion. J Neurolog Sci 1991; 104: 13–18.

12

Sleep and Nocturnal Delirium in the Dementias

Alzheimer's Disease, Multi-Infarct Dementia, and Parkinson's Disease

Donald L. Bliwise
Emory University School of Medicine
and Wesley Woods Geriatric Hospital
Atlanta, Georgia

TECHNICAL CONSIDERATIONS FOR POLYSOMNOGRAPHY IN DEMENTED POPULATIONS

Conducting clinical polysomnography in patients with dementia represents a considerable technological challenge at several different levels. First, it should be clear what diagnostic question underlies the basis for referral and the necessity for the study. Viable reasons for polysomnography of a demented patient in the laboratory include but are not limited to: 1) differential diagnosis of abnormal nocturnal behavior (e.g., REM vs. non-REM parasomnias vs. nocturnal paroxysmal dystonia vs. agitation arising out of the waking state), 2) elucidation of the basis for uncontrollable excessive daytime sleepiness to an extent out of proportion to the patient's age, and 3) evaluation of breathing disorder in sleep as a possible cause of excess disability or, conceivably, dementia in a geriatric patient (Bliwise, 1996). Less compelling reasons for studying such patients in the sleep laboratory would be confirmation of specific dementia diagnoses or to assist in the differential diagnosis of dementia versus depression (see "Sleep in Alzheimer's Disease" below).

Once the decision to perform nocturnal polysomnography has been made, the value of including daytime testing with the multiple sleep latency test (MSLT) or the maintenance of wakefulness test (MWT) should also be carefully considered, particularly if daytime hypersomnolence is at issue. For example, we have recently noted that a surprising number of patients with narcolepsy present in their later years, often having undergone extensive radiological workups to evaluate possible ischemic events and/or other presumed autonomic dysfunction (Rye et al., 1998). Additionally, use of the MSLT in patients with Parkinson's disease (PD) has shown that some may present with multiple REM-sleep onsets on the MSLT (Dihenia et al., 1997; Johnston et al., 1998). Both phenomenological and neurobiological parallels between narcolepsy and PD have been noted (Johnston et al., 1998) that may involve similar elements of disruption in striatal/dopaminergic circuits and brainstem centers impacting upon REM atonia (Rye, 1997).

Managing the demented patient in the sleep laboratory requires particular interpersonal and technical skills on the part of the polysomnographic technologist. In many cases, it is important for the technologist to understand that the patient is likely to benefit from a highly structured environment. It is also essential that the technologist realize that demented patients may be less aware of what is happening to them and less able to recall otherwise rational explanations of procedures that may have been given only several minutes earlier. Often, having the primary or nighttime caregiver of the patient accompany him or her to the laboratory (and, if necessary, actually spend the night in an adjacent bedroom) is helpful. Reassurance for and questions of the caregiver can be answered, thus allowing the patient, although incapable of fully understanding the explanations, to feel comfortable with the people performing the recording procedures and laboratory environment. Finally, the technologist should be aware that at any point during the night the demented patient may arouse and attempt to leave not only the bed but also the facility. We have noticed this even in patients who do not have an explicit history of ''sundowning'' per se (see below). The unfamiliarity of the nocturnal environment can be quite disruptive for the mentally compromised patient who awakens in the middle of the night in what are otherwise strange surroundings. The technologist who is used to quiet ''down time'' once ''lights out'' has occurred may find that studying a demented patient in the sleep laboratory is quite demanding.

A particularly difficult aspect of performing polysomnography in demented patients is the discrimination of traditionally defined sleep stages. Although in their original manual describing the arbitrary rules for scoring of discrete sleep stages Rechtschaffen and Kales (1968) left open the possibility of alternative stage scoring criteria, they certainly never envisioned the possibility that those definitions of state would themselves subject to change. Yet, as our conceptualization of dissociative states has advanced from an experimental model of absence of REM-sleep atonia in a feline pontine lesion preparation (Henley and Morrison,

1974) to a parallel recognition in human disease (Schenck et al., 1986, 1987), our view of what constitutes REM sleep has been dramatically altered. The well-accepted notion of REM sleep without atonia has since broadened into a concept of dissociative states in general (Mahowald and Schenck, 1991) and the demonstration of pontine lesions present in such patients on MRI (Culebras and Moore, 1989) provides a structural basis for this state.

In scoring sleep in demented patients, the likelihood of encountering diffuse slow (<2 Hz) activity on the central EEG lead during behaviorally defined wakefulness makes difficult the discrimination of non-REM sleep, specifically initial stage 1. We encourage careful behavioral observations by the technologist with precise notations on the recording, since such observations may enhance appreciation of state; elsewhere we (Bliwise et al., 1990a,b; 1995) have even shown the value of behavioral observations per se of sleep–wake state in dementia in the absence of polysomnography.

Figure 1 shows the exaggerated (i.e., exceptionally slow, often less than 0.5 Hz) delta activity during deep non-REM sleep in a 69-year-old woman with

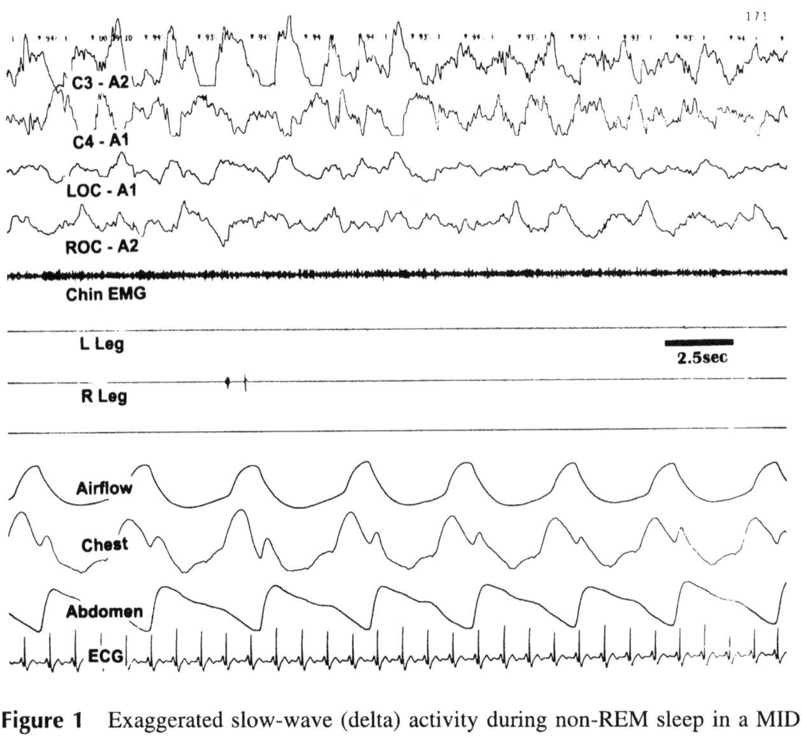

Figure 1 Exaggerated slow-wave (delta) activity during non-REM sleep in a MID patient.

multi-infarct dementia. Similarly, Figure 2 demonstrates the transition from waking to stage 1 sleep in a 91-year-old woman with prior stroke; the presence of somewhat slower alpha band activity (7–8 Hz), as well as delta frequencies, makes for difficult differentiation of the point of sleep onset, although the decreases in mentalis electromyogram (EMG) and alterations in respiration may be clues to the impending change in state.

Discrimination of not only non-REM but also REM sleep is hampered by such slow activity. Figures 3 (Alzheimer's disease) and 4 (multi-infarct dementia) show REM sleep in two of these three patients. Because of the difficulties in identifying the EEG of REM sleep in Alzheimer's disease (AD) and vascular dementias, reliance on a high-quality, low-impedence surface EMG from the mentalis assumes added importance, although in the case of parkinsonian syndromes such EMG recordings may have their own distinctive characteristics (see below). Similarly, two monopolar leads (right and left outer canthus) for recording electro-oculogram (EOG) referenced to the opposite mastoid can assume yet greater importance in identifying REM in AD, though density of eye movements in REM tends to be decreased in AD (Bliwise, 1993).

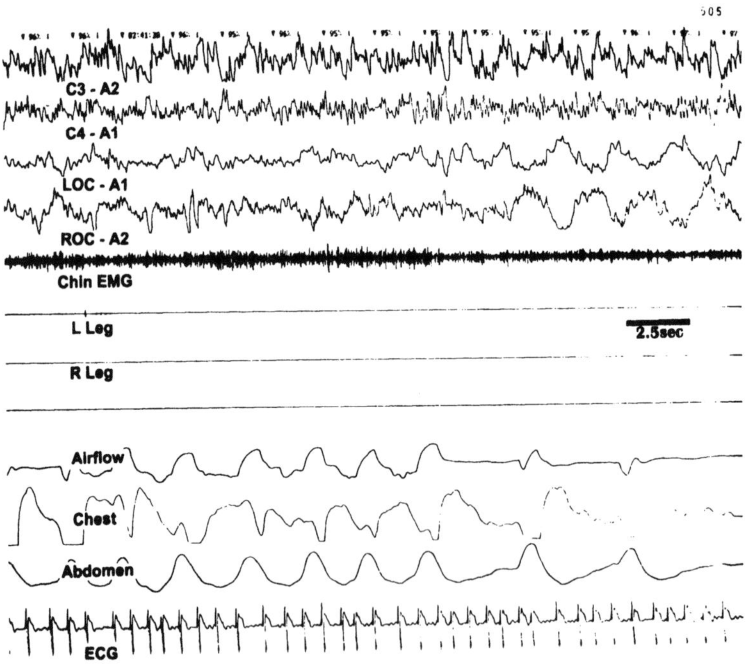

Figure 2 Transition from waking to stage 1 in a stroke patient.

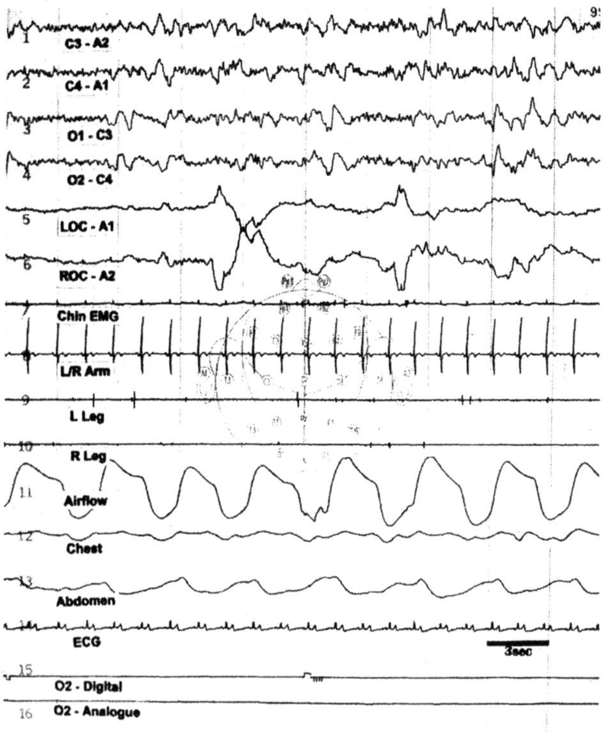

Figure 3 REM sleep in an AD patient showing continuing slow-wave (delta) activity in the EEG.

Insofar as non-REM sleep stages are concerned, the presence of widespread delta frequencies in the EEG of many dementia patients has led some investigators to propose the benefit of scoring ''indeterminate'' non-REM sleep rather than attempting to discern customary non-REM sleep stages in these recordings (Reynolds et al., 1985). Such alternative scoring may also be advisable, given deterioration in other EEG sleep landmarks as well, such as sleep spindles. Our recent experience with scoring non-REM sleep in PD patients (Williams et al., 1998), underscores the necessity of scoring non-REM sleep in this manner (see below).

In PD, the dissociation of muscle atonia from REM sleep makes for a particularly difficult challenge in identifying REM sleep. The development of PD has been shown in some cases to be heralded years earlier by REM-sleep behavior disorder (RSBD) (Schenck et al., 1996). This pattern has been suggested in the

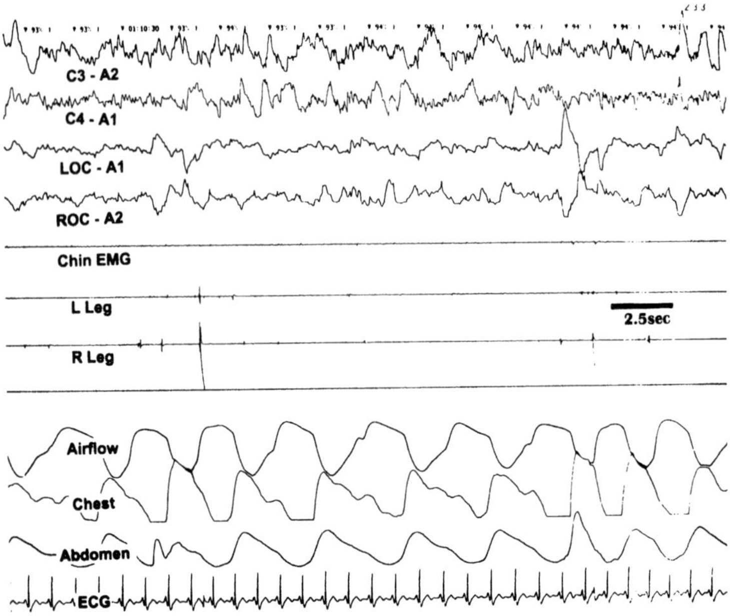

Figure 4 REM sleep in an MID patient showing continuing slow-wave (delta) activity in the EEG.

development of Lewy body dementia (Turner et al., 1997) as well other neurodegenerative conditions such as multisystem atrophy (Tachibana et al., 1997). The suspension of typical REM-sleep atonia in full-fledged disease again represents a challenge to conventional notions of state. The manual by Rechtschaffen and Kales (1968) relies heavily on the absence of muscle tone in the mimetic musculature to derive stage scoring of REM sleep, particularly when the EEG shows mixed-frequency (4–7 Hz), low-voltage activity and eye movements are relatively sparse. Without muscle atonia as an "anchor," it becomes considerably more difficult to define whether the state under question more closely resembles waking or REM sleep. The clinical phenomonology of dream-enactment behaviors (often resembling waking behavior) only underscores this issue.

Given these challenges to the reliable discrimination of state in patients with neurodegenerative disease, we had three experienced scorers each independently score polysomnograms from 10 PD patients (Williams et al., 1998). The patients had moderate to advanced disease and all were treated with Sinemet. A variety of medications including serotonin-reuptake inhibitors, dopamine agonists, and benzodiazepines were also used. Sleep apnea was minimal in this group. The three scorers were all experienced in technical aspects of polysomnography in dementia patients in general, and in PD patients in particular. Data were analyzed for all possible scorer pairs. Results indicated that when non-REM sleep stages were collapsed so that scorers were compared only on their reliability to discriminate waking/REM/non-REM, relatively high levels of agreement were obtained. On the basis of 8395 epochs, the average scorer pair agreement was 87% with the majority of disagreements occurring among wakefulness versus non-REM sleep (average = 8.3%). When non-REM sleep was broken down into its component stages, however, average pair agreement was considerably lower (72%), suggesting that scorers had considerable difficulty achieving reliability among the various non-REM stages, undoubtedly reflecting discriminations made more difficult because of diffuse slow activity in the EEG.

SLEEP IN ALZHEIMER'S DISEASE

Sleep in AD has been studied relatively extensively using both polysomnographic and actigraphic techniques. More detailed description of this literature has been offered elsewhere (Bliwise 1993, 1994a), but, in brief, it appears that sleep efficiencies and the proportion of stages 3–4 sleep decrease in association with the extent of severity of the dementia. REM sleep (as a proportion of total sleep) has also been shown to be negatively correlated with level of dementia on the Mini-Mental State Exam (Vitiello et al., 1990). Other aspects of REM sleep have been reported to be altered in AD as well, such as decreased density of eye-movement activity and an increased latency to the first REM sleep period (REM latency). These changes in REM would be predicted by the dependency of REM sleep on cholinergic systems in the CNS and the widespread cholinergic deterioration that is the neurochemical hallmark of AD.

More recent sophisticated signal processing of the EEG during REM sleep in AD patients has revealed that 3–7 Hz spectral power recorded occipitally during REM distinguished very mild AD patients from elderly controls (Prinz et al., 1992). Furthermore, Petit et al. (1992) noted that asymmetry of temporal regions in REM sleep better distinguished AD patients from controls relative to the degree of asymmetry in the waking state.

During the 1980s, a series of studies suggested that polysomnographic measurements of sleep architecture might have utility in making the differential diagnosis between late-life depression and early AD. In fact, some of these studies suggested that elderly patients with affective disorders had worse sleep (e.g., poorer sleep continuity, early-morning awakening) relative to AD patients. Other data implied that recovery effects following sleep deprivation might differentiate the two types of patient groups, as well as patients whose clinical presentation had a mixed component of both cognitive loss and affective features. For example, aged depressed patients showed an absence of REM-sleep rebound following REM-sleep deprivation but AD patients showed increases in REM-sleep activity after undergoing the same procedure. While these results have proven interesting experimentally, the practical value of examining sleep architecture polysomnographically before and after sleep deprivation or even for a single baseline night in the laboratory for the purpose of making this differential has not gained acceptance as a common utility for polysomnography. For example, differences in definition in the latency to the first REM period of the night may have a major impact upon the values obtained (Bliwise et al., 1989b), and at least one well-documented case of AD was characterized by both *short* REM-sleep latency and *abundant* REM sleep (Bliwise et al., 1990c).

Considerable debate remains regarding whether sleep apnea may have any role in AD. While the topic remains controversial (see Bliwise, 1993, 1994a), evidence suggesting neuropsychological morbidity associated with sleep apnea continues to accrue (Kim et al., 1997; Dealberto et al., 1996). Given plausible mechanisms linking sleep apnea to alterations in brain perfusion (Qureshi et al., 1997b, Fischer et al., 1992) and some data linking sleep apnea and stroke (see below), it is not inconceivable that sleep apnea may be associated with a form of reversible dementia (Bliwise, 1996).

SLEEP IN MULTI-INFARCT DEMENTIA

MID, or vascular dementia, encompasses a number of heterogeneous conditions broadly defining cerebrovascular disease, including: frank ischemic stroke, hemorrhagic stroke, and ischemic-hypoxic lesions. Often included in the diagnosis of vascular dementia are a wide array of other related syndromes, including Binswanger's disease, hyalinosis (small-vessel swelling), subcortical white-matter dementia, lacunar dementia, and leukoencephalopathy. A definition of vascular dementia developed by the NINDS/AIREN working group (Roman et al., 1993) incorporated specific criteria including the presence of dementia (confirmed neuropsychologically), presence of cerebrovascular disease (confirmed with CT/MRI), clinical examination (sensory loss, muscle weakness, other focal findings), and history (stepwise course). Of historical interest is that the Hachinski rating scale (Hachinski et al., 1975; Rosen et al., 1980), which for many years was considered the standardized way of distinguishing vascular dementia from AD, incorporated nocturnal confusion as an item more characteristic of MID than of AD [see section below, "Clinical Presentations: Nocturnal Delirium ('Sundowning') as a Common Final Behavioral Pathway of Dementia Syndromes"].

The number of published polysomnographic studies examining sleep in MID and/or examining differences in the sleep between AD and MID patients is quite limited, far more so than in the case of studies of AD or PD individually. Differences in sleep architecture have been reported between MID and AD, but these appear to be trivial (Allen et al., 1987). Several descriptive studies using wrist actigraphy and/or behavioral observations, however, have suggested that vascular-dementia patients have greater disruption of their circadian rhythms (poorer nocturnal sleep and decreased daytime alertness) relative to other dementias such as AD (Aharon-Peretz et al., 1991; Meguro et al., 1995; Mishima et al., 1997). This may be due in part to greater disruption of the body temperature cycle in MID (Mishima et al., 1997), which synchronizes the timing of sleep/wakefulness across the 24-hour day (Bliwise, 1999). The study of Meguro et al. (1995) is particularly interesting in demonstrating a higher proportion of daytime sleep and lower proportion of nighttime sleep (assessed behaviorally) in patients with CT scans showing white-matter lucencies in regions such as the internal/outer capsule, thalamus, and periventricular white matter.

Some literature has suggested a higher prevalence of sleep apnea in patients with ischemic stroke (Bassetti et al., 1996; Mohsenin and Valor, 1995); however, interpretation of these data remains equivocal since it is unclear whether the higher rates of disordered breathing during sleep preceded the stroke or might be a result of it. Nonetheless, the fact that several case-control studies have suggested a greater likelihood of snoring in patients prior to their stroke relative to patients hospitalized for other reasons, and that prospective epidemiological data have also suggested that snoring may be a risk factor for stroke (Palomaki et al., 1992), raises the suspicion that sleep apnea may indeed be a risk factor for vascular dementias (including MID and frank stroke). Snoring has been shown to adversely affect prognosis subsequent to ischemic stroke (Spriggs et al., 1992), and, in the National Health and Nutrition Examination Survey (NHANES), symptoms of sleep apnea, such as excessive napping and prolonged nocturnal sleep times, also predicted stroke in multivariate models (Qureshi et al., 1997a). Although formal controlled clinical trials have yet to occur, these data would suggest tangible benefit in the diagnosis and treatment of sleep apnea in patients otherwise at risk for cerebrovascular disease and, conceivably, in individuals who have already incurred such an adverse event.

SLEEP IN PARKINSON'S DISEASE

As in AD and MID, sleep architecture is usually disturbed in PD, with decreased stages 3/4 and lower sleep efficiencies noted. Total sleep times, as recorded in the laboratory in PD across a wide variety of studies, have generally been reported to be lower than in AD, although few good comparisons actually exist. REM sleep is often greatly suppressed in advanced PD, an effect that is usually attributable to the REM-sleep-suppressing effects of L-dopa, a finding well recognized in normals for over 25 years (Gillin et al., 1973). Curiously, the nocturnal REM suppression in the majority of PD patients may occur in the context of an apparently large number of REM-sleep onsets on MSLT in about 20% of PD patients (Dihenia et al., 1997), a finding that was borne out in another case of an adolescent PD patient with apparent secondary narcolepsy who had four of five REM-sleep onsets on the MSLT (Johnston et al., 1998).

Sleep in PD may be characterized by excessive movement (Rye and Bliwise, 1997). To some extent, this runs counter to the prevailing notion that tremor and movement decline during sleep in parkinsonism, a finding originally reported by Stern et al. (1968). Despite the fact that Parkinson himself noted that movement originated in sleep in his patients (see Rye and Bliwise, 1997), some contemporary studies have suggested that the apparent sleep-related movement that occurs in PD actually consists of microawakenings occurring prior to the movement (Fish et al., 1991). While the latter study has several distinct methodological difficulties (e.g., scoring of movement and EEG were not made independently), data from others (Lapierre and Montplaisir, 1992; Schenck et al., 1996; Silber et al., 1993) and our group (Irbe et al., 1994; Rye and Bliwise, 1997; Bliwise et al., 1998; Rye, 1997) suggest that tremor and movement often arise directly from sleep and persist during sleep. Figures 5 and 6 demonstrate the abundant amount of muscle activity in various muscle groups (mentalis, extensor digitorum, flexor carpi ulnaris, gastrocnemius, tibialis anterior) seen in a PD patient in REM and non-REM sleep, respectively, with periodic leg-movement activity conspicuous during non-REM sleep. This basis for the abundant motor activity in sleep in PD

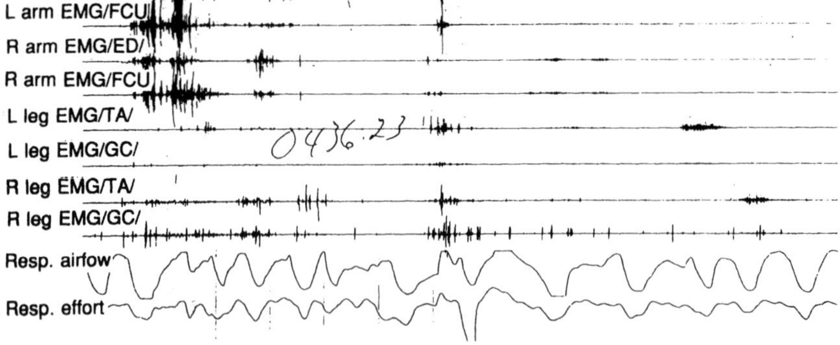

Figure 5 Excessive motor activity during REM sleep in a PD patient.

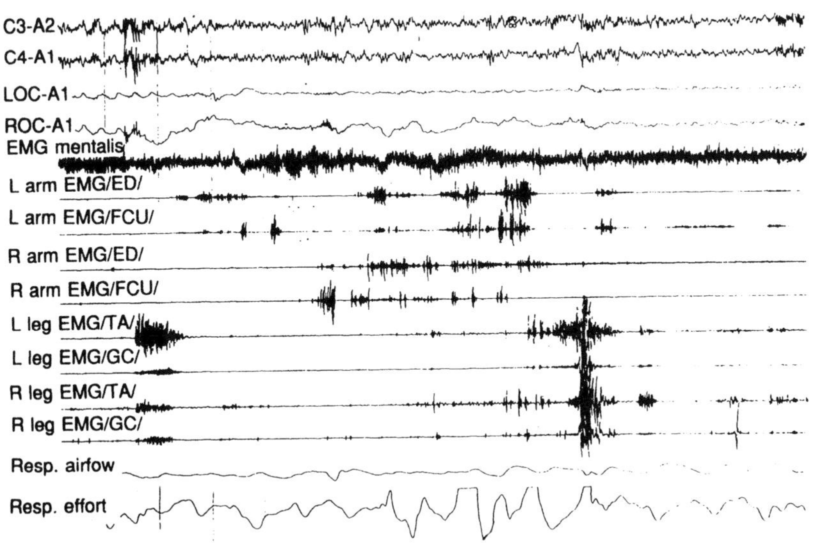

Figure 6 Excessive motor activity during non-REM sleep in a PD patient.

remains uncertain, although similarity of neural substrates for sleep regulation and control of movement, primarily involving pathways between the basal ganglia and brainstem regions involved in motor control, have recently been elucidated (Rye 1997; Rye and Bliwise, 1997).

Of considerable interest in this regard is the observation that a sizable proportion of patients with idiopathic RSBD who show high rates of EMG activity in mini (2.5-second) recording epochs (Lapierre and Montplaisir, 1992) develop PD within about 10 years (Schenck et al. 1996). Together with data suggesting abundant, similarly scored EMG activity in patients with PD (Irbe et al., 1994), this phenomenon suggests that release of motor inhibition, particularly during REM sleep, may be suspended in patients with PD. The extent of periodic leg movement in parkinsonian patients who were unmedicated exceeded the rates of movement seen in patients receiving L-dopa/carbidopa, AD patients, or aged controls (Bliwise et al., 1998).

Sleep apnea appears to be no more common in idiopathic PD than in age-matched controls, and in fact may even be somewhat less prevalent owing to the relative lack of obesity in most idiopathic PD patients. Parkinsonian patients with ''Parkinson plus'' syndromes and/or with accompanying autonomic dysfunction may represent a different situation since these patients often have sleep apnea (Apps et al., 1985; Guilleminault et al., 1981; McNicholas et al., 1993).

CLINICAL PRESENTATIONS: NOCTURNAL DELIRIUM ("SUNDOWNING") AS A COMMON FINAL BEHAVIORAL PATHWAY OF DEMENTIA SYMDROMES

Cases of dementia coming to the attention of sleep clinicians invariably present with a symptomatic picture of agitated, disruptive, and/or combative behavior during the night, a syndrome that has over the years been labeled "sundowning." Such phenomena are not unique to dementia, as nocturnal delirious states have been shown to characterize many infectious, metabolic, and toxic conditions. Nonetheless, sundowning is thought to occur in a large proportion of demented patients at some point in their illness, although the stage of disease when the condition manifests is still debated (Zarcone et al., 1998). The relatively solid behavioral evidence suggesting that such phenomena indeed have a temporal proclivity was recently reviewed (Bliwise, 1996) and, although timing estimates vary slightly from study to study, most studies place the time of maximal agitation in such patients between 5 and 9 P.M., or, in some studies, slightly later during at night.

The mechanistic basis for this phenomenon remains uncertain, although, on the basis of its temporal course, several possibilities have been proposed. Sociological perspectives have emphasized that agitated behavior is primarily a consequence of environmental factors such as interruptions by staff (Schnelle et al., 1993) or even expectations of staff, as evidenced by use of antipsychotic medication prior to shift change (Exum et al., 1993). Medically oriented perspectives, however, place the origin of such behavior on patient-related factors, such as confusion occurring upon awakening from sleep. For example, spontaneous awakenings may lead to confusion and agitation (Bliwise et al., 1993). Alternatively, the episodes might consist of behavioral responses to specific events occurring during sleep, such as delirium induced by transient nocturnal hypoxia accompanying sleep apnea episodes. As a case in point, there is some evidence that AD patients who desaturate during the night are considerably more confused upon awakening in the morning than AD patients who do not have sleep apnea (Bliwise et al., 1989a; Moldofsky et al., 1983). A third possibility is that sundowning could represent episodes of dream-enactment behavior occurring during the nighttime hours following awakenings specifically from REM sleep. A final explanation may be that such episodes are the result of dysfunction of the circadian timing system, perhaps occurring during periods of exaggerated activity in the course of the normal fluctuation of the body-temperature cycle or even as an aberration of the body-temperature cycle itself (Bliwise, 1993). A modicum of evidence exists for each of these perspectives (Bliwise 1994b; 1996); however, it is likely that sundowning behavior represents a common endpoint to a wide variety of conditions, and its treatment probably involves careful consideration of any or all such alternatives.

TREATMENTS

Nonpharmacological treatments deserving of consideration in the treatment of agitated demented patients include avoidance of daytime napping, enhanced exposure to outdoor light, particularly during the late afternoon and early evening, and induction of physical activity to the extent that such behavior is possible given the patient's level of frailty and level of incapacity. Daytime dozing, so endemic to nursing homes and often considered a part of the ennui of nursing-home life, may be a particularly pernicious phenomenon with adverse consequences for nighttime sleep. In one study in severely demented nursing-home patients with presumed AD (Bliwise et al., 1990a), we noted that excessive sleep during the day was invariably related to poor sleep the subsequent night. Similarly, disturbed sleep at night was inversely related to excessive sleep the following day. These data suggest a vicious cycle of sleep–wake regulation apparent in such patients, a cycle that with appropriate environmental interventions, such as restriction of daytime naps, may be modifiable (Friedman et al., 1991). Coincidentally, the data also imply that, despite a profound level of dementia, homeostatic regulation of the sleep–wake cycle appears to be maintained, at least in these patients, largely with the presumptive diagnosis of AD, as opposed to patients with PD, who may show disruption of homeostatic regulation in the relationship between daytime alertness and sleep the preceding night (Dihenia et al., 1997).

Pharmacological management for the nocturnal agitation accompanying dementia has typically employed antipsychotic medication, such as haloperidol and thioridazine at low doses (typically 0.5–1.0 mg and 25 mg, respectively), with varying degrees of success (McGaffigan and Bliwise, 1997). However, typical side effects (extrapyramidal symptoms and orthostatic hypotension, respectively) necessitate careful monitoring. More recently, use of selective dopamine antagonists such as clozapine, a D_4-selective antagonist, and risperidone, a selective D_2 and serotonin type 2 antagonist, has been reported to be of some value in demented patients with nocturnal agitation, particularly those involving dopamimetic-induced psychosis (McGaffigan and Bliwise, 1997). Typical initial dosages range from 12.5 to 25.0 mg for clozapine to 1 to 2 mg for risperidone. Newer antipsychotic medications such as olanzapine (typical dosage 1–15 mg) (Wolters et al., 1996) have been suggested to have some utility as well. Some studies have reported beneficial effects on sleep of melatonin (2 mg) in institutionalized nondemented patients (Haimov et al., 1995); however, its value in treating disturbed sleep and agitation in dementia remains uncertain. Singer et al. (1995;

1997) have presented preliminary data from ongoing double-blind crossover, placebo-controlled clinical trials of 0.5 and 10 mg in which only the higher dosages (10 mg) showed any suggestion of a positive effect. Caution may be indicated in the use of melatonin in patients with cerebrovascular disease, however, since animal models indicate that it may promote vasoconstriction of peripheral vessels (Krause et al., 1995).

ACKNOWLEDGMENT

This work was supported by AG-10643 and NS-35345.

REFERENCES

Aharon-Peretz J, Masiah A, Pillar T. Sleep-wake cycles in multi-infarct dementia and dementia of the Alzheimer type. Neurology 1991; 41:1616–1619.

Allen SR, Seiler WO, Stahelin HB, Spiegel R. Seventy-two hour polysomnographic and behavioral recordings of wakefulness and sleep in a hospital geriatric unit: comparison between demented and nondemented patients. Sleep 1987; 10:143–159.

Apps MCP, Sheaff PC, Ingram DA, Kennard C, Empey DW. Respiration and sleep in Parkinson's disease. J Neurol Neurosurg Psychiatry 1985; 48:1240–1245.

Bassetti C, Aldrich MS, Chervin RD, Quint D. Sleep apnea in patients with transient ischemic attack and stroke: a prospective study of 59 patients. Neurology 1996; 47:1167–1173.

Bliwise DL. Sleep in normal aging and dementia. Sleep 1993; 16:40–81.

Bliwise DL. Sleep in dementing illness. In: Oldham JM, Riba MB, eds. Review of Psychiatry. Vol 13. Washington, DC: American Psychiatric Press, 1994a:757–776.

Bliwise DL. What is sundowning? J Am Geriatr Soc 1994b; 42:1009–1011.

Bliwise DL. Is sleep apnea a cause of reversible dementia in old age? J Am Geriatr Soc 1996; 44:1407–1409.

Bliwise DL. Sleep and circadian rhythm disorders in aging and dementia. In: Turek F, Zee P, eds. Neurobiology of Sleep and Circadian Rhythms. New York: Marcel Dekker, 1999.

Bliwise DL, Yesavage JA, Tinklenberg J, Dement WC. Sleep apnea in Alzheimer's Disease. Neurobiol Aging 1989a; 10:343–346.

Bliwise DL, Tinklenberg J, Yesavage JL, Davies H, Pursley AM, Petta DE, Widrow L, Guilleminault C, Zarcone VP, Dement WC. REM latency in Alzheimer's Disease. Biolog Psychiatry 1989b; 25:320–328.

Bliwise DL, Bevier WC, Bliwise NG, Edgar DM, Dement WC. Systematic 24-hour behavioral observations of sleep/wakefulness in a skilled nursing facility. Psychol Aging 1990a; 5:16–24.

Bliwise DL, Carroll JS, Dement WC. Predictors of observed sleep/wakefulness in residents in long term care. J Gerontol: Med Sciences 1990b; 45:M126–M130.

Bliwise DL, Nino-Mucia G, Forno LS, Viseskul C. Abundant REM sleep in a patient with Alzheimer's Disease. Neurology 1990c; 40:1281–1284.

Bliwise DL, Yesavage JA, Tinklenberg JR. Sundowning and rate of decline in mental function in Alzheimer's Disease. Dementia 1992; 3:335–341.

Bliwise DL, Carroll JS, Lee KA, Nekich JC, Dement WC. Sleep and sundowning in nursing home patients with dementia. Psychiatry Res 1993; 48:277–292.

Bliwise DL, Hughes M, McMahon P, Kutner N. Observed sleep/wakefulness and severity of dementia in an Alzheimer's disease special care unit. J Gerontol: Med Sciences 1995; 50A:M303–306.

Bliwise DL, Rye DB, Yesavage JA, Pursley AM, Williams ML, Ansari FP. Periodic leg movements in sleep in elderly patients with parkinsonism. Sleep 1998; 21(suppl): 196.

Culebras A, Moore JT. Magnetic resonance findings in REM sleep behavior disorder. Neurology 1989; 39:1519–1523.

Dealberto MJ, Pajot N, Courbon D, Alperovitch, A. Breathing disorders during sleep and cognitive performance in an older community sample: the EVA study. J Am Geriatr Soc 1996; 44:1287–1294.

Dihenia BH, Rye DB, Bliwise DL. Daytime alertness in Parkinson's disease. Sleep Res 1997; 26:550.

Exum ME, Phelps BJ, Nabers KE, Osborne JG. Sundown syndrome: is it reflected in the use of PRN medications for nursing home residents? Gerontologist 1993; 33:756–761.

Fischer AQ, Chaudary BA, Taormina MA, Akhtar B. Intracranial hemodynamics in sleep apnea. Chest 1992; 102:1402–1406.

Fish DR, Sawyers D, Allen PJ, Blackie JD, Lees AJ, Marsden CD. The effect of sleep on the dyskinetic movements of Parkinson's disease, Gilles de la Tourette syndrome, Huntington's disease and torsion dystonia. Arch Neurol 1991; 48:210–214.

Friedman L, Bliwise DL, Yesavage JA, Salom SR. A preliminary study comparing sleep restriction and relaxation treatments for insomnia in older subjects. J Gerontol: Psycholog Sciences 1991; 46:P1-P8.

Gillin JC, Post RM, Wyatt RJ, Goodwin FK, Snyder F, Bunney WE Jr. REM inhibitory effect of L-dopa infusion during human sleep. Electroencephalogr Clin Neurophysiol 1973; 35:181–186.

Guilleminault C, Briskin JG, Greenfield MS, Silvestri R. The impact of autonomic nervous system dysfunction on breathing during sleep. Sleep 1981; 4:263–268.

Hachinski VC, Iliff LD, Zilhka E, DuBoulay GH, McAllister VL, Marshall J, Russell RW, Symon L. Cerebral blood flow in dementia. Arch Neurol 1975; 32:632–637.

Haimov I, Lavie P, Laudon M, Herer P, Vigder C, Zisapel N. Melatonin replacement therapy of elderly insomniacs. Sleep 1995; 18:598–603.

Hajak G, Klingelhofer J, Shulz-Varszegi M, Sander D, Staedt J, Conrad B, Ruther E. Cerebral perfusion during sleep-disordered breathing. J Sleep Res 1995; 4(suppl 1): 135–144.

Henley K, Morrison AR. A re-evaluation of the effects of lesions of the pontine tegmentum and locus coeruleus on phenomena of paradoxical sleep in the cat. Acta Neurobiol Exp 1974; 34:215–232.

Irbe D, Rye DB, Bliwise DL. Sinemet in advanced Parkinson's Disease (PD): effects on sleep-related movements and tremor. Sleep Res 1994; 23:368.

Johnston LH, Dihenia BH, Watts RL, Bliwise DL, Rye DB. Parkinson's disease presenting with secondary narcolepsy in an adolescent with an unaffected monozygotic twin. Sleep 1998; 21 (suppl):173.

Kim HC, Young T, Matthews CG, Weber SM, Woodard AR, Palta M. Sleep disordered breathing and neuropsychological deficits: a population-based study. Am J Respir Care Med 1997; 156:1813–1819.

Krause DN, Barrios VE, Duckles SP. Melatonin receptors mediate potentiation of contractile responses to adrenergic nerve stimulation in rat caudal artery. Eur J Pharmacol 1995; 276:207–213.

Lapierre O, Montplaisir J. Polysomnographic features of REM sleep behavior disorder: development of a scoring method. Neurology 1992; 42:1371–1374.

Mahowald MW, Schenck CH. Status dissociatus: a perspective on states of being. Sleep 1991; 14:69–79.

McGaffigan S, Bliwise DL. The treatment of sundowning: a selective review of pharmacological and non-pharmacological studies. Drugs Aging 1997; 10:10–17.

McNicholas WT, Rutherford R, Grossman R, Moldofsky H, Zamel N, Phillipson EA. Abnormal respiratory pattern generation during sleep in patients with autonomic dysfunction. Am Rev Respir Dis 1983; 128:429–433.

Meguro K, Ueda M, Kobayashi I, Yamaguchi S, Yamazaki H, Oikawa Y, Kikuchi Y, Sasaki H. Sleep disturbance in an elderly patient with cognitive impairment, decreased daily activity and periventricular white matter lesions. Sleep 1995; 18 (suppl 2):109–114.

Mishima K, Okawa M, Satoh K, Shimizu T, Hozumi S, Hishikawa Y. Different manifestations of circadian rhythms in senile dementia of Alzheimer's type and multi-infarct dementia. Neurobiol Aging 1997; 18(suppl 1):105–109.

Mohsenin V, Valor R. Sleep apnea in patients with hemispheric stroke. Arch Phys Med Rehabil 1995; 76:71–76.

Moldofsky H, Goldstein R, McNicholas W, Lue F, Zamel N, Phillipson E. Disordered breathing during sleep and overnight intellectual deterioration in patients with pathological aging. In: Guilleminault C, Lugaresi E, eds. Sleep/Wake Disorders: Natural History Epidemiology and Long-Term Evolution. New York: Raven Press, 1983:143–150.

Palomäki H, Partinen M, Erkinjuntti T, Kaste M. Snoring, sleep apnea syndrome and stroke. Neurology 1992; 6:75–82.

Petit D, Montplaisir J, Lorrain D, Gauthier S. Spectral analysis of the rapid eye movement sleep electroencephalogram in right and left temporal regions: a biological marker of Alzheimer's Disease. Ann Neurol 1992; 32:172–176.

Prinz PN, Larsen LH, Moe KE, Vitiello MV. EEG markers of early Alzheimer's disease in computer selected tonic REM sleep. Electroencephalogr Clin Neurophysiol 1992; 83:36–43.

Qureshi AI, Giles WH, Croft JB, Bliwise DL. Habitual sleep patterns and risk for stroke and coronary disease: a ten-year follow-up from NHANES I. Neurology 1997a; 48:904–991.

Qureshi AI, Winter WC, Shahrukh S, Bliwise DL. Overnight change in vasomotor reactivity of the middle cerebral artery as a function of sleep apnea and stage upon awakening. Sleep Res 1997b; 26:476.

Rechtschaffen A, Kales A, eds. A Manual of Standardized Terminology, Techniques, and Scoring System for Sleep Stages of Human Subjects. Washington, DC: U.S. Government Printing Office, 1968.

Reynolds CF III, Kupfer DJ, Taska LS, Hoch CC, Spiker DG, Sewitch DE, Zimmer B, Marin RS, Nelson JP, Martin D, Morycz R. EEG sleep in elderly depressed, demented, and healthy subjects. Biol Psychiatry 1985; 20:431–442.

Roman GC, Tatemichi TK, Erkinjuntti T, Cummings JL, Masdeu JC, Garcia JH, Amaducci L, Orgogozo J-M, Brun A, Hofman A, Moody DM, O'Brien MD, Yamaguchi T, Grafman J, Drayer BP, Bennett DA, Fisher M, Ogata J, Kokmen E, Bermejo F, Wolf PA, Gorelick PB, Bick KL, Pajeau AK, Bell MA, DeCarli C, Culebras A, Korczyn AD, Bogousslavsky J, Hartmann A, Scheinberg P. Vascular dementia: diagnostic criteria for research studies report of the NINDS-AIREN International Workshop. Neurology 1993; 43:250–260.

Rosen WG, Terry RD, Fuld PA, Katzman R, Peck A. Pathological verification of ischemic score in differentiation of dementias. Ann Neurol 1980; 7:486–488.

Rye DB. Contributions of the pedunculopontine region to normal and altered REM sleep. Sleep 1997; 20:757–788.

Rye DB, Bliwise DL. Movement disorders specific to sleep and the nocturnal manifestations of waking movement disorders. In: Watts RL, Koller WC, eds. Movement Disorders: Neurologic Principles and Practice. New York: McGraw-Hill, 1997: 687–713.

Rye DB, Dihenia B, Weissman JW, Epstein CM, Bliwise DL. Presentation of narcolepsy after 40. Neurology 1998; 50:459–465.

Schenck CH, Bundlie SR, Ettinger MG, Mahowald MW. Chronic behavioral disorders of human REM sleep: a new category of parasomnia. Sleep 1986; 9:293–308.

Schenck CH, Bundlie SR, Patterson AL, Mahowald MW. Rapid eye movement sleep behavior disorder: a treatable parasomnia affecting older adults. JAMA 1987; 257: 1786–1789.

Schenck CH, Bundlie SR, Mahowald MW. Delayed emergence of a parkinsonian disorder in 38% of 29 older men initially diagnosed with idiopathic rapid eye movement sleep behavior disorder. Neurology 1996; 46:388–393.

Schnelle JF, Ouslander JG, Simmons SF, Alessi CA, Gravel MD. The nighttime environment, incontinence care, and sleep disruption in nursing homes. J Am Geriatr Soc 1993; 41:910–914.

Silber MH, Dexter DD, Ahlskog JE, Hauri PJ, Shepard JW. Abnormal REM sleep motor activity in untreated Parkinson's Disease. Sleep Res 1993; 22:274.

Singer C, McArthur A, Hughes R, Sack R, Kaye J, Lewy A. High dose melatonin administration and sleep in the elderly. Sleep Res 1995; 24A:151.

Singer CM, Moffit MT, Colling ED, Hughes RJ, Cutler NL, Sack RL, Lewy AJ. Low dose melatonin administration and nocturnal activity levels in patients with Alzheimer's disease. Sleep Res 1997; 26:752.

Spriggs DA, French JM, Murdy JM, Curless RH, Bates D, James OF. Snoring increases the risk of stroke and adversely affects prognosis. Q J Med 1992; 303:555–562.

Stern M, Roffwarg H, Duvoisin R. The parkinson tremor in sleep. J Nerv Ment Dis 1968; 147:202–210.

Tachibana N, Kimura K, Kitajima K, Shinde A, Kimura J, Shibasaki H. REM motor dysfunction in multiple system atrophy: with special emphasis on sleep talk as its early clinical manifestation. J Neurol Neurosurg Psychiatry 1997; 63:678–681.

Turner RS, Chervin RD, Frey KA, Minoshima S, Kuhl DE. Probable diffuse Lewy body disease presenting as REM sleep behavior disorder. Neurology 1997; 49:523–527.

Vitiello MV, Prinz PN, Williams DE, Frommlet MS, Ries RK. Sleep disturbances in patients with mild-stage Alzheimer's disease. J Gerontol: Med Sci 1990; 45:M131-M138.

Williams ML, Irbe D, Ansari FP, Rye DB, Bliwise DL. Stage scoring reliability for nocturnal polysomnography in patients with Parkinson's disease. Sleep 1998; 21(suppl): 171.

Wolters EC, Jansen EN, Tuynman-Qua HG, Bergmans PL. Olanzapine in the treatment of dopaminomimetic psychosis in patients with Parkinson's disease. Neurology 1996; 47:1085–1087.

Zarcone V, Friedman L, Kraemer HC, Noda A, Wicks D, Bliwise DL, Sheikh J, Tinklenberg J, Yesavage J. A follow-up study of actigraphic measures in home-residing Alzheimer disease patients. Sleep 1998; 21(suppl):52.

13

Obstructive and Nonobstructive Sleep Apnea

The Neurological Perspective

Christian Guilleminault and Ali G. Bassiri
Stanford University Medical School
Palo Alto, California

INTRODUCTION

Disorders of breathing during sleep comprise many different syndromes and frequently pose diagnostic and therapeutic challenges for the neurologist. The consequences of such disorders vary from motor vehicle and industrial accidents during waking hours (1,2) to death from arrhythmias or myocardial infarction during sleep (3–9). Despite these well-recognized and well-documented consequences, a survey of a university-based neuromuscular disorders clinic revealed that less than 5% of the patients with breathing disorders during sleep were appropriately treated, and one died during a home-ambulatory recording performed as part of the survey (10).

Classically, breathing disorders during sleep are divided into two categories: 1) disorders of the upper airway and 2) disorders of diaphragmatic and/or other inspiratory muscle dysfunction. In the mid 1960s, this division led to creation of the terms "apnea," which refers to the cessation of air flow at the nose and the mouth, and "hypopnea," which refers to a reduction in airflow accompanied with a drop in oxygen saturation (11,12). "Obstructive apneas" are apneas due to an obstruction along the upper airway, and "central apneas" are apneas secondary to cessation of inspiratory muscle contraction. "Mixed apneas" are a combination of both, usually a central apnea followed by an obstructive component as inspiration resumes (the opposite chain of events is rarely seen in very young infants). Both central and obstructive hypopneas both involve a reduction in airflow accompanied by oxygen desaturation and may be difficult to distinguish from each other. Central hypopneas, however, are associated with a decreased respiratory effort, while obstructive hypopneas are associated with a maintained or decreased effort.

''Abnormal (increased) breathing effort'' refers to an increase in inspiratory effort during one breath while asleep, and is currently measured by monitoring intrathoracic pressure swings via esophageal manometry. The latter measures esophageal pressure (Pes), which reflects intrathoracic (pleural) pressure. Abnormal breathing effort does not result in a drop in oxygen saturation as measured by noninvasive equipment. Increased respiratory effort is often due to increased upper-airway resistance. Accurate calculations of resistance, however, require the measurement of tidal volume and hence airflow via a pneumotachometer, and the measurement of pressure via esophageal manometry. Such dual monitoring disturbs sleep and, for practical purposes, increased effort as monitored by esophageal manometry is taken to indicate the presence of increased airway resistance. A succession of at least three breaths with progressively increasing breathing effort is referred to as a ''crescendo.'' Such ''crescendos,'' frequently terminating with arousals on the electroencephalogram, are the hallmark of the upper-airway resistance syndrome (UARS) (13).

Disorders with abnormalities located in the upper airway can lead to crescendos, hypopneas, or any of obstructive, central, and mixed apneas. Disorders with abnormalities involving the inspiratory muscles can also rarely lead to the three types of apneas or hypopneas. Hence, polygraphic techniques may not always distinguish between disorders of uppper-airway resistance and inspiratory muscle dysfunction. With this fact in mind, we shall consider the two major locations of breathing abnormalities during sleep: the upper airway and the inspiratory muscles.

Upper-Airway Obstruction During Sleep

The disorders of upper-airway obstruction are the obstructive sleep apnea syndrome (OSAS), the pure obstructive sleep hypopnea syndrome, and the UARS. It is likely that these disorders represent different degrees of severity along the same spectrum of breathing disorders, and the division into three distinct syndromes is based as much on specific polygraphic features as on the technical capabilities of the monitoring equipment used. It is important to note that the severity of the symptoms does not necessarily imply one syndrome over the other.

Prevalence

Current data on prevalence is limited to studies carried out in the United States and Europe mainly on caucasian adults with OSAS. There are no similar data on UARS. In the Wisconsin sleep cohort study of white-collar workers, the prevalence of OSAS was 9% in women and 24% in men aged 30 to 60 years (14). This data was extrapolated to the general population to yield a prevalence of 2% in women and 4% in men (14). Similar results of 1.9% in women and 3.7% in men were obtained in a community-based survey in the British Isles (15). In comparison with other neurological disorders, for every 100,000 individuals in the United States, 3000 have OSAS, 2000 migraines, 650 epilepsy, 250 dementia, 200 Parkinson's disease, 60 multiple sclerosis, 40 narcolepsy, and 20 polyneuropathy (16).

Pathophysiology

The site of the increased resistance in upper airways that leads to obstruction almost always occurs between the caudal region of the soft palate and the epiglottis. This anatomical compromise is further increased during sleep due, in part, to the decrease in the tone of the upper-airway dilator muscles (17). Airway collapse occurs mostly at end expiration when the positive airway pressure has dissipated and when contraction of upper-airway dilators has not yet started. Other factors compromising the airway include the supine position and incoordination between the upper-airway dilator muscles and the diaphragm. The latter is due to the relative difference in the strengths of the upper-airway dilators and the diaphragm seen in some neuromuscular disorders.

Craniofacial abnormalities that can culminate in the long face syndrome (long and narrow facial appearance, retro- and micrognathia, and high-arched and narrow hard palate), as well as obesity associated with peripalatal fat pads are features that are commonly associated with OSAS. Both may be present in varying degrees in patients with OSAS.

Finally, one research group has found that chronic snoring and the associated vibration may induce a progressive XIIth nerve peripheral neuropathy (18,19). This may theoretically further exacerbate OSAS by affecting the function of the upper-airway muscles. If this is true, snoring in the absence of apneas may not be as benign as commonly believed.

Clinical Features

Symptoms Snoring of variable severity is very common and may be the presenting complaint. Perception of snoring by bed partners indicate that a worsening of sound level occurs over time. On the other hand, snoring may be absent in some patients with abnormally narrow upper airways, particularly if the soft palate is short and the narrowing is located predominantly behind the tongue.

Sleep fragmentation is another consequence of OSAS, which may occasionally be consciously perceived by the patient as nocturnal awakening. Such disrupted sleep may lead the patient to complain of insomnia or nonrestorative sleep (20). It may also be associated with sleepwalking and night terrors if sleep fragmentation is prominent during sleep stage 3 and 4, or repetitive unpleasant dreams (themes commonly reported include drowning, choking, or being smothered) if fragmentation is in REM sleep.

Nocturia and enuresis (more frequent in children) are common as are reports of restlessness and diaphoresis. Bruxism at times associated with biting of the buccal mucosa or tongue, dry mouth, and drooling are signs of mouth-breathing during sleep. Patients with OSAS frequently report awakening with a gasping or choking sensation which may be accompanied by tachycardia. Finally, patients may awaken with gastroesophageal reflux.

Daytime symptoms include headaches, erectile dysfunction of decreased libido, fatigue, memory deficits, and personality or mood changes.

Symptoms of OSAS may be exacerbated by weight gain, nighttime alcohol consumption, use of CNS depressants, sleep deprivation, and chronic nasal congestion as may be seen with environmental allergies.

Signs A complete physical examination is required in every patient with possible OSAS with particular attention to the body-mass index, neck circumference, and the upper airway.

A low-lying soft palate, large uvula, excess pharyngeal tissue, and enlarged tonsils may all be indicators of a narrow upper airway (21). A high-arched and narrow hard palate also tends to be associated with a small posterior space behind the genioglossus muscles and indicates possible compromise of the region. Retrognathia, often accompanied by a dental overbite (also called an overjet) and micrognathia, may be associated with posterior positioning of the tongue and upper-airway compromise. Macroglossia and obstructed nasal passages may exacerbate obstruction. Temporomandibular joint clicks, laxity, tenderness, or crepitus may indicate that the jaw may fall posteriorly during sleep and further obstruct the airway.

Craniofacial anomalies such as the long-face syndrome (22), cleft palate (particularly if repaired with flap surgeries), any of the neurocristopathies (such as the Pierre Robin syndrome), or spinal deformities such as kyphoscoliosis (23) all predispose to OSAS.

Finally, medical diseases such as hypothyroidism, Hodgkin's disease, Down's syndrome, Prader-Willi syndrome, peripheral neuropathies of the XIIth nerve, or myopathies of the genioglossus or geniohyoid muscles may all contribute to upper-airway narrowing or incoordination between the diaphragm and the upper-airway dilator muscles (which usually contract just before the diaphragm) and lead to OSAS.

Diagnostic Tests

The diagnosis of OSAS is definitively established by nocturnal polysomnography. Many recommendations have been published regarding polysomnography and the diagnosis of OSAS. It is important to keep in mind two facts: 1) increasing the length of the test or the number of the variables monitored decreases the risk of erroneous findings, and 2) there is a balance between the number and the degree of invasiveness of variables monitored and the amount of sleep achieved.

In clinically obvious cases, fewer parameters need to be monitored, and the severity of the OSAS may be determined based on the severity and frequency of apnea and hypopneas, oxygen desaturations, sleep fragmentation, and any cardiac arrhythmias. Such monitoring may be carried out in an ambulatory setting. Less obvious cases require formal polysomnography in a sleep laboratory. Such elaborate testing allows the accurate assessment of respiratory efforts (which may be performed by esophageal manometry if available) and the detection of the upper-airway resistance syndrome. The choice of ambulatory versus laboratory testing should be based on the clinical assessment and the likelihood of OSAS. If other sleep disorders, such as periodic limb movement syndrome, are suspected, polysomnography is preferred.

Classically polysomnography monitoring includes channels for EEG, eye movements, chin and anterior tibilalis EMG, cardiac-rhythm strip, airflow, respiratory effort, respiratory noise (snoring, oxygen saturation, and body position). Video monitoring may complement polysomnography if desired.

Inspiratory Muscle Dysfunction During Sleep

Inspiratory muscle dysfunction may lead to central apnea (absence of muscle contraction for $\geq$10 seconds) or central hypopneas (decrease in contractions for $\geq$10 seconds), which are associated with sleep arousals or oxygen desaturation. Such muscle dysfunction may follow lesions of the peripheral or central nervous system and may involve the sensory, the integrative and executive, or the motor component of the nervous pathway (20).

The Sensory Component

The classic disorder in this category is the congenital central alveolar hypoventilation syndrome (CCHS, also called Ondine's curse) (24,25). It is usually detected in the first few days of life and is characterized by repetitive central apneas, CO_2 retention, and respiratory arrest. In most cases the abnormality is present only during sleep and it is usually less marked during REM stage. Rarely, in older infants with the mild form of the disease, hypoventilation is seen exclusively during stages 3 and 4 non-REM sleep. In some cases, hypercapnia may be also be present while awake, and repetitive cries and agitation normalize the CO_2 levels via the associated tachypnea.

The primary defect in CCHS is thought to be a dysfunction of central chemoreceptors. There is usually a blunted (but not absent) response to hypercapnia. Abnormal responses to experimentally induced hypercapnia and hypoxia during sleep and wake have been demonstrated. Such abnormalities may partly explain the frequently observed central apnea and hypopneas, and the accompanying hypercapnia (as measured by transcutaneous electrodes) during sleep in these patients.

We have observed abnormal heart rates in some of our patients, which may indicate that CCHS is part of a more generalized syndrome of autonomic dysfunction (25). Supporting this notion is the higher incidence of ganglioblastoma and Hirschsprung's disease in CCHS patients. In fact, the presence of one should prompt a search for the other disorder.

Several other syndromes are associated with familial or acquired autonomic dysfunction and central sleep apnea and hypopnea, again with a predominance in non-REM sleep (26–29). These include familial dysautonomia (Riley-Day syndrome), insulin-dependent diabetes mellitus, chronic uremia, Shy-Drager syndrome, and other chronic neuropathies. The most common polygraphic finding is seen during non-REM sleep and involves a decreased tidal volume for one or two breaths without an appreciable change in CO_2 levels. Shy-Drager syndrome is unique in that a combination of both upper-airway abnormality and central hypoventilation is observed (27,29). The upper-airway component is secondary to a vocal-cord palsy with abnormal closure resulting in obstructive hypopneas. Sleep-related hypoventilation has been observed in patients after cervical cordotomy for intractable cancer pain (30). The resulting bilateral lesions of the ventrolateral tracts of the cervical spine lead to severe hypoventilation, repetitive central apneas, and sleep fragmentation. In all these cases, sudden death during sleep has been observed.

The Integrative and Executive Component

As opposed to CCHS, acquired alveolar hypoventilation during sleep is classically secondary to bilateral posterolateral medullary lesions (31–33). These acquired hypoventilation syndromes are often present during wakefulness and usually worsen during sleep, particularly in non-REM stages. They are seen more commonly now, probably because of improved survival from the initial neurological insult. These lesions are usually secondary to vascular pathology (31–33), but may be a consequence of bilateral brainstem lesions, epidural or subdural hematomas (34), intracranial abscess, encephalitis, or acute intratumoral hemorrhage. Degenerative and metabolic diseases such as Leigh disease (35) may be responsible for impairment of the medullary respiratory neuronal network.

Occasionally, no underlying etiology can be found in a patient with an acquired central hypoventilation syndrome. Often such patients are overweight and the syndrome occurs during an acute lung infection or on a trip to high altitudes. It is thought that these subjects have an undiagnosed upper-airway resistance syndrome that leads to an unrecognized sleep fragmentation, in association with a genetically determined blunted hypoxic and hypercapnic response. The sleep fragmentation further blunts their CO_2 response, and the acute exacerbating event leads to hypercapnia and central apneas during sleep. One of our patients, who was suffering from an upper-respiratory-tract infection, experienced acute respiratory arrest after repetitive apneas witnessed by her husband during a trip to a destination 7000 feet above sea level.

The Motor Component

Disorders of the motor component are the most common neurological causes of central apnea and hypopneas. A significant percentage of these disorders, however, remain undiagnosed, increasing the morbidity and mortality.

A common cause of death in amyotrophic lateral sclerosis (ALS) is worsening of central alveolar hypoventilation with increasingly repetitive and prolonged apnea and hypopneas, and consequent cardiac arrhythmia and arrest during sleep (10). Nocturnal alveolar hypoventilation has also been reported in poliomyelitis, especially in patients who have had the disease for over 15 years (38). This is particularly true in those who developed initial bulbar involvement with good recovery of respiratory function. In these patients, the longest apneic events occurred during REM sleep because of the combined effects of REM-sleep atonia and pathological phrenic-nerve output due to medullary impairment. Varying degrees of hypercapnia and reduced tidal volumes are observed, most prominently in REM sleep.

Poliomyelitis may also cause atrophy of respiratory accessory and thoracoabdominal muscles, leading to kyphoscoliosis and restrictive chest-wall disease. Such sequelae will affect ventilation while awake as well as asleep. Finally, the VIIth, XIIth, and motor branch of the Vth nerve may become affected and result in tongue-muscle dysfunction and maxillomandibular instability. Upper-airway resistance will increase due to such muscular impairment, and combined with the decreased respiratory efforts, will produce a mixed pattern of obstructive and central apnea and hypopneas seen during REM and non-REM stages. It is important to determine the different components of sleep-related breathing disorders. Interestingly, treatment of one type (e.g., the obstructive component by positive pressure) may unmask the other. It should also be noted that exacerbations of the above disorders occurs (e.g., with infections) and may require management in an intensive care unit.

Most of the other disorders have a significant worsening of the alveolar hypoventilation during REM and, less commonly, non-REM sleep stages. Hereditary motor-sensory neuropathies and patients with unilateral lesions of the lower motor neurons, or of the roots or trunk of the phrenic nerve are at risk of repetitive central apnea and hypopneas. Similarily, patients with myasthenia gravis commonly experience REM-sleep breathing abnormalities, hypercapnia, and even acute respiratory failure. These patients usually have generalized myasthenia and have not been been prescribed slow release pyridostigmine bromide at bedtime (39). Hence, their muscle weakness reappears while asleep and exacerbates their breathing abnormalities, especially during the longer REM stage in early morning. Increases in body weight will exacerbate the hypoventilation.

In all these neuromuscular disorders, reports of nocturnal sleep disruption, with or without dyspnea, as well as daytime fatigue and sleepiness should raise the possibility of a sleep-related breathing abnormality. Myopathies are associated with a decreased tidal volume, which is worsened during REM sleep due to the atonia (40). The longest apneas are noted during the phasic component of REM sleep, when rapid eye movements are detected. Sleep-related complaints may be the initial manifestations of patients with maltase deficiency, and the only abnormality may be brief (5 to 7 seconds) repetitive bouts of central hypopnea during REM sleep. This is explained by the rapid onset of significant diaphragmatic impairment, which usually occurs before the atrophy of other skeletal muscles (20).

In myotonic dystrophy, the initial presentation may also be sleep-related, with such symptoms as sleep fragmentation, insomnia, and daytime sleepiness (41). The first polysomnography may not reveal many abnormalities; however, utilization of esophageal manometry may increase its sensitivity. Patients with myotonic dystrophy have a combination of airway resistance and intermittent central apnea and hypopneas. The upper-airway resistance is the consequence of impaired mandibular growth very early in life. Mandibular growth requires proper function of its supporting muscles. Obstructive and central breathing abnormalities are present in both REM and non-REM sleep. During REM sleep, the respiratory accessory muscles become atonic and the diaphragm becomes the sole muscle of inspiration. Any diaphragmatic lesions will manifest as central apnea and hypopneas, particularly during the phasic periods of REM, when atonia is augmented.

Most of the literature has emphasized a lack of direct relationship between awake respiratory-muscle dysfunction and the severity of sleep-related breathing abnormalities. A recent survey performed at a neuromuscular disorders clinic showed that 42% of the patients had an apnea–hypopnea index of more than 15 events per hour and 80% had an index of more than five events per hour (10). However, only one of the 60 nonselected subjects was diagnosed with a sleep breathing disorder. Systematic monitoring of patients at risk may be the best diagnostic solution, and the cost associated with treating exacerbations, including potential intensive care unit stays, may justify the cost of such an approach.

Abnormal Upper-Airway Resistance and Central Sleep Apnea

A group of patients have been identified in whom all neurological, cardiac, and metabolic causes of central sleep apnea have been eliminated but esophageal manometry indicates the presence of intermittent increase in respiratory effort and hence a narrow upper airway.

Because some of these subjects have low CO_2 partial pressures while awake, one hypothesis is that the different sensitivities of the chemoreceptors during awake (or arousal) and sleep may be responsible for the repetitive central apneas that may occur after very brief arousals. Postarousal hyperventilation would further decrease the CO_2 content just before resuming sleep and the resulting hypocapnia would predispose to central apneas (41).

Not all patients have low CO_2 partial pressures during awake states or post-arousal hyperventilation. However, nasal continuous positive-airway pressure (n-CPAP) completely eliminates these central apneas. Hence, in these patients, there may be a mechanism by which upper-airway resistance somehow induces central apneas (41).

Finally, one must remember that apnea during sleep may be associated with metabolic, cardiac, pulmonary, and other medical diseases.

Treatment

Upper-Airway Obstruction

Many treatment options exist, and the exact knowledge of the site of obstruction is important in some of these modalities. Unfortunately, there is not an ideal test for identifying the site of obstruction during sleep. This lack of identification is of little practical importance with n-CPAP; however, it assumes significance when surgical options are considered.

Nasal CPAP is now well established as an effective treatment modality for obstructive sleep apnea (42). Its drawbacks include claustrophobia, rhinitis, air leakage, local skin reactions, problems with appearance and intimacy between bed partners, and the inconvenience of traveling with the machine. These factors lead to poor compliance, especially in younger patients (43).

Dental appliances may be tried in patients with mild to moderate apnea who are intolerant of n-CPAP (44). Although no definitive predictions of success can be made, patients with obstruction predominantly behind the base of the tongue may be better candidates for such appliances. The drawbacks of dental appliances include their tendency to fall out of the mouth during sleep, worsening of temporomandibular joint dyslocations with or without pain, and incomplete control of the breathing problem.

Surgical procedures, such as uvulopalatopharyngoplasty (UPPP) with or without tonsillectomy and turbinectomy, have had variable results. One of the problems has been the lack of good follow-up data. Newer surgical techniques include various osteotomies for tongue advancement, and maxillomandibular advancement procedures, either of which can be combined with UPPP to improve outcome. These procedures require general anesthesia and are dependent on the experience of the surgeon. Another technique, posterior glossectomy, is a difficult procedure with a clear risk of morbidity, and best left to well-trained surgeons. The recent introduction of radio-frequency ablation for soft-tissue reduction is exciting, although long-term results are not yet available.

Treatment of upper-airway disorders is thus very much debated, and factors influencing the choice of treatment include the personal preference of the treating physician, age of the patient, severity of the disease, patient preferences, and the availability of well-trained surgeons.

Inspiratory Muscle Dysfunction

Central apneas are often poorly treated, despite the fact that good treatment often exists. The underlying disorder should be optimally treated, as in patients with myasthenia gravis (39). One should also assess the likelihood of near future tracheostomy and permanent mechanical ventilation while considering noninvasive treatment options. All treatment modalities aim to assist—or, in advanced cases, replace—the patient's ventilatory capability (45–47).

If hypoventilation is not significant during awake states, and problems are mainly nocturnal, nasal ventilation, such as bilevel positive airway pressure (BiPAP), may be considered. If this treatment becomes ineffective, usually due to progression of the disease, one may resort to nasal intermittent positive ventilation (n-IPPV) (45–47). The final option, however, is tracheostomy with initially nocturnal and eventually continual mechanical ventilation.

Diaphragmatic pacing is reserved for a small group of patients who have significant hypoventilation during awake and sleep states. Experience with this modality is not as common as the other options, and in the United States, 70 patients per year receive a diaphragmatic pacemaker (48).

CONCLUSION

Disorders of obstructive and central sleep apnea are challenging to both diagnose and treat. Treatment, however, may influence mortality, and the newer modalities such as noninvasive nasal ventilation and newer surgical techniques may allow the neurologist the opportunity to significantly improve the patient's quality of life.

Sleep is a new and rapidly growing field, and the neurologist's role in both research and patient care remains of paramount importance.

REFERENCES

1. Aldrich MS. Automobile accidents in patients with sleep disorders. Sleep 1989; 12: 487.
2. American Thoracic Society. Sleep apnea, sleepiness, and driving risk. Am J Respir Crit Care Med 1994; 150:1463–1471.

3. Koskenvuo M, Kaprio J, Telakivi T. Snoring as a risk factor for ischemic heart disease and stroke in men. Br Med J 1987; 294:16–19.
4. Hung J, Whitford EG, Parsons RW, Hillman DR. Association of sleep apnoea with myocardial infarction in men. Lancet 1990; 336:261–264.
5. Saito T, Yoshikawa T, Sakamoto Y, Tanaka K, Inoue M, Ogawa R. Sleep apnea in patients with acute myocardial infarction. Crit Care Med 1991; 19:938–941.
6. Koehler U, Schafer H. Is obstructive sleep apnea (OSA) a risk factor for myocardial infarction and cardiac arrhythmias in patients with coronary heart disease (CHD)? Sleep 1996; 19:283–286.
7. Hillman DR. Sleep apnea and myocardial infarction. Sleep 1993; 16:S23–S24.
8. Hoffstein V, Mateika S. Cardiac arrhythmias, snoring, and sleep apnea. Chest 1994; 106:466–471.
9. Guilleminault C, Connolly S, Winkle R. Cardiac arrhythmia during sleep in 400 patients with obstructive sleep apnea. Am J Cardiol 1983; 52:490–494.
10. Labanowski M, Schmidt-Nowara W, Guilleminault C. Sleep and neuromuscular diseases: frequency of sleep disordered breathing in a neuromuscular disease clinic population. Neurology 1996; 47:1173–1180.
11. Gastaut H, Tassinari C, Duron B. Etude polygraphique des manifestations episodique (hypnique et respiratoires) du syndrome de Pickwick. Rev Neurol 1965; 112: 568–576.
12. Gastaut H, Tassinari CA, Duron B. Polygraphic study of the episodic diurnal and nocturnal (hypnic and respiratory) manifestations of the Pickwick syndrome. Brain Res 1965; 2:167–186.
13. Guilleminault C, Stoohs R, Clerk A, Cetel M, Maistros P. A cause of excessive daytime sleepiness: the upper airway resistance syndrome. Chest 1993; 104:781–787.
14. Young T, Palta M, Dempsey J, Weber S, Badr S. The occurrence of sleep-disordered breathing among middle-aged adults. N Engl J Med 1993; 328:1230–1235.
15. Ohayon MM, Guilleminault C, Priest RG, Caulet M. Snoring and breathing pauses during sleep: telephone interview survey of a United Kingdom population sample. Br Med J 1997; 314:860–863.
16. Kurtzke JF. The current neurologic burden of illness and injury in the United States. Neurology 1982; 32:1207–1214.
17. Orem J. Neuronal mechanisms of respiration in REM sleep. Sleep 1980; 3:251–267.
18. Friberg D, Ansved T, Borg K, Larsson H, Norlander B, Svanborg E. Histological indications of progressive ''snorer disease'' in an upper airway muscle. Am J Respir Crit Care Med. 1998; 157:586–593.
19. Friberg D, Gazelius B, Hokfelt T, Norlander B. Abnormal afferent nerve endings in the soft palatal mucosa of sleep apneics. Regulatory Peptide. 1997; 71:29–36.
20. Guilleminault C, Stoohs R, Quera-Salva MA. Obstructive and non-obstructive apneas during sleep and neurological disorders. Neurology 1992; 42(suppl 6):53–60.
21. Miljeteig H, Mateika S, Haight JS, et al. Subjective and objective assessment of UPPP for the treatment of snoring and obstructive sleep apnea. Am J Respir Crit Care Med 1994; 150:1286–1291.
22. Shapiro PA. Effects of nasal obstruction on facial development. J Allergy Clin Immunol 1988; 81:967–975.

23. Guilleminault C, Kurland G, Winkle R, et al. Severe kyphoscoliosis, breathing, and sleep (the "Quasimodo" syndrome during sleep). Chest 1980; 79:626–630.
24. Guilleminault C, McQuitty J, Ariagno RL, et al. Six infants with congenital alveolar hypoventilation syndrome. Pediatrics 1982; 70:684–694.
25. Guilleminault C, Challamel MJ. Congenital central hypoventilation syndrome (CCHS): independent syndrome or generalized impairment of the autonomic nervous system. In: Guilleminault C, Korobkin R, eds. Progress in Perinatal Neurology. Vol 1. Baltimore: Williams and Wilkins, 1981:107–215.
26. Guilleminault C, Briskin JG, Greenfield MS, et al. The impact of autonomic nervous system dysfunction on breathing during sleep. Sleep 1981; 4:263–278.
27. Briskin JG, Lehrman KL, Guilleminault C. Shy-Drager syndrome and sleep apnea. In: Guilleminault C, Dement WC, eds. Sleep Apnea Syndromes. New York: Alan R Liss, 1978:317–322.
28. Severinghaus JW, Mitchell RA. Ondine's curse: failure of respiratory center automaticity while asleep. Clin Research 1962; 10:122.
29. Lehrman KL, Guilleminault C, Schroeder JS, et al. Sleep apnea syndrome in a patient with Shy-Drager syndrome. Arch Intern Med 1978; 138:206–209.
30. Krieger AJ, Rosomoff HL. Sleep induced apneas: a respiratory and autonomic dysfunction syndrome following bilateral percutaneous cervical cordotomy. J Neurosurg 1974; 32:277–283.
31. Levin B, Margolis G. Acute failure of autonomic respirations secondary to unilateral brainstem infarct. Ann Neurol 1977; 1:583–586.
32. Devereaux MW, Kleane JR, Davis RL. Automatic respiratory failure associated with infarction of the medulla. Arch Neurol 1973; 29:46–52.
33. Guilleminault C, Quera-Salva M, Nino-Murcia G, et al. Central sleep apnea and partial obstruction of the upper airway. Ann Neurol 1987; 21:465–469.
34. Quera-Salva MA, Guilleminault C. Post-traumatic central sleep apnea in a child. J Pediatr 1987; 110:906–909.
35. Cummiskey J, Guilleminault C, Davis R, et al. Automatic respiratory failure: sleep studies and Leigh's disease. Neurology 1987; 37:1876–1878.
36. McNicholas W, Rutherford R, Grossman R, et al. Abnormal respiratory pattern generation during sleep in patients with autonomic dysfunction. Am Rev Respir Dis 1983; 128:429–433.
37. Bradley TD, McNicholas WT, Rutherford R, et al. Clinical and physiological heterogeneity of the central sleep apnea syndrome. Am Rev Respir Dis 1986; 134:217–221.
38. Guilleminault C, and Motta J. Sleep apnea syndrome as a long sequela of poliomyelitis. In: Guilleminault C, Dement WC, eds. Sleep Apnea Syndromes. New York: Alan R Liss, 1978:309–315.
39. Quera-Salva MA, Guilleminault C, Troche G. Breathing disorders during sleep in myasthenia gravis. Ann Neurol 1992; 31:86–92.
40. Smith PE, Calverly PMA, Edwards RHT. Hypoxemia in Duchenne muscular dystrophy. Am Rev Respir Dis 1988; 137:884–888.
41. Guilleminault C, Cummiskey J, Motta J, Lynne-Davis P. Respiratory and hemodynamic study during wakefulness and sleep in myotonic dystrophy. Sleep 1978; 1:19–32.

42. Sullivan CE, Issa FG, Berthon-Jones M, et al. Reversal of obstructive sleep apnea by continuous positive airway pressure applied through the nares. Lancet 1981; i:862–864.
43. Reeves-Hoche MK, Meck R, Zwillich CW, et al. Nasal CPAP: an objective evaluation of patient compliance. Am J Respir Crit Care Med 1994; 149:149–154.
44. Schmidt-Nowara W, Lowe A, Wiegand L, Cartwright R, Perez-Guerra F, Menn S. Oral appliances for the treatment of snoring and obstructive sleep apnea: a review. Sleep 1995; 18:501–515.
45. Kerby GR, Mayer LS, Pingleton SK. Nocturnal positive pressure ventilation via nasal mask. Am Rev Respir Dis 1985; 131:41–45.
46. Ellis ER, Bye PTR, Bruderer JW, et al. Treatment of alveolar hypoventilation in a six year old girl with intermittent positive pressure ventilation through a nose mask. Am Rev Respir Dis 1987; 136:188–191.
47. Ellis ER, Bye PTR, Bruderer JW, et al. Treatment of respiratory failure during sleep in patients with neuromuscular disease. Am Rev Respir Dis 1987; 135:148–152.
48. Chervin RD, Guilleminault C. Diaphragmatic pacing for respiratory insufficiency. J Clin Neurophysiol 1997; 14:369–377.

14

Sleep and Stroke

Heikki Palomäki
University of Helsinki
Helsinki, Finland

Markku Partinen
Haaga Neurological Research Center
and University of Helsinki
Helsinki, Finland

CEREBROVASCULAR DISORDERS

Stroke is a major health problem in all developed countries. Although it is more often disabling than life-threatening, it ranks third among the leading causes of death, surpassed only by coronary heart disease and cancer (1). It consumes major amounts of the resources of acute-care hospitals and long-term care institutions.

In the Framingham study (1), ischemic brain infarction covers nearly 80% of all strokes, while intracerebral hemorrhage and subarachnoid hemorrhage together account for roughly 20%. Atherosclerosis appears to be the basic pathological condition responsible for most acute occlusive cerebrovascular events. As would be expected, several important determinants of atherosclerosis are associated with ischemic stroke. The most important risk factors of brain infarction are age, male gender, arterial hypertension, various abnormal cardiac conditions, diabetes mellitus and cigarette smoking. In addition to these established risk factors, however, several other factors may potentially increase the risk of suffering a stroke.

There is accumulating evidence suggesting a link between sleep-disordered breathing and cerebrovascular diseases. This association may be confounded by several factors because many of those determinants of stroke or atherosclerosis named above may also show connections with sleep-related breathing disorders. Adding to the complexity, sleep is often disturbed after a cerebrovascular accident, and among poststroke sleep disorders, respiratory dysfunctions occur frequently.

In this chapter we evaluate the epidemiological, clinical, and laboratory data on the interrelationship between snoring, sleep apnea, and stroke, as well as sleep disorders as a consequence of stroke. Also, in the latter case, emphasis is given to respiratory dysfunctions. Because of the natural distribution of stroke subtypes, we pay special attention to ischemic stroke.

Snoring, Obstructive Sleep Apnea, and Risk of Stroke

The History of Sleep-Disordered Breathing: How Valid Is It?

The reliability of snoring histories obtained by interviewing patients and their relatives may be questioned, and the importance of validating questionnaire information by direct recording is obvious. In a laboratory study addressing this problem (2), the reliability of snoring data obtained using a standardized questionnaire was demonstrated. Results of all-night polysomnographic registrations, with monitoring of snoring, respiration, oxygen saturation, and body movements, showed that those who reported being habitual snorers were in fact heavy snorers. On the other hand, 13% of those who believed they were never-snorers were simply unaware of their snoring (2). Thus, a self-reported snoring history appears to be valid and certainly unlikely to represent an overestimate. Nevertheless, the history of snoring should be graded as follows: 1) always or almost always (habitually), 2) often, 3) occasionally, or 4) never. It may reasonably be assumed that the influences and consequences of snoring may be dependent not only on its heaviness but also on its frequency.

When the estimates of snoring are based on questionnaire data, response errors are always possible. It is well known that those providing their own snoring histories are more likely to underestimate their snoring than are those with whom they sleep. Breathing arrests connected to snoring are also more often recognized by partners than by snorers themselves. Therefore, all attempts should be made to ascertain the snoring history from bed partners. In many cases, the presence of an obstructive sleep apnea syndrome (OSAS) can be suspected on the basis of sleep-related symptoms. To make firm conclusions about the detrimental effects of sleep-related breathing arrests on cerebral circulation, however, the frequency and type of apneic episodes should always be ascertained by polysomnographic recordings.

Snoring and the Risk of Stroke

The association between a history of snoring and stroke from 10 studies is shown in Table 1.

Table 1 Studies of the Association Between Stroke and History of Snoring

Study (ref.)	*n* (Patients/ controls)	Gender	Design	Snoring frequency	Stroke type	Odds ratio or relative risk (95% confidence interval)	Controlling for confounders
Partinen and Palomäki, 1985	50/100	M	CC	H, O/Occ, N H/O, Occ, N	BI	OR = 2.8 (1.3–5.8) OR = 10.3 (3.5–30.1)	A, G
Koskenvuo et al., 1987	4388/—	M	P	H, O/N	—[a]	RR = 2.1 (1.2–3.6)	A, H, BMI, S, AC
Schmidt-Nowara et al., 1990 (8)	1222/—	M, F	CS	H, O/Occ, N	—	OR = 0.6 (0.2–2.0)	A, G, BMI, S
Palomäki, 1991 (12)	177/177	M	CC	H, O/Occ, N	BI	OR = 2.1 (1.3–3.5)	A, G, H, CHD, DM, BMI, S, AC
Qizilbash et al., 1991	105/300	M, F	CC	—	TIA, BI	OR = 0.7 (0.4–1.2)	A, G, H, CHD, DM, S, AC, PCV
Spriggs et al., 1992 (4)	400/400	M, F	CC	H, O/Occ, N	—[b]	OR = 1.7 (1.3–2.2)	A, G, H, CHD, DM, BMI, S, AC, AF, PS
Smirne et al., 1993 (5)	164/330	M, F	CC	H, O/Occ, N	—	OR = 1.9 (1.2–2.9)	A, G, H, DM, BMI, S, AC, DL
Jennum et al., 1994 (10)	804/—	M, F	P	H/Occ, N	—	RR = 1.3 (0.7–2.3)	G, H, DM, BMI, S, AC, DL, SC, PA, C
Olson et al., 1995 (9)	441/—	M, F	CS	"Self-report of regular snoring"	—[c]	OR = 1.3 (0.7–2.4)	A, G, BMI, S, AC
Neau et al., 1995 (6)	133/133	M, F	CC	H/O, Occ, N	BI	OR = 2.9 (1.3–6.8)	A, G, H, DM, CA

[a] Coronary heart disease or stroke, stroke not defined; [b] subarachnoid hemorrhage excluded; [c] self-report of coronary artry disease, "blocked arteries," or stroke.

OR = odds ratio; RR = relative risk; M = male; F = female; CC = case-control; CS = cross-sectional; P = prospective.

BI = brain infarction, TIA = transient ischemic attack

Snoring frequency: H = always or almost always (habitual); O = often; Occ = occasionally (or infrequently); N = never.

Controlling for confounders: A = age; G = gender; H = hypertension (or blood-pressure values); CHD = coronary heart disease; DM = diabetes mellitus (or glucose values); BMI = body mass index; S = smoking; AC = alcohol consumption; AF = atrial fibrillation; DL = dyslipidemia; PCV = packed cell volume; PS = previous stroke; SC = social class; PA = physical activity; C = catecholamines; CA = cardiac arrhythmia.

In our earlier review dealing with sleep-disordered breathing and stroke (3), we identified seven studies of the association between snoring and cerebrovascular disorder. The frequency of snoring was reported in five of six case-control studies, and in all of them cerebrovascular disease was found to be significantly associated with snoring. The risk was greater in those who snored always, almost always, or often than in those who snored occasionally or never. The odds ratios (OR) relating to snoring and cerebrovascular disease were of the order of two to three (3). In one cohort study, the adjusted relative risk of snoring for combined ischemic heart disease and undefined stroke was 2.1.

Later case-control studies of the connection between snoring and stroke yielded results in accordance with those reported above (4–6). After adjusting for several potential confounders, the ORs of snoring "often" for stroke were 1.7 (4) and 1.9 (5). The OR for "habitual" snoring in relation to ischemic brain infarction was 2.9 (6). All these risk estimates were significant. Among stroke victims and control subjects, the percentages of those who reported snoring at least "often" ranged between 48 and 58, and between 30 and 38, respectively.

Zaninelli et al. (7) investigated the influence of snoring on morbidity and mortality from cardiovascular disease over 5 years. An increase in morbidity and mortality from heart disease and stroke was found in snorers with other risk factors compared with nonsnorers with other risk factors. No difference was noted between snorers and nonsnorers without additional risk factors. It was concluded that the prognosis in patients with traditional determinants of cardiovascular disease who snored was worse than in nonsnorers, but that snoring was not itself an independent predictive risk factor.

In a population-based sample of 1222 Hispanic-Americans (8), the age-adjusted prevalence of regular loud snoring was 27.8% in men and 15.3% in women. After adjustment for age, gender, obesity, and smoking, there was no significant effect of snoring on stroke (OR = 0.6). In another community study including 441 subjects (9), a category of "occlusive vascular disease" was defined by self-report of coronary artery disease or of "blocked arteries" or stroke. After adjustments, no significant association with occlusive vascular disease existed between snorers and nonsnorers (OR = 1.3). The authors concluded that the association of snoring with vascular disease is due at least partly to confounding. There were few cases of stroke in that study, however, and the large proportion of self-reported regular snorers (66%) suggests an attenuated effect of snoring on stroke; in some cases snoring history may have been contaminated by occasional snoring. Jennum et al. (10) studied the connection between snoring and stroke in a six-year follow-up study in a 70-year-old population. Although a significantly higher stroke incidence was found among those who snored "always or almost always" (relative risk = 1.8), no significant association could be found after several additional risk factors were controlled for (relative risk = 1.3). Accordingly, snoring history did not emerge as an independent risk factor of stroke in this elderly population. On the other hand, this does not rule out the influence of snoring on the risk of stroke in middle-aged or younger populations.

Hence, results from case-control and population-based studies seem to be diverging. It should be remembered that in most community studies there have been relatively few stroke cases. Direct comparison of the results is also impossible if the classification of snoring history has not been uniform across studies. It may be generalized that the influence of snoring on cerebrovascular disorders is dependent on its frequency, and habitual snoring (always or almost always) probably carries substantial risk. Habitual snoring is also more often connected to breathing arrests than is occasional snoring.

Obstructive Sleep Apnea Syndrome and the Risk of Stroke

Sporadic obstructive apneic episodes often occur in loud snorers, in particular during light and rapid-eye-movement (REM) sleep when supine (11). On the basis of observations of the natural history of loud, habitual snoring, it has been suggested that snoring and OSAS represent extremes of the same fundamental disturbance: sleep-related stenosis of the upper airways (11). Subjects who develop OSAS have usually been loud snorers for years (11). Heavy snoring invariably accompanies OSAS.

Consequently, it might be expected that patients with OSAS are more prone to vascular accidents than snorers not subject to sleep-related respiratory pauses. On the basis of data available, this is the case. In a study of 177 male stroke victims and controls (12), nine patients (5.2%) and two controls (1.2%) were suspected of having OSAS because they had histories of snoring with apneic periods, suffered from excessive daytime sleepiness, and were overweight. Suspected OSAS was associated strongly with ischemic stroke (OR = 8). Accordingly, the connection between snoring and cerebrovascular disease may be due to the increased likelihood of OSAS in those who snore frequently. Snoring on its own, without apnea, obesity, and sleepiness, did not increase the likelihood of suffering stroke (12).

In studies published later, overnight polysomnographic recordings were performed to determine whether sleep apnea was more prevalent in patients with transient ischemic attacks (TIAs) or stroke than in control subjects (13–15). The differences were clear and significant. In each study, approximately 70% of patients with TIA or stroke were diagnosed as having sleep apnea, whereas the respective proportions in control subjects ranged from only 15% to 19%. The proportions of patients who presented with sleep apnea were nearly equal in TIA or stroke groups (13,14).

At this stage, the real influence of sleep-disordered breathing on the long-term risk of cerebrovascular events still remains open. Longitudinal studies are required to ascertain whether a causal relationship exists between snoring, sleep apnea, and stroke. Some follow-up data already suggest that patients suffering from nocturnal breathing arrests may be prone to vascular accidents. In this context, active treatment of OSAS has also been beneficial. In a follow-up study carried out at Stanford University, California, 71 or 198 patients with OSAS were subjected to tracheostomy, whereas the other 127 patients received only recommendations to lose weight (16). After 7 years, a considerable effect attributable to treatment was evident. As compared with the tracheostomized group, the morbidity from cardiovascular and cerebrovascular disorders among patients treated conservatively was greater (16). Although patients treated conservatively presented fewer vascular problems at entry, the rate among them of vascular deaths during follow-up was higher: there were 14 deaths in the group treated conservatively but only one among tracheostomized patients (16).

In their 5-year study of 400 patients mentioned earlier, Zaninelli et al. (7) also studied the contribution of sleep apnea to morbidity from heart disease and stroke. Of 18 sleep apnea patients who also had other risk factors for cardiovascular disease, 17 suffered a cardiovascular event. Ten of 12 sleep apnea patients without other obvious risk factors also suffered a vascular event.

From available data, there appears to be increased risk of cerebrovascular morbidity as risk of OSAS increases. At present, the findings of the studies cited above are in keeping with the statement that for simple snoring without obstructive sleep apnea aggressive treatment to prevent vascular problems is not justified (17). It should be kept in mind, however, that snoring and OSAS may be regarded as a continuum of sleep-disordered breathing, and those with asymptomatic heavy snoring may progressively become symptomatic OSAS patients (11).

Circadian Variation of Stroke Onset and Risk of Stroke in Sleep

The risk of suffering stroke is not evenly distributed throughout the day (18). Moreover, different subtypes of stroke seem to follow a different circadian periodicity. Intracerebral hemorrhage and subarachnoid hemorrhage typically have their onset during daily activities, whereas ischemic stroke more often occurs at night or is linked to awakening or getting up from bed (Figure 1) (18). While sleep seems to protect against hemorrhagic strokes, this is not the case with ischemic cerebrovascular events.

On the basis of findings from several studies (see Ref. 18 for review), the morning peak for ischemic stroke onset is between 6 A.M. and 8 A.M., or between 8 A.M. and 10 A.M. during holidays. A peak between 10 A.M. and noon has been found in some studies (18).

In a retrospective study, the day was divided into four periods of 6 hours each. Brain infarction occurred most frequently between midnight and 6 A.M. (19). In one study of 24 consecutive patients, retinal infarction of embolic origin was found to occur frequently during sleep (20). Neau et al. (6) reported that 46.6% of their patients with brain infarction suffered a sleep-related stroke, that

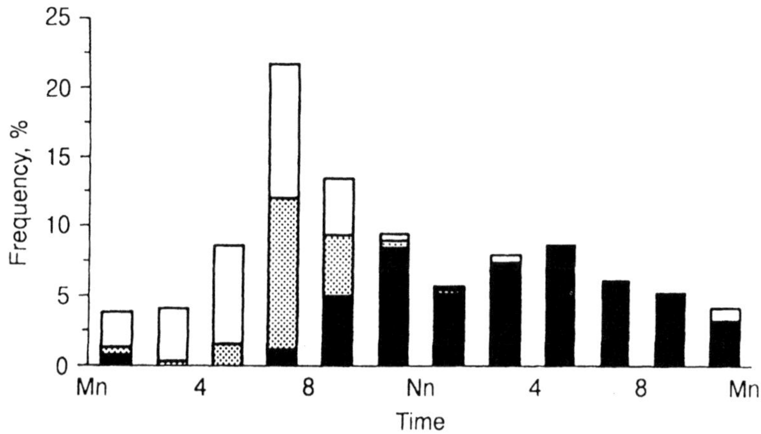

Figure 1 Frequency in two-hour intervals of onset of ischemic stroke. Black columns: patients (n = 294) having been awake for more than 2 hours before the onset of stroke; white columns: patients (n = 160) whose stroke onset was observed on awakening; gray columns: patients (n = 102) being stricken within 2 hours after awakening. Mn = midnight; Nn = noon. (From Ref. 18.)

is, stroke occurring during sleep or within 30 minutes after awakening. In the study by Dyken et al. (15), more than 50% of stroke victims were stricken during sleep.

Although there are some conflicting findings (18), ischemic cerebrovascular events seem to occur at an unexpectedly high rate during sleep or immediately after awakening. The risk reaches a peak early in the morning. This pattern closely resembles that for acute events related to myocardial ischemia.

Potential Determinants of the Circadian Periodicity of Ischemic Stroke

In most investigations, attempts to identify factors responsible for the circadian periodicity of cerebrovascular ischemia have been unsuccessful. In one of them, the risk-factor patterns of sleep-related ischemic strokes were compared with those of strokes occurring during daytime activities (21). In 167 male patients, 35.3% suffered brain infarction during sleep and it was noticed on waking. The percentage was 41.9 when the first 30 minutes after awakening were included. History of snoring was a significant factor in relation to circadian variation of stroke onset: snorers suffered brain infarction more often during sleep than did nonsnorers (adjusted OR = 2.7). This study showed that snoring may carry the most substantial risk in relation to nocturnal strokes. On the other hand, in two other studies, snoring did not differentiate between sleep-related or daytime strokes (4,6).

The finding of excess of nocturnal and early-morning brain infarction in snorers reflects a similar distribution of sudden cardiovascular death and snoring in men (22). In the latter study, habitual snoring was significantly related to early-morning death from cardiovascular causes. No similar variation in time of death was found in snorers who died for other reasons.

Although no mechanisms explaining circadian variation of ischemic vascular events have been determined, a number of potential triggering factors have temporal distribution resembling those of ischemic episodes.

Blood-pressure values follow a prominent circadian rhythm. Lowest values occur at night and early in the morning, and highest values occur before noon (23). Nocturnal and early-morning hypotension in precipitating cerebral ischemia have been suggested as causes of circadian variation in brain infarction, but no real evidence for this has been recorded. It is doubtful that hypotension plays an important role in the risk of brain infarction. The results of a study in patients who were resuscitated after cardiac arrest also suggest that hypotensive episodes are not a major cause of brain infarction (24).

Rapid increases in blood pressure may lead to a rupture of areas of atherosclerotic plaque. Such a mechanism has been postulated in relation to myocardial infarction (25). It can result in development of thrombi and dislodging of embolic material in distal arteries. Other concomitant mechanisms favoring thrombus formation also exist. Among them, hematocrit values and blood viscosity have been shown to peak in the morning (26). There is a marked reduction in activity of tissue-type plasminogen activator at night and in the morning, and fibrinolytic activity is low at these times (27). Furthermore, platelet activity increases in the morning. This has also been suggested as a mechanism precipitating myocardial infarction and sudden cardiac death in the morning hours (28).

Accordingly, a number of physiological processes that may cause rupture of atherosclerotic plaques and hypercoagulable state are accentuated in the morning (25). Circadian changes in the balance between thrombosis and thrombolysis may consequently lead to thrombus formation and propagation at that time. Although the morning has frequently been suggested to be the peak time of onset of ischemic vascular disease, it has also been suggested that similar physiological mechanisms trigger onset of disease at other times (25). With respect to the way in which snoring and sleep apnea could precipitate ischemic stroke, this is of interest because there may be connections between sleep-related breathing disturbances and suggested mechanisms leading to early-morning stroke.

Possible Mechanisms Explaining the Connection Between Sleep-Disordered Breathing and Ischemic Stroke

High catecholamine concentrations and sympathetic nervous tone have been found in patients with OSAS (29). In such patients, high sympathetic activity has been suggested to result in high daytime blood pressure, and cardiovascular catastrophe in hypertensive individuals during sleep (30). Because of connections with cardiac arrhythmia, sleep-related breathing disturbances may also increase the risk of cardioembolic strokes (31). In accordance with these findings, snoring, and arterial hypertension have been suggested as additive risk factors for sleep-related brain infarction (6,21), and snoring has been found to be in especially strong association with cardiogenic embolism (12). Some patients with OSAS may be prone to paradoxical embolism owing to changes in intrathoracic pressure associated with obstructive sleep apnea (31).

Alterations in cerebral blood flow are known to occur in relation to sleep apnea (31). In elderly patients with sleep-related breathing disorders, sympathetic reflexes can be impaired, leading to marked hypotensive periods and a risk of circulatory failure in connection with apnea (32). Although hypotension as a precursor of brain infarction may be infrequent, these phenomena could be important in the pathophysiology of sleep-related stroke in some cases.

Platelet aggregability may be enhanced by high sympathetic tone. In a small study including 10 male stroke patients, those with increased platelet thromboxane B2 release in the morning experienced significantly more oxygen-desaturation periods during sleep than those without increased values (33). There seems to be no unequivocal evidence for increased platelet activation and aggregation in OSAS, however.

High hematocrit and blood-viscosity levels secondary to sleep-related hypoxemia could play a role in some cases. On the other hand, polycythemia is not common in patients with OSAS (34), and no difference was found in the mean hematocrit between regular snorers and other subjects (4).

In most patients suffering from ischemic cerebrovascular disease, the underlying process is atherosclerosis leading to stenosis or occlusion or cervicocranial arteries. Experimental evidence links hypoxemia with atherosclerosis (35). Apneic episodes in connection with oxygen desaturations could therefore increase the long-term risk of ischemic stroke by accelerating the atherosclerotic process. Sleep-related breathing disturbances may thus have connections with hemodynamic disturbances and, perhaps, coagulability of the blood. Theoretically, these mechanisms could act as immediate triggers for acute cerebrovascular disorders. There might also be long-term systemic effects on the process of atherosclerosis. At present, no established mechanisms have been demonstrated.

SLEEP IN ACUTE STROKE AND IN STROKE RECOVERY

Sleep is frequently disturbed after neurological disorders, including stroke. Data on poststroke sleep disturbances are, however, scarce and somewhat conflicting.

At the acute stage, patients with ischemic hemispheral lesions have shown a significant suppression of REM sleep (36–38). This reduction has been correlated with the severity of neurological deficit (38), and it has been more pronounced in deep lesions (38) or lesions of the right hemisphere (36). The attenuation of REM sleep may normalize over days or weeks (37,38), but it may be present even months after stroke (39). REM-sleep alteration may also be predictive of neurological outcome: the early presence of REM sleep and normal non-REM–REM cycles has been suggested to be a good prognostic sign (38). In convalescing hemispheric stroke patients, the time spent in slow-wave sleep may be increased (40) but an opposite finding has also been reported (39). Loss of stage 2 sleep after a large hemispheric stroke has been associated with an unfavorable prognosis for survival (41). Findings concerning sleep disturbances after brainstem infarction have also been inconsistent, but REM and non-REM sleep reduction are repeatedly observed (42–44).

The thalamus seems to have a key role in both arousal control and sleep production. Thalamic stroke may be accompanied by daytime drowsiness, with no major alterations in nocturnal sleep (45,46). Sleep architecture may parallel the degree of hypersomnia: in 12 patients with paramedian thalamic stroke, those with severe hypersomnia showed most prominent reductions in nocturnal non-REM sleep (stages two to four) (47). It was postulated that both deficient daytime arousal and disturbances in nocturnal sleep architecture may operate in hypersomnia following paramedian thalamic stroke (47).

Poor sleep quality in patients convalescing from stroke may be connected to mood disorders, and depression is a well-known consequence of stroke. In a prospective study of poststroke depression (48), patients were rated using the Hamilton Depression Scale (49), three items of which relate to insomnia (early, middle, and late insomnia). Seventy-five percent of 191 patients rated positive for one or more kinds of insomnia at least once during 1-year follow-up. Although insomnia in stroke victims appears to be common, it has received little attention so far.

Respiratory dysfunctions occur frequently after stroke (50). Depending on the extent and localization of the vascular lesion, breathing may be impaired in different ways. Central respiratory centers are located in the brainstem (51). After infratentorial strokes, apneusis (apnea during sustained inspiration), central sleep apnea, and failure of automatic breathing (Ondine's curse), as well as obstructive and mixed sleep apnea are observed (50). In hemispheric ischemic strokes, a Cheyne-Stokes breathing pattern may occur. It is more frequent with bilateral than with unilateral lesions (50).

In some uncontrolled series of patients with ischemic stroke, high percentages of sleep-disordered breathing were observed (52–54). Among breathing disturbances, obstructive sleep apnea (apnea–hypopnea index of 10 or more per hour) was the most common. It was reported to be present in 72% (52) and 54% (54) of patients. Prevalence and severity of disturbed breathing were similar between patients with supratentorial and infratentorial stroke (54). In a case-control study conducted by Mohsenin and Valor (39), patients with hemispheric stroke had significantly more respiratory events per hour than control subjects. Although patients with prior history of sleep-related breathing disturbances were excluded, eight of the 10 patients were found to have significant sleep apnea. Obstructive apneas comprised the majority of respiratory events.

Associations between stroke and sleep-related breathing disorders are thus complicated: while snoring and OSAS have been suggested as risk factors for stroke, sleep-disordered breathing may also be a consequence of cerebrovascular disorder. In this context, it is worth referring to an earlier, well-documented case history (55) of a patient who had breathing arrests following a vertebrobasilar stroke. He exhibited repeated episodes of transient coma, left-sided hemiplegia, bilateral Babinski's signs, and ophthalmoplegia, with each episode occurring while sleeping. Polysomnographic recordings revealed that obstructive apneic periods consistently preceded the attacks. This suggests that obstructive—possibly symptomatic—apneic events were triggers for further brainstem ischemia (55).

Spriggs et al. (4) assessed the outcome of stroke patients in relation to snoring. Patients were followed up for six months after their strokes. Snoring adversely affected prognosis: those who snored regularly had higher short- and long-term mortalities than nonsnorers (4). Similarly, Good et al. (53) discovered an association between overnight arterial oxyhemoglobin desaturations, higher 1-year mortality rate, and worse functional outcome in stroke patients undergoing rehabilitation. In their study, the frequent history of snoring also suggested that sleep-disordered breathing preceded the stroke in most patients. Dyken et al. (15) found obstructive sleep apnea in 71% of patients with a recent stroke. The four-year mortality rate for patients with stroke was 20.8%; all patients who died had obstructive sleep apnea.

Sleep apnea should probably be regarded as a precursor rather than a sequel of stroke. In support of this, the occurrence of sleep apnea has been shown to be nearly equal in both TIA patients and those who have suffered complete strokes (13,14). Regardless of whether it precedes or follows a cerebrovascular accident, sleep-disordered breathing may increase the risk of unfavorable outcome after stroke. Sleep-related mechanisms precipitating first-ever strokes or myocardial ischemia may also operate in the convalescing period. Additionally, breathing disorders during sleep may result in daytime somnolence, decreased attention, and difficulties in cognitive performance, which are all factors that potentially hamper the rehabilitation process.

REFERENCES

1. Wolf PA, Cobb JL, D'Agostino RB. Epidemiology of stroke. In: Barnett HJM, Mohr JP, Stein BM, Yatsu FM, eds. Stroke: Pathophysiology, Diagnosis, and Management. 2nd ed. New York: Churchill-Livingstone, 1992:3–27.

2. Telakivi T, Partinen M, Koskenvuo M, Salmi T, Kaprio J. Periodic breathing and hypoxia in snorers and controls: validation of snoring history and association with blood pressure and obesity. Acta Neurol Scand 1987; 76:69–75.
3. Palomäki H, Partinen M, Erkinjuntti, T, Kaste M. Snoring, sleep apnea syndrome, and stroke. Neurology 1992; 42(suppl 6):75–82.
4. Spriggs DA, French JM, Murdy JM, Curless RH, Bates D, James OFM. Snoring increases the risk of stroke and adversely affects prognosis. Q J Med 1992; 84:555–562.
5. Smirne S, Palazzi S, Zucconi M, Chierchia S, Ferini-Strambi L. Habitual snoring as a risk factor for acute vascular disease. Eur Respir J 1993; 6:1357–1361.
6. Neau JP, Meurice JC, Paquereau J, Chavagnat JJ, Ingrand P, Gil R. Habitual snoring as a risk factor for brain infarction. Acta Neurol Scand 1995; 92:63–68.
7. Zaninelli A, Fariello R, Boni E, Corda L, Alicandri C, Grassi V. Snoring and cardiovascular disease. Int J Cardiol 1991; 32:347–351.
8. Schmidt-Nowara WW, Coultas DB, Wiggins C, Skipper BE, Samet JM. Snoring in a Hispanic-American population: risk factors and association with hypertension and other morbidity. Arch Intern Med 1990; 150:597–601.
9. Olson LG, King MT, Hensley MJ, Saunders NA. A community study of snoring and sleep-disordered breathing: health outcomes. Am J Respir Crit Care Med 1995; 152:717–720.
10. Jennum P, Schultz-Larsen K, Davidsen M, Christensen NJ. Snoring and risk of stroke and ischaemic heart disease in a 70 year old population: a 6-year follow-up study. Int J Epidemiol 1994; 23:1159–1164.
11. Lugaresi E, Cirignotta F, Gerardi R, Montagna P. Snoring and sleep apnea: natural history of heavy snorers disease. In: Guilleminault C, Partinen M, eds. Obstructive Sleep Apnea Syndrome: Clinical Research and Treatment. New York: Raven Press, 1990:25–36.
12. Palomäki H. Snoring and the risk of ischemic brain infarction. Stroke 1991; 22: 1021–1025.
13. Voll CL, Mosewich R, Senthilselvan A. Sleep apnea in symptomatic ischemic cerebrovascular disease: a prospective study [abstr]. Neurology 1992; 42(suppl 3):60.
14. Bassetti C, Aldrich MS, Chervin RD, Quint D. Sleep apnea in patients with transient ischemic attack and stroke: a prospective study of 59 patients. Neurology 1996; 47: 1167–1173.
15. Dyken ME, Somers VK, Yamada T, Ren Z-Y, Zimmerman MB. Investigating the relationship between stroke and obstructive sleep apnea. Stroke 1996; 27:401–407.
16. Partinen M, Guilleminault C. Daytime sleepiness and vascular morbidity at seven-year follow-up in obstructive sleep apnea patients. Chest 1990; 97:27–32.
17. Rees J. Snoring. Tackle obesity, smoking, and alcohol consumption first. Br Med J 1991; 302:860–861.
18. Haapaniemi H, Hillbom M, Numminen H, Juvela S, Palomäki H, Kaste M. Early-morning increase in the onset of ischemic stroke. Cerebrovasc Dis 1992; 2:282–286.
19. Marshall J. Diurnal variation in occurrence of strokes. Stroke 1977; 8:230–231.
20. Bruno A, Biller J, Adams HP, Corbett JJ. Retinal infarction during sleep and wakefulness. Stroke 1990; 21:1494–1496.

21. Palomäki H, Partinen M, Juvela S, Kaste M. Snoring as a risk factor for sleep-related brain infarction. Stroke 1989; 20:1311–1315.
22. Seppälä T, Partinen M, Penttilä A, Aspholm R, Tiainen E, Kaukiainen A. Sudden death and sleeping history among Finnish men. J Intern Med 1991; 229:23–28.
23. Millar-Craig MW, Bishop CN, Raftery EB. Circadian variation of blood-pressure. Lancet 1978; i:795–797.
24. Torvik A, Skullerud K. How often are brain infarcts caused by hypotensive episodes? Stroke 1976; 7:255–257.
25. Muller JE, Tofler GH, Stone PH. Circadian variation and triggers of onset of acute cardiovascular disease. Circulation 1989; 79:733–743.
26. Kubota K, Sakurai T, Tamura J, Shirakura T. Is the circadian change in hematocrit and blood viscosity a factor triggering cerebral and myocardial infarction? Stroke 1987; 18:812–813.
27. Kluft C, Jie AFH, Rijken DC, Verheijen JH. Daytime fluctuations in blood of tissue-type plasminogen activator (t-PA) and its fast-acting inhibitor (PAI-1). Thromb Haemost 1988; 59:329–332.
28. Tofler GH, Brezinski D, Schafer AI, Czeisler CA, Rutherford JD, Willich SN, Gleason RE, Williams GH, Muller JE. Concurrent morning increase in platelet aggregability and the risk of myocardial infarction and sudden cardiac death. N Engl J Med 1987; 316:1514–1518.
29. Fletcher EC, Miller J, Schaaf JW, Fletcher JG. Urinary catecholamines before and after tracheostomy in patients with obstructive sleep apnea and hypertension. Sleep 1987; 10:35–44.
30. Somers VK, Mark AL, Abboud FM. Sympathetic activation by hypoxia and hypercapnia—implications for sleep apnea. Clin Exp Hypertens A 1988; 10(suppl 1): 413–422.
31. Shephard JW Jr. Hypertension, cardiac arrhythmias, myocardial infarction, and stroke in relation to obstructive sleep apnea. Clin Chest Med 1992; 13:437–458.
32. McGinty D, Beahm E, Stern N, Littner M, Sowers J, Reige W. Nocturnal hypotension in older men with sleep-related breathing disorders. Chest 1988; 94:305–311.
33. Palomäki H, Kaste M. Association of thromboxane B2 production to hypoxemic periods during sleep in male stroke patients. J Stroke Cerebrovasc Dis 1993; 3:145–149.
34. Douglas NJ. The sleep apnoea/hypopnoea syndrome and snoring. Br Med J 1993; 306:1057–1060.
35. Gainer JL. Hypoxia and atherosclerosis: re-evaluation of an old hypothesis. Atherosclerosis 1987; 68:263–266.
36. Korner E, Flooh E, Reinhart B, Wolf R, Ott E, Krenn W, Lechner H. Sleep alterations in ischemic stroke. Eur Neurol 1986; 25(suppl 2):104–110.
37. Hachinski VC, Mamelak M, Norris JW. Clinical recovery and sleep architecture degradation. Can J Neurol Sci 1990; 17:332–335.
38. Giubilei F, Iannilli M, Vitale A, Pierallini A, Sacchetti ML, Antonimi G, Fieschi C. Sleep patterns in acute ischemic stroke. Acta Neurol Scand 1992; 86:567–571.
39. Mohsenin V, Valor R. Sleep apnea in patients with hemispheric stroke. Arch Phys Med Rehabil 1995; 76:71–76.

40. Culebras A, Miller M. Absence of sleep-related elevation of growth hormone level in patients with stroke. Arch Neurol 1983; 40:283–286.
41. Hachinski V, Mamelak M, Norris JW. Sleep morphology and prognosis in acute cerebrovascular lesions. In: Meyer JS, Lechner H, Reivich M, eds. Cerebral Vascular Disease. Amsterdam: Excerpta Medica, 1977:69–71.
42. Markand ON, Dyken ML. Sleep abnormality in patients with brain stem lesions. Neurology 1976; 26:769–776.
43. Autret A, Laffont F, de Toffol B, Cathala H-P. A syndrome of REM and non-REM sleep reduction and lateral gaze paresis after medial tegmental pontine stroke. Arch Neurol 1988; 45:1236–1242.
44. Schafer D, Bianchi O, Greulich W, Schafer C, Schafer T, Schlafke ME. Sleep and breathing disorders in patients with brain stem lesions. Wien Med Wochenschr 1996; 146:296–298.
45. Catsman-Berrevoets CE, Harskamp F. Compulsive pre-sleep behaviour and apathy due to bilateral thalamic stroke. Neurology 1988; 38:647–649.
46. Guilleminault C, Quera-Salva MA, Goldberg MP. Pseudohypersomnia and pre-sleep behaviour with bilateral paramedian thalamic lesions. Brain 1993; 116:1549–1563.
47. Bassetti C, Mathis J, Gugger M, Lövblad KO, Hess CW. Hypersomnia following paramedian thalamic stroke: a report of 12 patients. Ann Neurol 1996; 39:471–480.
48. Vestergaard K, Mohr-Drewes A, Andersen G, Jorgensen-Taagholt S. Post-stroke sleep disorder treated with the selective serotonin reuptake inhibitor citalopram—a case study. Eur J Neurol 1996; 3:164–168.
49. Hamilton M. A rating scale for depression. J Neurol Neurosurg Psychiatry 1960; 23:56–62.
50. Vingerhoets F, Bogousslavsky J. Respiratory dysfunction in stroke. Clin Chest Med 1994; 15:729–737.
51. Simon RP. Respiration. In: Asbury AK, McKhann GM, McDonald WI, eds. Diseases of the Nervous System: Clinical Neurobiology. Vol I. Philadelphia: WB Saunders, 1986:651–664.
52. Kapen S, Park A, Goldberg J, Wynter J. The incidence and severity of obstructive sleep apnea in ischemic cerebrovascular disease [abstr]. Neurology 1991; 41(suppl 1):125.
53. Good DC, Henkle JQ, Gelber D, Welsh J, Verhulst S. Sleep-disordered breathing and poor functional outcome after stroke. Stroke 1996; 27:252–259.
54. Bassetti C, Aldrich MS, Quint D. Sleep-disordered breathing in patients with acute supra- and infratentorial strokes: a prospective study of 39 patients. Stroke 1997; 28:1765–1772.
55. Rivest J, Reiher J. Transient ischemic attacks triggered by symptomatic sleep apneas [abstr]. Stroke 1987; 18:293.

15

Sleep, Epilepsy, and Sudden Death

Christine Quinto
Saint Vincents Hospital
New York, New York

Sudhansu Chokroverty
Saint Vincents Hospital and
New York Medical College
New York, New York

INTRODUCTION

The existence of a reciprocal relationship between sleep and epilepsy was observed centuries ago. Hippocrates allegedly described ''fears, rages, deliria, leaps out of bed, and seizures during the night'' (1). Aristotle also noted that most epilepsies began during sleep. However, it was not until the late 19th century that physicians took interest in this apparent relationship of epilepsy to the sleep–wake cycle. At around this time, Fere (2) observed that most of his epileptic patients had attacks between the hours of 8 P.M. and 8 A.M. In addition to corroborating Fere's observations, later investigators also noted that seizures occurred at certain times of the night (3–5).

The advent of electroencephalography in 1929 validated these clinical observations with neurophysiological correlates. In 1947, Gibbs and Gibbs (6) found that paroxysmal discharges on EEG occurred twice as often during sleep as in the waking state. This finding was duplicated by numerous investigators over the next several years (7–10).

With the firm establishment of the intimate relationship between paroxysmal EEG discharges and sleep came the search for the physiological and biochemical basis for this association. In this chapter we discuss the effect of sleep on epilepsy and vice versa. We also discuss the diagnostic and therapeutic approaches toward sleep-related epilepsy. Finally, we attempt to elucidate the mechanisms underlying sudden death in epilepsy.

BASIC MECHANISMS OF EPILEPSY

Epilepsy is a state of recurrent seizures. During a seizure, abnormal synchronized neuronal discharges arise either locally from a population of cortical neurons (partial) or diffusely from both hemispheres (generalized). Experimental models of partial epilepsy are produced by applying chemicals such as penicillin directly to, or by stimulating a focal area of, cortical tissue. Generalized epilepsy models are created by systemic injections of convulsants or by electric shock (11).

The hallmark of the interictal state is the spike-and-wave discharge that correlates on a cellular level to the paroxysmal depolarization shift (PDS), a prolonged high-amplitude depolarization that is followed by a hyperpolarization (12,13). Maintenance of the interictal state, and thus prevention of ictal precipitation, is determined by strong inhibitory influences. It is the breakdown of these inhibitory interictal mechanisms plus excessive synchronizing thalamocortical afferent input that leads to the development of an ictus (11).

Neuronal epileptogenesis is dependent on both genetic and acquired factors that maintain increased neuronal hyperexcitability and increased neuronal synchronization (11).

BASIC MECHANISMS OF SLEEP

We now know that there are two sleep states in humans: synchronized, or non-rapid-eye-movement (non-REM), sleep and desynchronized, or rapid-eye-movement (REM), sleep, each of which is determined by a different set of physiological mechanisms (14).

In non-REM sleep, nonspecific thalamic nuclei provide diffuse synchronized afferent input to the cortex and are responsible for the rhythmicity of sleep spindles (15). This same diffuse cortical synchronization leads to active ictal activation in susceptible individuals. Hence, non-REM sleep is a known convulsant.

On the other hand, REM sleep appears to behave like an anticonvulsant because during this state there is inhibition of thalamocortical synchronizing mechanisms (16). In addition, there is a tonic reduction of interhemispheric transmission through the corpus callosum, preventing generalization of epileptiform discharges (17).

A variety of neurotransmitters have been implicated in the initiation of sleep and the generation of the non-REM–REM cycle. It appears that during

REM sleep there is cholinergic hyperactivity and aminergic hypoactivity (14,18). During wakefulness, noradrenergic and dopaminergic neurons prevail.

RELATIONSHIP BETWEEN SEIZURES AND SLEEP

In the following section we describe the effect of sleep on both interictal EEG discharges and clinical seizures (19).

Generalized Epilepsies

Primary Generalized Grand Mal Seizure

The interictal EEG discharges of primary generalized grand mal epilepsy are generally observed in non-REM sleep and disappear in REM sleep (20–22). They are usually prominent at sleep onset and during the first part of the night. On occasion, the discharges are activated during non-REM sleep in the late part of the night and are thought to result from reduced serum levels of antiepileptic medications (20). These observations correlate with the clinical occurrence of generalized seizures almost exclusively in non-REM sleep, most frequently 1–2 hours following sleep onset and at 5–6 A.M. (23–25). Interictal discharges may be fragmented or may appear as polyspikes or focal spikes during non-REM sleep.

In a study of 171 patients, Billiard et al. (26) found exclusively nocturnal seizures in only 8%. Passouant et al. (27) called the seizure occurring exclusively during sleep "l'epilepsie morpheique" and considered this a benign form of epilepsy. In most of these patients, daytime EEG remains normal; they rarely go on to develop waking epilepsies and do so only after 2 years from onset (28).

Petit Mal (Absence) Epilepsy

Absence seizures are most common in childhood. They are generally brief, lasting only a few seconds, and are manifested by blinking, staring, or other minor facial movements. Absence seizures are commonly observed in the waking state and may be difficult to diagnose during sleep. Niedermeyer (29) noted fluttering of the eyelids in association with the typical 3-Hz spike-and-wave discharges during sleep. Observations of petit mal status during REM sleep have been reported (30–32).

The interictal EEG discharges of absence epilepsy are found in all stages of non-REM sleep, particularly during the first sleep cycle, and are generally absent in REM sleep (26,33,34). Just as in generalized grand mal epilepsy, alterations of spike-and-wave discharge morphology during the different stages of non-REM sleep have been reported: regular or irregular spike-and-wave discharges in non-REM stages 1 and 2, and irregular polyspikes and slow waves during non-REM stages 3 and 4 (33). In addition, fragmentation or focalization of spikes can be seen over the frontal regions during non-REM sleep.

Juvenile Myoclonic Epilepsy

Juvenile myoclonic epilepsy usually starts in adolescence and is characterized by the presence of myoclonic, generalized tonic-clonic, and absence seizures, although not all seizure types may be present in the same patient. Seizures usually occur shortly after awakening in the morning, with the duration of the attack longer upon awakening from non-REM than from REM sleep (35). Occasionally these attacks may occur on awakening in the middle of the night or later in the afternoon (7).

Interictal discharges in these patients are prominent at sleep onset and on awakening but are virtually nonexistent during the rest of the night (20). According to Touchon (36), induced awakening is a better facilitator than spontaneous awakening in these patients.

Lennox-Gastaut Syndrome

Lennox-Gastaut syndrome comprises a combination of seizures: tonic, myoclonic, generalized tonic-clonic, atonic, and atypical absence (37). Information about the effect of sleep on the clinical seizures in this syndrome is lacking in the literature (38). Tonic seizures, however, are typically activated by sleep and are much more frequent during non-REM sleep than during wakefulness (39). They are never seen during REM sleep (40).

The typical EEG finding in Lennox-Gastaut syndrome is the slow spike and wave (1.5–2.5 Hz). These spike-and-wave discharges characteristically increase in non-REM sleep (38). They may be intermixed with trains of fast spikes of 10–25 Hz lasting for 2 to 10 seconds. On occasion, bursts of electrodecremental activity may alternate with bursts of polyspikes, giving rise to a burst-suppression-like pattern (38). According to Markand (41), prognosis is better in patients with a significant increase of interictal EEG abnormalities during sleep.

West Syndrome (Infantile Spasms)

West syndrome usually begins between 4 and 12 months of age. The characteristic seizure is brief (1 second long) and consists of flexion at the neck, waist, arms, and legs. Spasms, usually occurring in series, are seen on arousal from sleep or prior to going to sleep (42,43). Less than 3% of spasms are noted during sleep.

The characteristic EEG finding is hypsarrhythmia characterized by irregular high-amplitude slow waves and spikes or sharp waves. The hypsarrhythmic EEG of wakefulness may change during non-REM sleep into a periodic, bilaterally synchronous, diffuse pattern interspersed with attenuated activity resembling "burst suppression" (44), and may even normalize during REM sleep. Occasionally, waking EEG may be normal but non-REM-sleep EEG may show the irregular high-voltage slow waves and spikes (45).

Partial Epilepsies

Partial seizures are noted more frequently during the day (21,28). During sleep, ictal phenomena are observed in both REM and non-REM stages (44,46-48).

Pure sleep epilepsies mostly present as focal seizures with or without secondary generalization (3,21). Examples include benign rolandic epilepsy and electrical status epilepticus during sleep, both of which are discussed later.

An increase of interictal EEG discharges during non-REM sleep and diminution or disappearance during REM sleep have been found both in surface and depth-electrode studies as well as in animal studies (47,49-51). Other investigators, however, have made conflicting observations, with reports of increased focal temporal discharges during REM sleep (36,48,52,53). It is important to note, though, that during non-REM sleep the discharges spread ipsilaterally and contralaterally from the primary focus while during REM sleep the discharges seem to focalize maximally (54–56).

Depth-electrode studies in human by Montplaisir et al. (57) and Lieb et al. (56) showed increased spike discharges during non-REM sleep and a reduction of the discharges during REM sleep. Depth-electrode studies also showed that during REM sleep the spike discharges became maximally focalized (56,57).

Lieb et al. (56) performed all-night depth-electrode recordings in 10 patients with medically refractory partial complex seizures and used computer-spike-recognition technique for depth-spike activities arising from medial temporal lobe sites. They found most frequent depth-spike activity during deep sleep in six and light sleep in three patients and an equal number during deep and light sleep in one patient. They did not find a strong relationship between temporal-lobe epilepsy and sleep pattern. Their findings that the discharge rates are greatest during non-REM sleep and are suppressed during REM sleep are in agreement with the previous reports of temporal-lobe epileptics. Similar findings have also been reported by Montplaisir and coworkers (57–59) and Passouant (60).

Malow et al. (61) studied the relationship of spikes to absolute delta log power (LDP), a continuous measure of sleep depth, in eight patients with partial epilepsy and found that in non-REM sleep, spikes were most likely to occur at higher levels of LDP (i.e., deep sleep), on the ascending limb of LDP, and with more rapid rises in LDP (i.e., deepening sleep). They suggested that processes underlying the deepening of non-REM sleep may contribute to spike activation in partial epilepsy.

Rossi et al. (62) obtained direct cerebral recordings (stereo EEG) by stereotactic implantation of stainless steel electrodes on preselected brain sites in 19 patients suffering from medically refractory partial epilepsy who were potential candidates for surgery. They found that interictal spiking increased at the onset of sleep, reaching maximum intensity during deep non-REM sleep, and returned to a lower level during REM sleep. The level in REM sleep was slightly lower as compared with the activity during wakefulness. They further noted that the spike rate was not influenced by spike location but was affected by the local level of epileptogenicity; i.e., the higher the epileptogenicity, the lower the variation. They further noted that the interictal spiking across sleep and wakefulness showed wide variation in different patients and in the different regions of the same patients.

In conclusion, non-REM sleep is the stage of augmentation of interictal focal and generalized EEG discharges. In REM sleep, generalized discharges are usually suppressed but focal discharges may persist.

Epileptic Syndromes Related to the Sleep–Wake Cycle

Benign Focal Epilepsy of Childhood with Rolandic Spikes

Benign focal epilepsy of childhood with rolandic spikes (BERS) (63,64) may account for almost one-quarter of all epilepsies in school-aged children. The clinical seizures, seen mostly during drowsiness and sleep, are simple partial in type. They usually begin in the face with variable secondary generalization. On occasion, there is speech arrest. Consciousness is preserved when seizures remain focal. The EEG shows centrotemporal or rolandic spikes or sharp waves. These discharges are present throughout the night in all stages of sleep. The prognosis is excellent, with cessation of seizures by the age of 15 to 20 years and without any neurological sequelae. The patients respond satisfactorily to anticonvulsants.

Juvenile Myoclonic Epilepsy of Janz

Originally described by Janz and Mathes (65), the electroclinical syndrome juvenile myoclonic epilepsy of Janz usually has its onset between 13 and 19 years and is manifested by massive bilaterally synchronous myoclonic jerks, which are most commonly seen in the morning shortly after awakening (66,67). The EEG is characterized by synchronous and symmetrical generalized spike-and-wave, and typically polyspike-and-wave, discharges. The excellent response to anticonvulsants makes this condition benign and easily distinguishable from the malignant syndrome of progressive myoclonus epilepsies.

Epileptic Syndrome with Generalized Tonic-Clonic Seizure on Awakening

This rare idiopathic syndrome affecting patients in the second decade of life is characterized by the occurrence of generalized tonic-clonic seizures on awakening from sleep (68). On occasion, absence or myoclonic seizures coexist. Photosensitivity and precipitation by sleep deprivation is characteristic. The interictal EEG reveals generalized spike-and-wave discharges.

Electrical Status Epilepticus During Sleep

Electrical status epilepticus during sleep (ESES), also known as continuous spike and waves during sleep (CSWS), is a rare childhood disorder characterized by generalized continuous spike-and-wave EEG discharges during slow-wave sleep (32,69). Patients display progressive behavioral disturbances, although the seizures disappear within months or years. Most of the patients have a prior history of epilepsy. The characteristic EEG finding consists of 2 to 2.5 cycles per second, with generalized spike-and-wave discharges seen during at least 85% of non-REM sleep. These discharges are suppressed during REM sleep, although occasional spikes and waves or focal frontal spikes have been reported. All-night polysomnographic study is necessary for diagnosis. During wakefulness a few bursts of generalized spike-and-wave discharges are seen in the EEG. In ESES, normal REM-non-REM cycling persists although non-REM sleep stages appear to be disrupted by the epileptiform discharges. Vertex sharp waves, K-complexes, and spindles are usually poorly formed. In general, these affected children have no sleep disturbances except for some difficulty awakening in the morning. However, a recent report by Ortega et al. (70) about a 7-year-old girl with ESES, hypersomnia, and secondary nocturnal enuresis suggests that ESES may be an intrinsic sleep disorder and not merely an EEG pattern.

Nocturnal Paroxysmal Dystonia

Initially described by Lugaresi and Cirignotta (71) and Lugaresi et al. (72), this entity—particularly the short-lasting (15 seconds to 2 minutes) variety consisting of dystonic motor phenomena occurring during sleep—is now increasingly recognized to be a form of frontal-lobe epilepsy (73–75). In addition to dystonic posturing, dyskinesias and vocalizations have been noted. These phenomena occur during non-REM sleep and usually lack interictal or ictal correlates but respond favorably to carbamazepine.

Autosomal Dominant Nocturnal Frontal-Lobe Epilepsy

Scheffer et al. (76) recently described an autosomal dominant form of frontal-lobe epilepsy in six families in which clusters of brief motor seizures occurred during sleep. The disorder usually started in childhood and persisted through adult life. Patients were of normal intellect and had normal neurological examination and neuroimaging. Response to carbamazepine was excellent. In most cases, interictal EEGs were normal, although one family with daytime attacks had epileptiform discharges. Videotelemetry during the attacks confirmed their epileptic nature.

Sleep Phenomena Resembling Epilepsy

Differentiating nocturnal seizures from nonepileptic sleep phenomena is usually difficult because of the inability of the patient and/or the bed partner to give a full history since both are asleep at the time of the event. In addition, certain sleep disorders, such as the non-REM parasomnias, have motor manifestations that may be mistaken for seizures. Examples of these disorders include night terror (pavor nocturnus), somnambulism (sleepwalking), somniloquy (sleep talking), teeth-grinding (bruxism), head-banging (jactatio capitis nocturnas), and nocturnal enuresis. Two other parasomnias occurring during REM sleep—REM-sleep behavior disorder and nightmares (dream-anxiety attacks)—may mimic complex partial seizures. In addition, periodic limb movements in sleep may be mistaken for motor seizures.

Characteristic clinical features combined with EEG and polysomnographic recordings are important to differentiate the abovementioned nocturnal events of nonepileptiform significance from true epileptic attacks. It should be noted, however, that the two conditions (epileptic and nonepileptic attacks) may coexist. Hence, video-EEG recordings to correlate behavior with EEG manifestations are crucial to establish the diagnosis. In addition, since some nonepileptiform sleep disorders respond to antiepileptic drugs, improvement after empirical anticonvulsant therapy does not necessarily mean that the condition in question is epileptic in nature.

Sleep Disturbances in Patients with Epilepsy

Sleep in epileptic patients has been reported to be altered in a large percentage of patients studied. Although the utility of sleep in the diagnosis of epilepsy is well established, the altered sleep characteristics in epileptics are not well known. One of the difficulties has been that most of the studies have been conducted in patients on anticonvulsants, thus adding the confounding effect of these medications on sleep architecture. Furthermore, well-designed longitudinal studies to determine the effect of epilepsy on sleep in the early versus the late stage of the illness are lacking. Despite these limitations, there is a general consensus regarding the effect of epilepsy on sleep and sleep structure. A variety of sleep disturbances have been observed in epileptics (47,52,77–79): a reduction in REM sleep, an increase in wake after sleep onset (WASO), increased instability of sleep states such as unclassifiable sleep epochs, an increase in non-REM stages 1 and 2, a decrease in non-REM sleep stages 3 and 4, a reduction in the density of sleep spindles, and an increase of sleep-onset latency.

WASO, sleep-stage shifts, and sleep fragmentation are found in all seizure types (23,78,80,81). Reduction of REM sleep and an increase in non-REM stages 1 and 2 are in part dependent on the type of epilepsy, and have been noted in patients with primary generalized or partial seizures with secondary generalization as compared with nonepileptic subjects (78). A decrease in REM sleep is characteristic of patients with complex partial seizures (80). Interestingly, absence of the REM rebound that usually follows REM deprivation has been noted in temporal-lobe epilepsy patients (23,80).

Touchon et al. (82), in a series of 15 patients with temporal-lobe seizures, found increased WASO, shifting of the sleep stages, and an increase of non-REM sleep stages 1 and 2. In a study of 23 patients with temporal-lobe epilepsy, Kohsaka (83) found significantly decreased sleep efficiency and increased awakenings in both treated and untreated patients. He also noted increased non-REM stage 4 in untreated patients compared to healthy controls. The site of the primary focus may determine the type of the sleep disturbances. Foci in the amygdalo-hippocampal region may lead to increased WASO and decreased sleep efficiency. On the other hand, frontal-lobe epileptics may show a specific reduction in stages 3 and 4 non-REM sleep.

Hoeppner et al. (84) studied self-reported sleep-disorder symptoms in epileptic patients and found significantly more symptoms (particularly frequent awakenings at night) in patients with simple and partial complex seizures than in those with generalized seizures who actually behaved like the control group. Patients with the most frequent seizures, irrespective of the type, had the most sleep disturbances. In similar questionnaire-based studies of children with tuberous sclerosis (TS), it was found that concurrent epilepsy was significantly associated with sleep disturbances (85,86).

It also appears that the severity of the seizure disorder is in part correlated with severity of the sleep deficits. Seizure occurrence during sleep accentuates sleep deficits that are more marked in primary generalized and partial seizures with secondary generalization than in other types. Several investigators reported difficulty in discriminating between the stages of sleep in patients with severe seizures because of disruptions in sleep architecture (23,78).

Although it is generally thought that sleep deficits in seizure disorders are secondary to the severity of the seizure disorder and are a direct result of seizures during sleep, Tanaka and Naquet (87) demonstrated that the progressive sleep deficits in amygdala kindling models persisted 1 month following discontinuation of kindling procedures. Their findings were supported by Shouse and Sterman (88), who, using similar amygdala kindling models, found progressive sleep disturbances that remained for a prolonged period following termination of amygdala stimulation. These findings suggest the "kindling" of a sleep disorder in addition to a seizure disturbance. Shouse and Sterman further stated that sleep abnormalities cannot be viewed as a simple or temporary side effect of epileptiform activity. It appears that a permanent change in sleep physiology occurs in epilepsy. Effective treatment of epilepsy with anticonvulsant medications or surgical methods normalizes sleep disturbances in human epilepsy.

EFFECT OF ANTICONVULSANTS ON SLEEP IN EPILEPTICS

The effects of anticonvulsant medications on sleep architecture have been intensively studied. In a literature review, Johnson (89) found that acute exposure to anticonvulsants may reduce REM and non-REM stages 3 and 4 and increase stage 2 non-REM sleep. However, acute and chronic drug trials in epileptics suggest that the main effects of anticonvulsants consist of sleep stabilization and that these improvements are concomitant with the reduction of seizures. Thus, the effects are due to the reduction of seizures and not to any specific effect of the anticonvulsants on sleep architecture.

In a survey of experimental epilepsy in animals, Wauquier et al. (90) observed that sleep fragmentation as obtained in epileptic animals as well as in humans may be the consequence of microarousals. Anticonvulsants may suppress microarousals because of their sedative properties and hence lead to stabilization of sleep fragmentation and normalization of sleep. On the other hand, anticonvulsants may normalize sleep because of a specific action on particular abnormal EEG patterns. Thus, despite the suggestion that anticonvulsants themselves may be partly responsible for the fragmentation and disruption of sleep architecture, the general consensus is that anticonvulsant medications normalize sleep architecture, most probably by reduction of the seizures.

Wolf et al. (91) reviewed the literature to assess the effect of barbiturates, phenytoin, carbamazepine, and valproic acid treatment on sleep. They noted significant reduction of REM sleep, a reduction in total awake time, and an increase in non-REM stage 2 sleep as the short-term effects of barbiturates. The long-term effects of barbiturates are somewhat similar or, in some cases, the sleep pattern returns to the premedication level.

Using a crossover design, Wolf et al. (91) performed a prospective polygraphic study of sleep in epileptic patients before and after medications. They studied phenobarbital, phenytoin, ethosuximide, valproic acid, and carbamazepine. The short-term effects of phenobarbital included reduction of WASO and REM sleep and increase of stage 2 non-REM sleep. There was no relationship with the serum drug levels. The short-term effects of phenytoin included no change in the percentage of WASO, but there was a decrease in non-REM sleep stages 1 and 2 and an increase in sleep stages 3 and 4; REM sleep remained unaltered. Again, there was no relationship with the serum drug levels. The long-term effects of phenytoin were in general a reversal of the short-term effects, consisting of an increase of non-REM sleep stages 1 and 2 and a decrease of stages 3 and 4. REM sleep, however, remained unaltered. The effects of ethosuximide included an increase in stage 1, a decrease in stages 3 and 4 sleep, and increased awakenings. Valproic acid similarly increased stage 1 but did not decrease stages 3 and 4 non-REM sleep.

Long-term phenytoin treatment by Hartmann (92) revealed a shortened sleep onset and an increase of light sleep in some subjects. Roder-Wanner et al. (93) noted a temporary increase of slow-wave sleep following phenytoin treatment.

Findji and Catani (94) reported an improvement of sleep organization and an increase of deep non-REM sleep in epileptic children after treatment with valproic acid. At high dosage, however, Harding et al. (95) observed a decrease of delta and REM sleep.

Manni et al. (96) performed an objective and subjective assessment of daytime sleepiness using MSLT, clinical, and psychometric data on 10 patients with generalized epilepsy treated chronically with phenobarbital, 10 patients with cryptogenic partial epilepsy treated with carbamazepine, and 10 healthy controls. They found that patients on phenobarbital had a greater daytime sleep tendency and did worse on the digit–symbol-substitution test compared to the other two groups. In a similarly designed study (97), they noted a shorter mean sleep latency in patients on phenobarbital compared with patients on sodium valproate and controls. Psychomotor functioning was also noted to be poor in patients on phenobarbital compared to controls, while patients on valproate were noted to have some attentional impairment and a tendency toward longer motor movement time. However, they did not find a correlation between the assessed parameters and serum drug concentrations.

It is evident from the preceding survey of the literature that more studies are needed to understand the interactions of the anticonvulsants, sleep, and epilepsy.

SUDDEN DEATH AND SEIZURES

Population-based studies have shown that patients with epilepsy have a two- to threefold greater risk of death compared with the general population (98). This increased mortality risk appears to be highest in the first year after diagnosis, and in most cases is related to the cause of the epilepsy itself. Other causes include convulsive status epilepticus, suicide, and accidents. However, a number of patients with epilepsy die suddenly with no apparent cause. This is the phenomenon of sudden unexpected death in epilepsy (SUDEP).

The incidence of SUDEP has been estimated to be between 1 in 110 and 1 in 370 deaths per epilepsy patient per year (99–101). The majority of deaths occur in males between the ages of 10 and 40 years. Other reported risk factors include more severe epilepsy, black race, alcohol abuse, poor compliance with antiepileptic medications, and the presence of structural lesions in the brain (98,99). Almost all reported cases involve patients suffering from generalized tonic-clonic seizures, with or without additional partial seizures (102). EEG findings are variable, and show a wide range of abnormalities. The most common place for death is the bedroom, with the majority occurring during sleep (102).

The pathogenesis of SUDEP is unclear, and there is controversy as to whether it is related to an unwitnessed seizure. Mechanisms implicated include neurogenic pulmonary edema, cardiac arrhythmias, and myocardial ischemia. Tigaran et al. (103) found episodes of ST-segment depression in eight patients with severe drug-resistant epilepsy, most of which coincided with video- and EEG-documented epileptic seizures. In earlier studies involving seizures provoked by either electroconvulsive therapy or pentylenetetrazol, premature ventricular contractions, bigeminy, premature atrial contractionns, and ventricular tachycardia were observed (104,105). Other cardiac findings reported in association with both generalized and partial seizures include bradycardia (106), tachycardia (106,107), and asystole (108).

The other suggested mechanism for SUDEP could be sleep-related respiratory dysrhythmia in epileptics. Nashef et al. (109) found episodes of apnea in 10 of 17 patients undergoing EEG-video recording. They observed apneic episodes in 20 of 47 clinical seizures (three secondary generalized, 16 complex partial, and one tonic). Most of the apneas were central in type, although obstructive apneas were also noted. Although an increase in heart rate was typical, bradycardia and sinus arrest were also observed. There are other reports of upper-airway obstructive, mixed, and central sleep apnea in patients with epilepsy, and of improvement in seizure control following treatment of sleep apnea (110–114).

Using a well-established sheep model of status epilepticus, Johnston et al. (115) demonstrated central apnea and hypoventilation in all eight animals studied, two of which died as a result. A third died of acute heart failure within 2 minutes of seizure onset. None of these animals exhibited malignant cardiac arrhythmias.

It is obvious from the preceding sections that a general consensus has yet to be reached regarding the pathogenesis of SUDEP. This phenomenon is still not widely recognized, and thus is frequently not accurately reported.

DIAGNOSTIC APPROACHES

The usefulness of sleep in the diagnosis of epilepsy is well established with regard to the use of all-night polysomnographic (PSG) recordings in patients with epilepsy. Broughton (116) listed the following important indications:

1. To differentiate between epileptic and nonepileptic nocturnal events
2. To clarify the classification in patients with known sleep epilepsies
3. To diagnose ESES
4. To diagnose benign epilepsy of childhood with rolandic spikes
5. To lateralize or localize the principal focus during REM sleep by use of stereo-EEG
6. To unmask the primary focus in a patient with secondary bilateral synchrony during REM sleep
7. In patients with hypsarrhythmia in which the waking EEGs may

rarely be normal but sleep EEG may reveal the abnormalities, and also for clarification of the focal abnormalities in such patients
8. To diagnose tonic seizures in patients with Lennox-Gastaut syndrome
9. To diagnose sleep apnea or other primary sleep disorders that may be mistaken for or associated with epilepsy
10. For investigation of patients complaining of excessive daytime somnolence that cannot be explained by the anticonvulsant medication

Two additional indications are to document nocturnal cardiac arrhythmias, which may be confused with—or even give rise to—seizures, and to document sleep disturbances and sleep-pattern changes in epileptics so that these disturbances may be treated to prevent chronic sleep deprivation, which may in turn have deleterious effects on epilepsy.

For the diagnosis of seizures occurring predominantly or exclusively in sleep, the use of split-screen videopolysomnography (VPSG) is essential. This technique combines video-EEG monitoring with standard polysomnographic recording. The video component helps characterize the spell in question while the extensive EEG coverage confirms its epileptic nature. The stage of sleep during which the spells occur helps identify the type of parasomnia.

Ambulatory 24-hour EEG recording and sleep scoring may reveal EEG discharges throughout the day and shed light on the relationship of these discharges to the circadian and ultradian rhythms. However, technical problems associated with these unattended recordings are serious limitations. Thus, in some patients, long-term video and EEG monitoring in an inpatient setting may be necessary. This procedure has the added benefit of being able to equate an ictal epileptiform discharge with its behavioral correlate.

Finally, neuroimaging studies are indispensable in investigating the presence of structural lesions that may serve as epileptogenic foci. Anatomical studies (computed tomography and magnetic resonance imaging) are usually performed in all adults with new-onset seizures and in children without any characteristic epileptic syndromes. Functional or physiological studies (single-photon emission computed tomography and positron emission computed tomography) may be able to identify seizure foci by revealing areas of cerebral hypermetabolism or hyperperfusion during an ictal episode and areas of hypometabolism during the interictal period.

THERAPEUTIC CONSIDERATIONS

Because disrupted sleep can worsen seizures, and seizures in turn can result in abnormal sleep architecture, we cannot overemphasize the importance of proper sleep hygiene in patients with seizure disorders. These patients should be encouraged to keep regular sleep and waking hours. Factors that have harmful effects on sleep initiation and maintenance such as caffeine and alcohol should be avoided. Any coexisting sleep disorder, such as obstructive sleep apnea, should be rigorously investigated and treated. Management of epilepsy itself is beyond the scope of this chapter, and the reader is referred to many excellent texts available outlining detailed management of epilepsy. For optimal patient care, both sleep specialists and epileptologists should participate in patient management.

REFERENCES

1. Passouant P. Historical aspects of sleep and epilepsy. In: Degen R, Niedermeyer E, eds. Epilepsy, Sleep and Sleep Deprivation. Amsterdam: Elsevier, 1985:67–73.
2. Fere L. Les Epilepsies et les Epileptiques. Paris: Alcan, 1890.
3. Turner WA. Epilepsy: A Study of the Idiopathic Disease. London: Macmillan, 1907.
4. Gallus R. Die allgemeinen Ursachen der Anfallshaufungen innerhalb grobgerer Gruppen von Kranken. Epilepsi (Leipzig) 1911; 3:46.
5. Amann R. Untersuchungen über die Veränderungen in der Häufigkiet der epileptischen Anfälle und deren Ursachen. Z ges Neurol Psychiatr 1914; 24:5.
6. Gibbs EL, Gibbs FA. Diagnostic and localizing value of electroencephalographic studies in sleep. Res Publ Assoc Res Nerv Ment Dis 1947; 26:366–376.
7. Janz D. The grand mal epilepsies and the sleep-waking cycle. Epilepsia 1962; 3: 69–109.
8. Passouant P. Influence des états de vigilance sur les epilepsies. In: Koella WP, ed. Sleep. Vol 3. Basel: S Karger, 1977:57–65.
9. Gastaut H, Batini C, Fressy J, et al. Etude electroencephalographique des phenomenes episodiques course du sommeil. In: Fischgold H, ed. Le Sommeil de Nuit Normal et Pathologique. Paris: Masson, 1965:239–254.
10. Cadilhac JC. Le Sommeil Nocturne des Epileptiques: Etude polygraphique. These de Medecine, Monsieur 1967:150.
11. Engel J Jr. Seizures and Epilepsy. Philadelphia: FA Davis, 1989:71–111.
12. Matsumoto H, Ajmone-Marsan C. Cortical cellular phenomena in experimental epilepsy: interictal manifestations. Exp Neurol 1964; 9:286–304.
13. Margerison JH, Corsellis JA. Epilepsy and the temporal lobes: a clinical, electroencephalographic and neuropathological study of the brain in epilepsy, with particular reference to the temporal lobes. Brain 1966; 69:499–530.
14. Chokroverty S. The assessment of sleep disturbances in autonomic failure. In: Bannister R, Mathias CJ, eds. Autonomic Failure. Oxford: Oxford University Press, 1992:422–461.
15. Steriade M. Brain electrical activity and sensory processing during waking and sleep states. In: Kryger MH, Roth T, Dement WC, eds. Principles and Practice of Sleep Medicine. 2nd ed. Philadelphia: WB Saunders, 1994:105–124.
16. Pompeiano O. Sleep mechanism. In: Jasper HH, Ward AA Jr, Pope A, eds. Basic Mechanisms of the Epilepsies. Boston: Little, Brown, 1969:453–473.
17. Berlucchi G. Callosal activity in unrestrained, unanesthetized cats. Arch Ital Biol 1965; 103:623.

18. Hobson JA, Lydic R, Baghdoyan HA. Evolving concepts of sleep cycle generation: from brain centers to neuronal populations. Behav Brain Sci 1986; 9:371–448.
19. Chokroverty S, Quinto C. Sleep and Epilepsy. In: Chokroverty S, ed. Sleep Disorders Medicine: Basic Science, Technical Considerations, and Clinical Aspects. 2nd ed. Boston: Butterworth-Heinemann, 1999:697–727.
20. Montplaisir J. Epilepsy and sleep: reciprocal interactions and diagnostic procedures involving sleep. In: Thorpy MJ, ed. Handbook of Sleep Disorders. New York: Marcel Dekker, 1990:643–661.
21. Billiard M. Epilepsy and the sleep-wake cycle. In: Sterman MB, Shouse MN, Passouant P, eds. Sleep and Epilepsy. New York: Academic Press, 1982:269–286.
22. Autert A, Laffon F, Roux S. Influence of waking and sleep stages on the interictal paroxysmal activity in partial epilepsy with complex seizures. Electroencephalogr Clin Neurophysiol 1983; 55:406–410.
23. Besset A. Influence of generalized seizures on sleep organization. In: Sterman MB, Shouse MN, Passouant P, eds. Sleep and Epilepsy. New York: Academic Press, 1982:339–346.
24. Gowers WR. Epilepsy and Other Chronic Convulsive Diseases. Vol 1. London: Williams Wood, 1885.
25. Langdon-Down M, Brain WR. Time of day in relation to convulsions in epilepsy. Lancet 1929; ii:1029–1032.
26. Billiard M, Besset A, Zachariev Z, et al. Relation of seizures and seizure discharged to sleep stages. In: Wolf P, Dam M, Janz F, et al. Advances in Epileptology. New York: Raven Press, 1987:665–670.
27. Passouant P, Latour H, Cadilhac J. L'épilepsie morphéplique. Ann Med Psychol 1951; 109:526–540.
28. D'Allesandro R, Santini M, Pazzagli P, et al. Pure sleep epilepsies: prognostic features. In: Nistico G, DiPerri R, Meinardi H, eds. Epilepsy: An Update on Research and Therapy. New York: Alan R Liss, 1983:235–239.
29. Niedermeyer E. Sleep electroencephalograms in petit mal. Arch Neurol 1965; 12: 625–630.
30. Gastaut H, Batini C, Broughton R, et al. An electroencepalographic study of nocturnal sleep in epileptic patients [abstr]. Electroencephalogr Clin Neurophysiol 1965; 18:96.
31. Gastaut H, Broughton R. A clinical and polygraphic study of episodic phenomenon during sleep. In: Wortis J, ed. Recent Advances in Biological Psychiatry. Vol 7. New York: Plenum Press, 1965:197–221.
32. Patry G, Lyagoubi S, Tassinari CA. Subclinical electrical status epilepticus induced by sleep in children. Ann Neurol 1971; 24:242–252.
33. Sato S, Dreifuss F, Penry JK. The effect of sleep on spike-wave discharges in absence seizures. Neurology (Minneapolis) 1973; 23:1335–1345.
34. Tassinari CA. Bureau-Paillas M, Dalla-Bernardina B, et al. Generalized epilepsies and seizures during sleep: a polygraphic study. In: Van Praag HM, Meinardi H, eds. Brain and Sleep. Amsterdam: De Erven Bohn, 1974:154–166.
35. Meier-Ewert K, Broughton R. Photomyoclonic response of epileptic subjects during wakefulness, sleep and arousal. Electroencephalogr Clin Neurophysiol 1967; 23:142–151.

36. Touchon J. Effect of awakening on epileptic activity in primary generalized myoclonic epilepsy. In: Sterman MB, Shouse MN, Passouant P, eds. Sleep and Epilepsy. New York: Academic Press, 1982:239–248.
37. Gastaut H, Roger J, Soulayrol R, et al. Childhood epileptic encephalopathy with diffuse slow spike-waves (otherwise known as Petit Mal variant) or Lennox syndrome. Epilepsia 1966; 7:139–179.
38. Dinner DS. Sleep and pediatric epilepsy. Cleve Clin J Med 1989; 56:S234–S239.
39. Gastaut H, Broughton R, Roger J, et al. Generalized convulsive seizures without local onset. In: Vinken PJ, Bruyn GW, eds. Handbook of Clinical Neurology. Vol 15. The Epilepsies. Amsterdam: Elsevier, 1974:107–129.
40. Erba G, Moschen R, Ferber R. Sleep-related changes in EEG discharge activity and seizure risk in patients with Lennox-Gastaut syndrome. Sleep Res 1981; 10: 247.
41. Markand ON. Slow spike-wave activity in EEG and associated clinical features: often called ''Lennox'' or ''Lennox-Gastaut'' syndrome. Neurology 1977; 27:746–757.
42. Kellaway P. Sleep and epilepsy. Epilepsia 1985; 26(suppl 1):S15–S30.
43. Gomez MR, Klass DW. Epilepsies of infancy and childhood. Ann Neurol 1983; 13:113–124.
44. Passouant P, Besset A, Carrier A, et al. Night sleep and generalized epilepsies. In: Koella WP, Levin P, eds. Sleep 1974. Basel: S Karger, 1975:185–196.
45. Jeavons PM, Bower BD. The natural history of infantile spasms. Arch Dis Child 1961; 36:17–21.
46. Cadilhac J. Complex partial seizures and REM sleep. In: Sterman MB, Shouse MN, Passouant P, eds. Sleep and Epilepsy. New York: Academic Press, 1982:315–324.
47. Kikuchi S. An electroencephalographic study of nocturnal sleep in temporal lobe epilepsy. Foli Psychiatr Neurol Jpn 1969; 23:59–81.
48. Epstein AW, Hill W. Ictal phenomena during REM sleep of a temporal lobe epileptic. Ann Neurol 1966; 15:367–375.
49. Niedermeyer E, Rocca U. The diagnostic significance of sleep electroencephalographs in temporal lobe epilepsy: a comparison of scalp and depth tracings. Eur Neurol 1972; 7:119–129.
50. Frank G. Epileptiform discharges during various stages of sleep. Electroencephalogr Clin Neurophysiol 1970; 28:95.
51. Angelieri F. Partial epilepsies and nocturnal sleep. In: Levin P, Koella WP, eds. Sleep 1974. Basel: S Karger 1975:196–203.
52. Passouant P, Cadihac J, Delange M. Indications apportées par l'étude du dommeil du nuit sur la physiopathologie des epilepsies. Int J Neurol 1965; 5:207–216.
53. Mayersdorf A, Wilder BJ. Focal epileptic discharges during all night sleep studies. Clin Electroencephalogr 1974; 5:73–87.
54. Montplaisir J, Laverdiere M, Saint-Hilaire JM. Sleep and focal epilepsy: contribution of depth recording. In: Sterman MB, Shouse MN, Passouant P, eds. Sleep and Epilepsy. New York: Academic Press, 1982:301–314.
55. Ross JJ, Johnson LC, Walter RD. Spike and wave discharges during stages of sleep. Ann Neurol 1966; 14:399–407.

56. Lieb J, Joseph JP, Engel J, et al. Sleep state and seizure foci related to depth spike activity in patients with temporal lobe epilepsy. Electroencephalogr Clin Neurophysiol 1980; 49:538–557.
57. Montplaisir J, Laverdiere M, Rouleau I, et al. Nocturnal sleep recording in partial epilepsy: a study with depth electrodes. J Clin Neurophysiol 1987; 4(4):383–388.
58. Montplaisir J, Laverdiere M, Saint-Hilaire JM, et al. Sleep and temporal lobe epilepsy: a case study with depth electrodes. Neurology (Minneapolis) 1981; 31:1352–1356.
59. Laverdiere M, Montplaisir J. Frequency of epileptic spike activity and sleep disturbances in temporal lobe epilepsy. Sleep Res 1984; 13:177.
60. Passouant P. Epilepsie temporale et sommeil. Rev Roum Neurol 1967; 4:151–163.
61. Malow BA, Kushwaha R, Lin X, Morton KJ, Aldrich MS. Relationship of interictal epileptiform discharges to sleep depth in partial epilepsy. EEG Clin Neurophysiol 1997; 102:20–26.
62. Rossi GF, Colicchio G, Polla P. Interictal epileptic activity during sleep: a stereo-EEG study in patients with partial epilepsy. Electroencephalogr Clin Neurophysiol 1983; 58:97–106.
63. Nayrac P, Beaussart M. Les pointes-ondes prerolandiques: expression EEG très particulière: étude electroclinique de 21 cas. Rev Neurol 1958; 99:201–206.
64. Beaussard M. Benign epilepsy of children with rolandic (centrotemporal) paroxysmal foci: a clinical entity—study of 221 cases. Epilepsia 1973; 13:795–811.
65. Janz D, Mathes A. Die propulsiv-petit-mal-epilepsie: Klinik and Verlauf der sog. Blitz-, Nick- und Salaamkrampfe. Basel: S Karger, 1955.
66. Janz D, Christian W. Impulsive petit mal. Dtsch Z Nervenheilkd 1957; 176:346–386.
67. Janz D. Epilepsy with impulsive petit mal (juvenile myoclinic epilepsy). Acta Neurol Scand 1985; 72:449–459.
68. Wolf P. Epilepsy with grand mal on awakening. In: Roger J, Dravet C, Bureau M, et al, eds. Epileptic Syndromes in Infancy, Childhood, and Adolescence. London: John Libbey, 1985:259–270.
69. Tassinari CA, Bureau M, Dravet C, et al. Electrical status epilepticus during sleep in children (ESES). In: Sterman MB, Shouse MN, Passouant P, eds. Sleep and Epilepsy. New York: Academic Press, 1982:465–479.
70. Ortega JJ, Belda VJ, Tripiana JL, Gil M, Salas R, Orenga JV, Serrano AL. Electrical status epilepticus during sleep. Revista de Neurologia 1996; 24(136):1551–1553.
71. Lugaresi E, Cirignotta F. Hypnogenic paroxysmal dystonia: epileptic seizure or a new syndrome? Sleep 1981; 4:129–138.
72. Lugaresi E, Cirignotta F, Montagna P. Nocturnal paroxysmal dystonia. J Neurol Neurosurg Psychiatry 1986; 49:375–380.
73. Sellal F, Hirsch E, Maquet P. Postures et mouvements anormaux paroxystiqueslors du sommeil: dystonie paroxystique hypnogenique ou epilepsie partielle? Rev Neurol (Paris) 1991; 147:121–128.
74. Meierkord H, Fish DR, Smith JM, Scott CA, Shorvon SD, Marsden CD. Is nocturnal paroxysmal dystonia a form of frontal lobe epilepsy? Mov Disord 1992; 7:38–42.
75. Oguni M, Oguni H, Kozam M, Fukuyama Y. A case with nocturnal paroxysmal

unilateral dystonia and interictal right frontal epileptic EEG focus: a lateralized variant of nocturnal paroxysmal dystonia? Brain Dev 1992; 14:412–416.

76. Scheffer IE, Bhatia KP, Lopes-Cendes I, Fish DR, Marsden CD, Andermann F, Andermann E, Desbiens R, Cendes F, Manson JI, Berkovic SF. Autosomal dominant frontal epilepsy misdiagnosed as sleep disorder. Lancet 1994; 343:515–517.
77. Montplaisir J, Laverdiere M, Saint-Hiliare JM. Sleep and epilepsy. In: Gotman J, Ives JR, Gloor P, eds. Long-Term Monitoring in Epilepsy (EEG suppl 37). Amsterdam: Elsevier, 1985:215–239.
78. Declerck AC, Wauquier A, Sijben-Kiggen R, et al. A normative study of sleep in different forms of epilepsy. In: Sterman MB, Shouse MN, Passouant P, eds. Sleep and Epilepsy. New York: Academic Press, 1982:329–337.
79. Delange D, Castan P, Cadihac J, et al. Study of night sleep during centrencephalic and temporal epilepsies [abstr]. Electroencephalogr Clin Neurophysiol 1962; 14: 777.
80. Baldy-Moulinier M. Temporal lobe epilepsy and sleep organization. In: Sterman MB, Passouant P, eds. Sleep and Epilepsy. New York: Academic Press, 1982:347–359.
81. Hamel AR, Sterman MB. Sleep and epileptic abnormalities during sleep. In: Sterman MB, Shouse MN, Passouant P. eds. Sleep and Epilepsy. New York: Academic Press, 1982:361–377.
82. Touchon J, Baldy-Moulinier M, Billiard M, et al. Organization du sommeil dans l'epilepsie recente du lobe temporal avant et après traitement par carbamazepine. Rev Neurol (Paris) 1987; 5:462–467.
83. Kohsaka M. Changes in epileptiform activities during sleep and sleep structures in temporal lobe epilepsy. Hokkaido J Med Sci 1993; 68(5):630-645.
84. Hoeppner J, Garron DC, Cartwright RD. Self-reported sleep disorder symptoms in epilepsy. Epilepsia 1984; 25:434–437.
85. Hunt A, Stores G. Sleep disorder and epilepsy in children with tuberous sclerosis: a questionnaire-based study. Develop Med Child Neurol 1994; 36:108–115.
86. Bruni O, Cortesi F, Gianotti F, Curatolo P. Sleep disorders in tuberous sclerosis: a polysomnographic study. Brain Dev 1995; 17:52–56.
87. Tanaka T, Naquet R. Kindling effect and sleep organization in cats. Electroencephalogr Clin Neurophysiol 1975; 39:449–454.
88. Shouse MN, Sterman MP. Sleep pathology in experimental epilepsy: amygdala kindling. In: Sterman MB, Shouse MN, Passouant P, eds. Sleep and Epilepsy. New York: Academic Press, 1982:151–164.
89. Johnson LC. Effects of anticonvulsant medication on sleep patterns. In: Sterman MB, Shouse MN, Passouant P, eds. Sleep and Epilepsy. New York: Academic Press, 1982:381–384.
90. Wauquier A, Clincake GHC, Declerck AC. Sleep alterations by seizures and anticonvulsants. In: Martins da Silva A, Binnie CD, Meinardi H, eds. Biorhythms and Epilepsy. New York: Raven Press, 1985:123–133.
91. Wolf DP, Roder-Wanner UU, Brede M, et al. Influences of antiepileptic drugs on sleep. In: Martins da Silva A, Binnie CD, Meinardi H, eds. Biorhythms and Epilepsy. New York: Raven Press, 1985:137–148.

92. Hartmann E. The effects of diphenylhydantoin (DPH) on sleep in man. Psychophysiology 1970; 7:316.
93. Roder-Wanner VV, Noachtar S, Wolf P. Response of polygraphic sleep to phenytoin treatment of epilepsy: a longitudinal study of immediate, short- and long-term effects. Acta Neurol Scand 1987; 76:157–167.
94. Findji F, Catani P. Readjustment des therapeutiques anticonvulsives chez l'enfant. L'Encephale 1982; 8:595–613.
95. Harding GFA, Alford CA, Powell TE. The effect of sodium valproate on sleep, reaction times and visual evoked potential in normal subjects. Epilepsia 1985; 26: 597-601.
96. Manni R, Ratti MT, Galimberti CA, Morini R, Perucca E, Tartara A. Daytime sleepiness in epileptic patients on long-term monotherapy: MSLT, clinical and psychometric assessment. Neurophysiol Clin 1993; 23:71-76.
97. Manni R, Ratti MT, Perucca E, Galimberti CA, Tartara A. A multiparametric investigation of daytime sleepiness and psychomotor functions in epileptic patients treated with phenobarbital and sodium valproate: a comparative controlled study. EEG Clin Neurophysiol 1993; 86: 322–326.
98. Cockerell OC. The mortality of epilepsy. Curr Opin Neurol 1996; 9:93–96.
99. Leestma JE, Walczak T, Hughes JR, Kalelkar MB, Teas SS. A prospective study on sudden unexpected death in epilepsy. Ann Neurol 1989; 26:195–203.
100. Terrence CF Jr, Wisotzkey HM, Perper JA. Unexpected, unexplained death in epileptic patients. Neurology 1975; 25:594–598.
101. Earnest MP, Thomas GE, Eden RA, Hossack KF. The sudden unexplained death syndrome in epilepsy: demographic clinical, and postmortem features. Epilepsia 1992; 33:310–316.
102. Brown SW. Sudden death and epilepsy. Seizure 1992; 1:71–73.
103. Tigaran S, Rasmussen V, Dam M, Pedersen S, Hogenhaven H, Friberg B. ECG changes in epilepsy patients. Acta Neurol Scand 1997; 96:72–75.
104. McKenna G, Engle RP, Brooks H, Dalent J. Cardiac arrhythmias during electroshock therapy: significance, prevention, and treatment. Am J Psychiatry 1970; 127: 530–533.
105. Mosier JW, White P, Grant P, Fisher JE, Taylor R. Cerebroautonomic and myographic changes accompanying induced seizures. Neurology 1957; 7:204–210.
106. Li LM, Roche J, Sander JWAS. Ictal ECG changes in temporal lobe epilepsy. Arq Neuropsiquiatr 1995; 53:619–624.
107. Massetani R, Strata G, Galli R, Gori S, Gneri C, Limbruno U, Di Santo D, Mariani M, Murri L. Alteration of cardiac function in patients with temporal lobe epilepsy: different roles of EEG-ECG monitoring and spectral analysis of RR variability. Epilepsia 1997; 38:363–369.
108. Howell SJL, Blumhardt LD. Cardiac asystole associated with epileptic seizures: a case report with simultaneous EEG and ECG. J Neurol Neurosurg Psychiatry 1989; 52:795–798.
109. Nashef L, Walker F, Allen P, Sander JW, Shorvon SD, Fish DR. Apnoea and bradycardia during epileptic seizures: relation to sudden death in epilepsy. J Neurol Neurosurg Psychiatry 1996; 60:297–300.

110. Wyler AR, Weymuller EA. Epilepsy complicated by sleep apnea. Ann Neurol 1981; 9:403–404.
111. Chokroverty S, Sachdeo R, Goldhammer T, et al. Epilepsy and sleep apnea [abstr]. Electroencephalogr Clin Neurophysiol 1985; 61:26P.
112. Vashista S, Ehrenberg B. Benefits of treating sleep-apnea in complex partial epilepsy [abstr]. Electroencephalogr Clin Neurophysiol 1988; 70:41P.
113. Devinsky O, Ehrenberg B, Barthlen GM, Abramson HS, Luciano D. Epilepsy and sleep apnea syndrome. Neurology 1994; 44:2060–2064.
114. Vaughn BV, D'Cruz OF, Beach R, Messenheimer JA. Improvement of epileptic seizure control with treatment of obstructive sleep apnea. Seizure 1996; 5:73–78.
115. Johnston SC, Siedenberg R, Min JK, Jerome EH, Laxer KD. Central apnea and acute cardiac ischemia in a sheep model of epileptic sudden death. Ann Neurol 1997; 42:588–594.
116. Broughton RJ. Epilepsy and sleep: a synopsis and prospectus. In: Degin R, Niedermeyer E, eds. Epilepsy, Sleep and Sleep Deprivation. Amsterdam: Elsevier, 1984: 317–356.

16

Narcolepsy, Idiopathic Hypersomnia, and Periodic Hypersomnias

Claudio Bassetti
University Hospital (Inselpital)
Bern, Switzerland

Michael S. Aldrich
University of Michigan Health System
Ann Arbor, Michigan

NARCOLEPSY

Historical Introduction

In 1880, Gélineau (1828–1906) coined the term narcolepsy (from the Greek ''seized by somnolence'') describing the association of imperative sleepiness with sudden loss of muscle tone (''astasia'') (1). Previous authors such as Willis (2), Caffé, and Westphal—who in 1877 gave the first description of a familial form of the disease (3)—had probably already recognized the syndrome. The term cataplexy (from the Latin ''to strike down with fear'') was proposed in 1908 by Heneberg. Hypnagogic hallucinations and sleep paralysis were first described in normal subjects in 1876 by Mitchell (4) and in 1848 by Maury, respectively, but were linked with narcolepsy only in the 1920s.

For several decades following Gélineau's report, narcolepsy was considered to be rare; up to 1924, only 25 cases had been published in the world literature (Redlich, quoted in Ref. 5). Furthermore, narcolepsy was also thought to be a nonspecific manifestation of sleepiness that could be caused by such different disorders as epilepsy, hysteria, and encephalitis (6). Following the communications of Löwenfeld in 1902 (7) and Adie in 1926 (8), and particularly reports of the first large series of patients in the 1930s by Redlich (9) and Daniels (10), narcolepsy was finally accepted as a disease "sui generis." In the 1950s, Yoss and Daly proposed the concept of the narcoleptic tetrad (sleepiness, cataplexy, sleep paralysis, and hypnagogic hallucinations) (11). In the 1960s, Vogel described the phenomenon of sleep-onset REM periods (12). In the 1970s, a canine model of the disease was found, and the 1980s saw the recognition of an association of narcolepsy with specific HLA antigens (13). The first treatment of narcolepsy was caffeine, suggested by Willis (2). Ephedrine and benzedrine were first used in the 1930s and methylphenidate in the 1950s. The positive effect of tricyclics on cataplexy, sleep paralysis, and hallucinations was first reported in the 1960s.

Epidemiology

The exact prevalence of narcolepsy remains unknown, with a reported variation from 0.0002% to 0.5% in different populations (14). Bedrich Roth's estimated prevalence of 0.02–0.05% in Caucasians was recently confirmed in the first study with polygraphic verification (15). Narcolepsy occurs in both sexes with a male/female ratio of 1–2:1, and in all races, with a lower prevalence suggested in Israeli Jews. Narcoleptics represent about 5–10% of patients seen in a sleep clinic (16). Rigorous clinical and paraclinical testing suggests a percentage of "true" familial narcolepsy of about 4–7% (17–20). Most relatives of narcoleptics reporting sleepiness do not have the classic variant of the disease. The risk of developing narcolepsy in children of narcoleptics is about 1%.

Clinical Features

Excessive daytime sleepiness and cataplexy are the key symptoms of narcolepsy (Tables 1 and 2). The narcoleptic tetrad is present in most series in only 10–15% of patients (21,22).

Excessive Daytime Sleepiness

Excessive daytime sleepiness (EDS), the most common initial symptom of the disease, is mandatory for the diagnosis of narcolepsy. Most patients with narcolepsy complain of continuous sleepiness, which episodically—typically at intervals of 2–3 hours or when the patient relaxes—becomes irresistible ("sleep attacks"). Nonspecific symptoms such as yawning, tingling or numbness of scalp and body, blurred vision, diplopia, hypoacusis and other perceptual abnormalities, pressure in the eyes, and twitching eyelid may precede or accompany sleep attacks. Involuntary naps may then occur in such unusual circumstances as talking, eating, standing, walking, driving in traffic, and even during coitus. Naps typically last less than 30 minutes and are easily terminated by external stimuli.

Table 1 Clinical and Paraclinical Features of Narcolepsy

- Symptoms
  - Narcoleptic tetrad (all four:10–15% of patients)
    - Excessive daytime sleepiness, ''sleep attacks''
    - Cataplexy
    - Sleep paralysis
    - Hypnagogic/hypnopompic hallucinations
  - Others
    - Disrupted sleep
    - Automatic behaviors
    - Impaired memory and concentration
    - Depression
    - Neurovegetative disturbances (headache, fainting spells, etc.)
    - Visual problems, impotence
- Nocturnal polysomnography
  - Short sleep latency
  - SOREMPs (40–50%)
  - Decreased sleep efficiency with increased number of arousals and awakenings
  - Increased motor activity in non-REM and REM sleep
  - Periodic limb movements in sleep (PLMS)
  - Central and obstructive sleep apnea
  - REM-sleep behavior disorder (RSBD)
- Multiple sleep latency tests (MSLT)
  - Mean sleep latency $\leq$5 minutes
  - Two or more SOREMPs
- Genetic studies
  - Positive HLA-DR15 (subtype of DR2)
    - 88–100% of Japanese and Caucasian narcoleptics
    - $\approx$60% of black American narcoleptics
    - $\approx$20-35% of normal population
  - Positive HLA-DQ6 (subtype of DQ1)
    - $\approx$95% or more in narcoleptics of all ethnic groups
    - $\approx$40–60% of normal population

They are often refreshing, and occasionally associated with dream experiences. Duration and time of naps may influence the refreshing effect of naps and postnap performances (''sleep inertia'') (23). Up to 80% of narcoleptics experience fluctuations of vigilance lasting from seconds to hours during which they can perform ''nonsense'' complex acts for which there is amnesia. During these so-called automatic behavior (''microsleep'') episodes, which usually happen during monotonous or repetitive activities, patients may write nonsense, drive to unexpected places, put clothes in the dishwasher, or make irrelevant remarks (5,24). Aware-

Table 2 Forms of Narcolepsy

Forms of Narcolepsy
Idiopathic narcolepsy
Narcolepsy with cataplexy (classic narcolepsy)
Narcolepsy without cataplexy (monosymptomatic narcolepsy)
REM-narcolepsy with two or more SOREMPs on MSLT
Non-REM narcolepsy with one or no SOREMP
Symptomatic narcolepsy
Associated with: brain tumor, stroke, encephalitis, multiple sclerosis, head trauma, neurodegenerative diseases

ness of drowsiness may be altered, and short-lasting involuntary episodes of sleep may be experienced in up to 20% of narcoleptics as "paroxysmal" loss of consciousness and mistaken for seizures or syncope (22).

Rarely, patients deny significant EDS (e.g., Epworth sleepiness scores are within normal limits) but complain of nonspecific symptoms (see above) which may be related to a fluctuating level of arousal and attempts to resist sleep (9). In a few narcoleptics, naps usually last >30–60 minutes and are unrefreshing. Occasionally, as recognized already by Gélineau (1), patients report sleep attacks following sudden emotions (5).

Cataplexy

Cataplexy is present in 60 to 100% of patients with narcolepsy, depending on the diagnostic criteria used (see below). The term cataplexy refers to a sudden bilateral paralysis of striated muscles—typically sparing ocular and (in most cases) respiratory muscles—triggered by sudden emotions, associated with normal consciousness, and lasting less than a few minutes. The frequency of attacks often correlates with their severity, and 35–75% of patients report one or more episodes per day (25). The loss of muscle tone is most commonly partial and may be unnoticeable to others. Patients describe closing of the eyelids, sagging of the jaw, loss of speech or dysarthria, dropping of the head, and buckling or unlocking of the knees. Only one-third of patients experience sudden and severe loss of muscle tone and collapse to the ground, usually without significant injury. Occasionally patients experience cataplexy as the inability to move (e.g., rising from a chair, so-called affective adynamia) (26). Loss of muscle tone can spread from cranial to upper- and lower-limb muscles and the patient may not be able to keep from falling. A few bursts of phasic motor activity can superimpose on muscle weakness and present as twitching or tic-like movements of facial (periocular, perioral) muscles, tremor and quivering of the affected limbs, sagging of the jaw, or stuttering that may be mistaken for a seizure. Associated symptoms of cataplexy may include unpleasent breathing difficulties (e.g., feeling of suffocation), short apneic episodes, sweating, and palpitations. The most common emotion provoking cataplexy is laughing (e.g., while telling or listening to a joke, also called gelolepsia), which is reported in more than 80% of cases (27). Other common triggering emotions are surprise, excitement [e.g., orgasmolepsia (28)], elation, or, less commonly, negative emotions such as anger, fear, and embarrassment. Sudden, unexpected, and surprising emotions are particularly prone to trigger cataplexy. The presence of other (particularly known) people, and a triumphant or aggressive character of the emotion also favor cataplexy. This may explain why cataplexy is typically reported in sport activities and hunting. Conversely, pain, crying, sorrow, or sudden noise rarely trigger cataplexy (5,29). Intentional muscle activation (e.g., clenching of fists, forced jaw closure) can prevent or abate the symptoms. In most patients, cataplexy lasts 1 minute or less, usually just a few seconds. Duration exceeds 2 minutes in 10–20% of patients (30) and 20 minutes in only 2% (25). Prolonged episodes of cataplexy may be associated with hallucinations or dreaming and lead to sleep.

Occasionally, the presentation of cataplexy is less typical. Nonspecific symptoms, such as those heralding "sleep attacks," (see above) may precede cataplexy. The loss of muscle tone may appear without cause and be provoked by a sudden movement or by the anticipation rather than by the emotion itself. In some patients, only one side of the body or single muscles may be involved (6,11,31,32). Some patients report that, along with the paralysis, they also experience twitching and an increase in muscle tone of one limb or body part, known as cataplectic hypertonia (9,22,33). Episodes rarely last more than 30 minutes in status cataplecticus, a condition often caused by sudden discontinuation of anticataplectic drugs or the use of prazosin. Episodes with overlapping features of EDS and cataplexy can also occur. Patients may describe exacerbation of cataplexy by sleepiness or resisting a sleep attack (5) and report associated symptoms usually accompanying a sleep episode, such as visual blurring, diplopia, or sensory disturbances. Exceptionally, narcoleptics may present urine or fecal incontinence as a manifestation of cataplexy (5,34).

Sleep Paralysis

Sleep paralysis (SP) refers to the inability and struggle to move and speak while in the process of falling asleep (hypnagogic SP) or awakening (hypnopompic SP). Rarely, SP may be experienced during the day, at times of relaxed wakefulness (5). SP (also called "catapléxie du réveil") has similarities with cataplexy but always involves the entire body. SP is reported by up to 80% of narcoleptics, and its frequency can vary from a few life events to daily episodes. SP is often accompanied by fear (e.g., of dying) and breathing problems such as a sense of suffocation, pressure over the chest, or shortness of breath. Fear may appear regularly and be uncontrollable in patients with frequent attacks of SP. Occasionally SP is accompanied by eye-fluttering, moaning, tingling or numbness of the involved limbs, and autonomic symptoms such as palpitations or sweating. The association of SP with fearful hallucinations is not uncommon and has been referred to as incubus or nightmares—the *halluzinatorisch-kataplektisches Angstsyndrom* described by Rosenthal (26). The episodes are more common in states of stress, irregular sleep, or sleep deprivation. Sleeping in an uncomfortable position may prevent the occurrence of SP (35). Some patients experience SP only in the prone position. Paralysis usually lasts less than 10 minutes, although a duration of 30 minutes has been reported (36). The patient often misestimates the true duration of the episodes. The attempt to resist SP may prolong the episode, whereas touching or speech can end (rarely, prolong) it. Exceptionally, some weakness or numbness of the limbs (a ''jelly feeling'') persists for a few minutes afterward.

Hallucinations

Hallucinations at sleep onset (hypnagogic) and at awakening (hypnopompic) are often reported by narcoleptics, and in up to 50% of cases they occur at least once weekly (25). During sleep-associated hallucinations, elements of the normal awake mentation are still present and the subject may realize the unreal character of the hallucinations. Visual hallucinations can be either simple (unformed sensations, geometric figures) or complex (faces, animals, landscapes), still or in motion, black and white or colorful (37). Somatosensory, kinetic, vestibular, gustatory, olfactory, and vegetative hallucinations such as the feelings of being touched, lifted, or deformed in one part of the body are less common. Often the patients incorporate daily scenes, or the hallucination may follow an illusion. However, fantastic and absurd contents with religious, mysterious, or sexual components are not infrequent. The hallucination of intruders or of the presence of a person or animal nearby, standing over the bed or lying underneath it, are particularly common (so-called psychic hallucinations). An emotional—often negative—component is frequent. Not uncommonly, hallucinations may have a psychotic character—e.g., feeling of snakes running along the back, worms moving beneath the skin or inside the head, laceration of one extremity, blood dripping from the heart (10,26). The fear and anxiety associated with hallucinations may be the most distressing symptoms of narcolepsy, and a few patients develop sleep-preventive measures (e.g., biting their own hands), rites, or even delusional systems in association with them. Hallucinations typically occur in association with nocturnal sleep, when they can be associated with SP. As for SP, hypnagogic and hypnopompic hallucinations may be exacerbated by sleeping in an unfamiliar environment. Less commonly, hallucinations occur during the day in isolation (''day dreaming'') or with cataplexy.

Sleep Disturbances

Sleep disturbances with frequent awakenings and light and nonrefreshing sleep are reported by 50–80% of narcoleptics. A few patients complain of severe sleep-onset insomnia (5). Terrifying, vivid, and bizarre dreams are common, and patients may be reluctant to report them. Motor dyscontrol in sleep is frequent in narcoleptics and may start in childhood as a first manifestation of the disease (38). In non-REM sleep, periodic and aperiodic limb movements, somnambulism, bruxism, sleep talking, and other motor parasomnias are often observed. In REM sleep, patients frequently act out their dreams [REM-sleep behavior disorder (RSBD)] (39). In some studies, narcoleptics were shown to have a higher prevalence of snoring and obstructive sleep apnea (OSA). Awakening is usually not problematic and patients feel refreshed. Occasionally, however, nighttime sleep is prolonged and awakening difficulties with sleep drunkenness are reported (40).

Other Disturbances

Other disturbances, including visual problems such as diplopia, blurring, micropsia, and porropsia (wrong estimation of distances), may be subjectively leading symptoms of narcolepsy and can herald a sleep attack or cataplexy. Headache, occasionally of migrainous type, is occasionally reported. Impotence is present in up to 25% of patients (40). Memory and concentration problems, noted in at least 50% of patients, are probably related to EDS and ''microsleep'' episodes. As a consequence of EDS and cataplexy, driving and occupational accidents, as well as declines in school and job performance, are frequent. Neurovegetative symptoms, including migraine, cold hands, Raynaud phenomena, and fainting spells, are also reported (41). Anxiety, depression (42), reduced self-esteem, and social withdrawal are more common than in the general population. In up to one-third of patients, a psychiatric diagnosis is first considered. These psychopathological traits are thought to be codetermined by the difficulties in coping with the symptoms of the disease, which are often attributed by family or friends to laziness or boredom. Cataplexy may inhibit social interaction. Rarely, narcoleptics can present with a hallucinatory syndrome that is indistinguishable from schizophrenia (26) apart from good response to treatment with stimulants. The association of narcolepsy with obesity and hypothyroidism reported in older publications reflects in some cases the inclusion of patients with other causes of EDS, such as OSA. An increased frequency of non-insulin-dependent diabetes mellitus has been found (43,44).

Evolution

Narcolepsy starts before the age of 25 years in 70–80% of patients, and the onset of EDS usually precedes the onset of cataplexy by months to years. In 5–15% of cases, narcolepsy starts before the age of 10, and in 5% of cases after the age of 50. In children, cataplexy seems to be present in over 80% of cases. The onset of narcolepsy may be difficult to recognize and assess retrospectively. First, EDS may present in childhood with irritability, hyperactivity, and attention-deficit symptoms. Second, hallucinations and cataplexy-like symptoms (e.g., during weeping or urination) can be physiological in infants and children under the age of 5. In about 10% of cases, the onset of cataplexy follows the onset of EDS by more than 10 years, with a maximum interval of over 50 years (33). Conversely, cataplexy can precede EDS in 10% of cases by a few months or, rarely, up to 28 years (21,45). SP, hallucinations, and motor dyscontrol in sleep usually follow the onset of EDS, although any of these can be the first symptom to appear. The onset of narcolepsy is often gradual. Sometimes precipitating events such as infection, surgery, psychosocial stress, minor head injury, pregnancy/childbirth, menarche, abrupt change of sleep–wake schedule, overexertion, or anesthesia are reported (36,46,47). EDS almost invariably persists over time, although a decline in severity is not rare and short remissions over a few months are possible (45,46). Disappearance of sleepiness is exceptional (25). Conversely, cataplexy, SP, and hallucinations may disappear in up to 37% of patients (46).

Pathophysiology

Neurophysiology

The hallmark of narcolepsy is the occurrence of REM sleep at the onset of sleep or within 15 minutes, hereafter referred to as sleep-onset REM periods (SOREMPs) (12). Since the amount of REM sleep is not greater in narcoleptics than in normals (48,49), SOREMPs probably result from a disinhibition rather than a true overactivity of REM-generating mechanisms. In fact, the pathophysiology of narcolepsy is not confined to REM sleep, but also involves wakefulness and non-REM sleep. During wakefulness, sleep attacks occur often at intervals of 90–120 minutes (ultradian rhythmicity), similar to the nocturnal non-REM/REM cycle and to the ultradian sleep–wake cycle of normal newborns (50). During sleep, intrusions of wakefulness with frequent arousals are often observed. Finally, in both wakefulness and sleep, features of the different states of being (wakefulness and REM and non-REM sleep) can intermingle and give rise to such clinical phenomena as sleepwalking, RSBD, SP, cataplexy, and hallucinations. Narcolepsy therefore appears to represent a disorder of state boundary control (51), whereas circadian, ultradian, and homeostatic regulatory sleep mechanisms appear essentially preserved (52,53). Whether or not narcoleptic symptoms represent an exaggeration of normal sleep mechanisms related to insufficient maturation of arousal or to non-REM-sleep mechanisms remains controversial (6,21).

Based on current evidence, it is likely that the neuronal mechanisms responsible for EDS and cataplexy differ. According to Broughton (54), EDS may arise from increased pressure for non-REM or REM sleep, from decreased arousal, or from all three. Narcoleptics are more sensitive to sleep deprivation than are normal subjects (52), but nighttime sleep is a bad predictor of daytime sleepiness (55). This observation, as well as that of EDS in narcoleptics with essentially unremarkable nighttime sleep, supports the hypothesis of a deficient arousal. The correlation between clinical characteristics of EDS and associated electrophysiological findings is not absolute, emphasizing the possibility of electroclinical dissociations in narcolepsy. The severity of EDS—as estimated by the multiple sleep latency test (MSLT)—appears to correlate with appearance of SOREMPs (56). Furthermore, naps associated with REM sleep appear to be linked to a more imperative sleepiness and a greater restorative effect (57). The report of dreaming, on the other hand, appears to be an unreliable indicator of SOREMPs (58).

Automatic behavior corresponds to fluctuations in the level of arousal with short periods of "subwakefulness" or non-REM sleep (microsleep). Cataplexy represents the intrusion in wakefulness of REM-atonia equivalents (in dogs, the neurophysiology of cataplexy and REM atonia appear to differ), with inhibition of muscle stretch reflexes, H-reflexes, and F-responses related to the activation of cells in the so-called inhibitory region of Magoun and Rhines in the medial medulla, which exerts a postsynaptic inhibitory influence on spinal alpha-motoneurons (35). It has been suggested that cataplexy may result from the activation by emotions of suprapontine structures (basal forebrain, amygdala, basal ganglia) leading through descending (cholinergic or dopaminergic) pathways to an abnormal trigger of REM-sleep atonia (35). Cataplexy may therefore represent the exaggeration or disinhibition of an "arrest and orienting" reaction physiologically triggered by sudden emotions and increased arousal (59). Current evidence suggests that cataplexy may arise from the interaction within a circuit connecting pontine tegmentum, basal forebrain, amygdala, and medial medulla. This hypothesis is supported by several observations, including: 1) narcoleptics exhibit abnormal startle responses (59), 2) modulation of emotions and startle responses can be impaired in both animals and humans following lesions of the amygdala (60), 3) the amygdala has a role in the regulation of REM sleep (61), 4) canine cataplexy can be triggered by stimulation of basal forebrain and pontine reticular formation (62), and 5) neurons that are active in canine cataplexy were identified in amygdala, basal forebrain, amygdala, and medial medulla (63–65). Hence, cataplexy can be conceptualized as a disorder of reactivity (rather than emotionality) and of the interaction between emotional, vegetative, and motor systems.

SP also seems to represent a dissociated manifestation of REM-sleep atonia. The preferential occurrence of SP at sleep onset probably reflects the combination of a higher level of arousal and a stronger motor inhibition occurring in the first REM period compared to REM periods appearing later in the night (66). The existence of SP without cataplexy in patients with and without narcolepsy and reports of SP without SOREMPs suggest that the pathogenesis of the two symptoms is not identical (67).

Hypnagogic and hypnopompic hallucinations are compared to dreaming in a half-awake state and are therefore often considered to represent intrusions of REM-sleep imagery. Indeed, hypnagogic and hypnopompic hallucinations often accompany SOREMPs and SP. Furthermore, similarities with dreaming in young children suggest that hypnagogic and hypnopompic hallucinations may correspond to a phylogenetically more archaic form of mental activity in REM sleep. Hypnagogic and hypnopompic hallucinations also occur, however, during the transition from wakefulness to non-REM sleep without SOREMPs in normal subjects and in narcoleptics (37). In these cases, hypnagogic and hypnopompic hallucinations may arise from an altered processing of stimuli from the internal and external world. The characteristics of sleep-associated mental activity vary with different depths and types of sleep, and a continuum between hypnagogic and hypnopompic hallucinations and dreaming appears to exist (37,68).

Neuropharmacology

Physiologically, wakefulness is accompanied by an increased firing of the ascending reticular activating system (ARAS), which uses noradrenaline, dopamine, histamine, serotonin, and acetylcholine as the main neurotransmitters. REM sleep is associated with a decrease of the firing rate of monoaminergic neurons in the raphe nuclei and locus coeruleus (REM-off cells) and an increase in the activity of cholinergic neurons in the dorsal mediolateral pontine tegmentum (REM-on cells). The presumed dysfunction of state boundary control in narcolepsy could result from an imbalance between REM-on and REM-off cells. Involvement of aminergic and cholinergic systems has been documented in both human and canine narcolepsy. Systemic administration or local injection in the pontine tegmentum of cholinergic agonists (via muscarinic receptors) facilitates the appearance of REM sleep (69), and increased numbers of cholinergic neurons are found (in the canine model of narcolepsy) in the mediolateral pontine tegmentum (70). Cholinergic stimulation in the basal forebrain can also lead to cataplexy (62). Hence, cataplexy may be related to hypersensitivity of the cholinergic system in different areas of the brain. A decrease of noradrenergic function in narcolepsy is suggested by the improvement of narcolepsy with blockade of aminergic uptake by stimulants and by the exacerbation of human and canine cataplexy by prazosin (71), a noradrenergic α_1-receptor antagonist. In addition, α_1- and α_2-adrenergic receptors in the amygdala and other regions of the brain may be altered in human and canine narcolepsy (72). Cataplexy can be improved by drugs modulating serotoninergic trasnmission (reuptake inhibitors such as clomipramine and fluoxetine) (73). Local administration of dopaminergic drugs into the ventral tegmental pons modulates (via D_2 and D_3 receptors) cataplexy in the narcoleptic canine (74). Activation of dopamine transmission in the mesolimbic system may be crucial for the alerting effect of stimulants, as also suggested by improvement of EDS in narcoleptics with L-dopa (75). It could also be involved in the triggering effect of cataplexy by sudden emotions (74). Furthermore, striatal dopamine D_2 receptors were increased in human autopsy studies (76,77), although these results were not replicated in PET studies in vivo (78,79).

Etiology

The existence of familial cases of narcolepsy, of a genetically determined canine model in which narcolepsy is transmitted as a single autosomal recessive gene, and of a strong association between the human leukocyte antigen (HLA) DR_2 and narcolepsy-cataplexy (13) points to a genetic substrate of the disease. The rarity of well-documented familial cases and the fact that two-thirds of monozygotic twins are discordant for narcolepsy underscore the importance of environmental factors (80). Despite the strong HLA association and the mild cerebrospinal fluid pleocytosis found in narcoleptic dogs at the time of onset of cataplexy, no evidence has been found to support the hypothesis of an autoimmune origin of narcolepsy. The onset of canine narcolepsy seems to coincide, however, with the expression of HLA by microglial cells, which are involved in cerebral immune-related mechanisms (81). Neuropathological studies in narcolepsy failed to reveal any histological changes with the exception of the recent description of degenerative changes in the medial septal and diagonal-band nuclei in narcoleptic dogs (82).

Caucasian and Japanese patients are positive for the haplotype DR15 (a subtype of HLA-DR2) in 88–100% of cases, whereas up to 40% of narcoleptic African-Americans are DR15-negative (83). It is currently thought that DQ6—which at the genomic level corresponds to the subregions DQB1*0602 and DQA1*0102 on chromosome 6—is a better marker for narcolepsy across all ethnic groups. Most DR2-negative Caucasians, however, are also negative for DQ6 (84). Several observations suggest that the contribution of HLA to the genetic predisposition to narcolepsy is limited (80,85). First, a significant proportion of the normal population is positive for the DR2 (20–35%) and DQ6 (40–60%) HLA alleles. Second, the existence of rare DQ6-negative cases of both idiopathic and symptomatic narcolepsy suggests that the narcoleptic gene may be closely linked but not identical to the DQ6 haplotype. Third, up to a third of familial cases of narcolepsy are negative for the DQ6 alleles (20,80). Fourth, even in DQ6-positive families, susceptibility does not seem to be related to this specific HLA haplotype (20).

Genetic factors may be more relevant for EDS, which is reported in the absence of cataplexy by 12–40% of family members of narcoleptics (20,85). On the other hand, the HLA DQB1*0602 is associated with clinical expression of cataplexy. Narcoleptics who are HLA DQB1*0602-positive have a higher prevalence of a more severe form of cataplexy, which starts later, more commonly involves facial muscles, and is more often triggered by positive emotions (30).

Symptomatic narcolepsy has been reported with brain tumors, multiple sclerosis, encephalitis (typically localized at the level posterior third of the III ventricle) (5), stroke, hypothalamic disorders, neurodegenerative diseases, and head trauma (86,87). Symptomatic narcolepsy is rare, can occur with brain lesions of different etiology and topography, is not invariably associated with the DR15/DQ6 haplotypes, and may resolve under specific treatment. The majority of cases of symptomatic narcolepsy in children is associated with Niemann-Pick disease type C (88,89). An autosomal dominant DR2-negative syndrome with cerebellar ataxia, sensorineural deafness, optic neuropathy, and familial narcolepsy with cataplexy was recently reported in a Swedish family (90). Familial narcolepsy has also been associated with diabetes and multiple sclerosis (which is also linked to the HLA DR15 haplotype) (44,91).

Diagnosis

The concept of a narcoleptic tetrad is somewhat misleading, since most patients do not present this combination of symptoms and only cataplexy is pathognomonic for narcolepsy. In patients with EDS and definite cataplexy (classic narcolepsy), the diagnosis usually does not pose any problems. The diagnosis of definite (''true'') cataplexy should be reserved for patients having bilateral, short-lasting episodes of muscle weakness following emotions associated with normal consciousness. Most episodes will lead to a noticeable loss of muscle tone, also involving facial muscles, and will be improved by treatment with tryciclic antidepressants. Polysomnography may be useful to determine the presence of OSA or periodic leg movements in sleep (PLMS), which may contribute to EDS and require specific treatment. Documentation of EDS and SOREMPs following a night spent in the sleep laboratory may help the identification of pseudonarcoleptics seeking stimulants. A brain MRI is usually unnecessary and should be performed only if symptomatic narcolepsy is suspected (92). In patients with EDS and uncertain (no definite) or no cataplexy (monosymptomatic narcolepsy), other causes of EDS must be considered, including OSA, PLMS, and insufficient-sleep syndrome (Table 3).

Although some authors have questioned the existence of monosymptomatic narcolepsy, its existence is suggested by three lines of evidence. First, in patients with narcolepsy, EDS and cataplexy can appear several years apart. In particular, cataplexy usually appears within 10 years from the onset of EDS, but in rare cases it follows EDS by more than 50 years. Second, in patients with the full narcoleptic tetrad, the frequency and severity of the different symptoms can vary considerably. For example, cataplexy can occur a hundred times daily or only a few times in a lifetime, and can vary from a mild feeling of weakness unnoticeable to others to severe atonic attacks with falls to the ground (25,45). Furthermore, cataplexy often decreases in severity several years after its appearance. Hence, depending on the severity and frequency of criteria chosen for the diagnosis of cataplexy, patients with EDS may be diagnosed as having classic or monosymptomatic narcolepsy. Third, patients with narcolepsy with cataplexy often have a positive family history of EDS but rarely of cataplexy (17), a phenomenon

Table 3 Differential Diagnosis of Excessive Daytime Sleepiness (Hypersomnia)

Common causes of hypersomnia
Sleep apnea syndrome (including upper-airway resistance syndrome)
Narcolepsy
Periodic limb movements in sleep (PLMS)
Insufficient sleep syndrome
Less common causes of hypersomnia
Idiopathic hypersomnia
Circadian rhythm disorders (including shift work)
Depression with "true" hypersomnia
Sedating medications
Withdrawal from stimulants
Periodic hypersomnias
Neurological disorders: encephalitis, encephalopathy, hydrocephalus, diencephalic tumor or stroke, multiple sclerosis, Lewy body disease, mytonic dystrophy, Prader-Willi syndrome
Hypothyroidism
Pseudohypersomnia
Depression
Chronic fatigue syndrome
Tiredness, apathy, or weakness associated with medical and psychiatric disorders
Malingering

that also suggests the existence of monosymptomatic forms of the disease. Narcolepsy without cataplexy but with two or more SOREMPs (monosymptomatic REM narcolepsy) represents about 10–30% of all cases of narcolepsy. An even milder form of narcolepsy, characterized by EDS without cataplexy and with at most a single SOREMP (monosymptomatic non-REM narcolepsy), even after repeated MSLTs, probably exists (16,28), as also suggested by follow-up studies in patients who develop or lose clinical or polygraphic REM phenomena over time. The differentiation from other causes of EDS, in particular from idiopathic hypersomnia, may become impossible, since sleep paralysis, hypnagogic hallucinations, sleep attacks, prolonged and unrefreshing nighttime sleep and naps, disrupted sleep, and confusional arousals may occur in both conditions (16,93).

Nocturnal Polysomnography

Nocturnal polysomnography (PSG) of narcoleptics usually documents a short sleep latency, SOREMPs in 40–50% of cases, excessive sleep disruption with frequent arousals, reduced total sleep time, and excessive motor activity in non-REM and REM sleep. The amount of REM and non-REM sleep is usually normal. Slow-wave sleep may be reduced or show a rapid fall in the first part of the night and an abnormal persistence over the rest of the night (49,94). Daytime sleep periods are common even in treated narcoleptics, who may underestimate the degree of residual EDS (95). The total amount of sleep in 24 hours is usually not increased (96). An increased number of apneas, particularly central apneas, has been reported in narcoleptics but not confirmed in all studies. PLMS have been found in 9–59% of patients with narcolepsy. RSBD has been described in 12% of narcoleptics and may be exacerbated by the use of tricyclic medications (39).

Multiple Sleep Latency Test

On initial evaluation, about 70% of patients with narcolepsy and cataplexy have a mean sleep latency of <5 minutes with two or more SOREMPs (97). Rarely—for example, in narcoleptics who are acutely anxious—results of the initial MSLT are entirely normal (97). Also, one or more SOREMPs can occur in narcoleptics with normal mean sleep latencies (98). The presence of one or more SOREMPs is associated in narcoleptics with a higher frequency of cataplexy, SP, and hypnagogic hallucinations (99). Up to 30% of all patients presenting with EDS, mean sleep latency of <5 minutes, and two or more SOREMPs have a condition other than narcolepsy (97). Hence, MSLT alone cannot diagnose or exclude narcolepsy.

Genetic Studies

Considering the high frequency of DR15 and DQ6 in the normal population, >99% of subjects with either of these two haplotypes do not have narcolepsy. On the other hand, the absence of the haplotype DR15 (in Caucasians and Japanese) or DQ6 (in all races) is found in up to 5–10% [a recent study (100) suggests an even higher percentage, around 25–30%] of patients with classic narcolepsy (83). In patients without cataplexy, this percentage may be even higher. Hence, the absence of the typical genetic markers does not exclude the diagnosis and their presence does not prove it.

Differential Diagnosis

Excessive Daytime Sleepiness

EDS is reported by about 2–5% [range 0.3–13% (101)] of the adult population. In all forms of EDS, sleep propensity is increased in the afternoon hours, in situations of boredom or limited physical activity, after large meals, in a warm environment, and after sleep deprivation. EDS must be distinguished from the increased sleep needs, fatigue, and lack of energy related to medical and psychiatric diseases. In such patients, drowsiness and naps are not reported and the MSLT is usually normal. A few subjects may feign EDS in order to obtain stimulants. More than 80% of patients with EDS have either OSA syndrome, narcolepsy, PLMS syndrome, or an insufficient-sleep syndrome. Less common causes of EDS include idiopathic hypersomnia, shift work, abuse of stimulants, and neurological disorders (Table 3). Although imperative sleepiness, short and refreshing naps, and onset of EDS in adolescence are suggestive of narcolepsy, the characteristics of EDS are not specific for its causes. In particular, sleep attacks and short and refreshing involuntary naps are not mandatory in narcoleptics and are conversely reported by patients with other forms of EDS, including OSA syndrome. "Sleep attacks" and "automatic behaviors" may sometimes suggest seizures; the history of drowsiness and blurred vision during these episodes, their occurence in boring situations, and the easy arousability usually clear the differential diagnosis.

Cataplexy-Like Experiences

Cataplexy-like experiences are reported by up to 29% of young adults evaluated by questionnaire and are reflected by such popular expressions as "*cela me coupe les jambes*" or being "weak with laughter," dropping of the jaw with surprise, buckling of the knees with fear, and loss of speech with anger (15,102). A continuum between "physiological" and "true" cataplexy may therefore exist, although a few authorities disagree and emphasize the differences between these two symptoms (29). In the absence of EDS, true cataplectic attacks can be observed as a rare familial disorder with or without SP (103) or in association with Niemann-Pick type C disease, Norrie syndrome, Prader-Willi syndrome, encephalitis lethargica, and brainstem lesions (89,104–107). The differentiation from drop attacks associated with vertebrobasilar ischemia or cryptogenic drop attacks in women, atonic-astatic seizures, myasthenia gravis, and periodic paralysis is usually not problematic because emotional provocation is not a feature of these disorders. In gelastic seizures, laughing is accompanied by falls; other clinical and EEG features of epilepsy are usually evident (108). Sporadic and familial startle syndromes are nonepileptic clonazepam-responsive disorders in which a startling stimulus, rather than a sudden emotion, can lead to loss of postural control with falling (109,110). Laughing syncope—so-called geloplegia of Oppenheim (111)—consists of a short loss of consciousness during bouts of laughing, probably related to similar mechanisms implicated in cough syncope.

Sleep Paralysis

SP can occur sporadically in up to 62% of normal subjects (Dahlitz and Parkes, 1993; Wing et al., 1994), more commonly in men than in women. Adolescents with irregular sleep schedules and sleep deprivation may be more prone to develop sporadic, benign SP episodes. In about 5% of cases, in females more than in males, SP occurs regularly and is familial (112). SP can also be experienced in patients with sleep disorders such as OSA associated with REM-sleep fragmentation. Some patients with schizophrenia, depression, anxiety, or chronic fatigue syndrome may wake from sleep or in the morning with anxiety, shortness of breath, and "paralysis" with inability to get out of bed after awakening (26). In these patients, however, musle weakness is only partial (e.g., inability to lift a finger or roll over). SP has also been described in patients with postencephalitic parkinsonism (26).

Hypnagogic and Hypnopompic Hallucinations

Hypnagogic and hypnopompic hallucinations are frequent in normal subjects—in up to 40% at least once per year (113)—particularly in children. They can also occur in sleep disorders other than narcolepsy (16,93,114). Hallucinations on awakening (hypnopompic) may be more suggestive of narcolepsy than hallucinations on going to sleep (hypnagogic) (113). The differentiation from other sleep-associated forms of mental activity (e.g., dreaming, nightmares) is not always clear. In hypnagogic and hypnopompic hallucinations, there is typically a partial preservation of wakefulness with awareness of the surroundings, recognition of the unreal character of the hallucinations, and the ability to make voluntary movements (115). Hallucinations associated with metabolic-toxic encephalopathies, thalamomesencephalic lesions (''peduncular hallucinosis'') (116), and disturbances of visual pathways (Charles Bonnet syndrome) (117) may appear periodically in association with sleep onset but are usually evident from the clinical context. Multimodal hallucinations with inappropriate affect, incapacity for relating to others, presence of formal thought disorders, and lack of insight point to a psychiatric origin.

Treatment

Narcolepsy is a lifelong disease that can be complicated by other sleep disorders, such as OSA, PLMS, and RSBD, as well as by psychosocial problems (118,119). Treatment is effective in at least two-thirds of patients. Complete control of symptoms, however, is rare and side effects are not uncommon. Individualized treatment with counseling, support, and regular follow-up are crucial.

Nonpharmacological Approaches

Education of the patient and family is important; good sleep hygiene and avoidance of sleep deprivation should be stressed. Risks of sleepiness related to driving and working in hazardous environments should be pointed out. One to three short naps per day of 10–60 minutes each may increase alertness and decrease the requirements for stimulants. Naps in midafternoon, when the maximal diurnal sleep propensity tends to occur in narcoleptics, appear to be particularly useful. However, not all patients benefit from regular naps, and some prefer to nap on an as-needed basis.

Pharmacological Treatment

Excessive daytime sleepiness The most commonly used stimulants are indirect sympathomimetic drugs such as methylphenidate [used by about 50% of narcoleptics in the United States (120)] pemoline, mazindol, and amphetamines. The arousing affect of stimulants—probably with the exception of modafinil (121)—may depend mainly on an increase in the synaptic availability of dopamine. A comparison of their relative efficacy has been estimated from available data (122). A reasonable approach is to maximize alertness at selected times of the day (work, school, driving) while minimizing side effects. Treatment efficacy should be evaluated clinically. Objective assessment is problematic because serum levels of stimulants do not correlate well with subjective effect, and normalization of sleepiness by MSLT criteria is rarely achieved. In fact, improvement in the ability to stay awake during the day is not always accompanied by an increase on the MSLT in the time to fall asleep.

In narcoleptics with mild to moderate sleepiness, pemoline (start with 18.75–37.5 mg in the morning, upper limit 150 mg/day) or mazindol (1–2 mg b.i.d., 8 mg/day) are usually tried first. Modafinil (50 mg b.i.d., 400 mg/day) is the best-tested treatment for narcolepsy and may become, because of its low side-effect profile, the preferred initial treatment in countries in which it is available (120,123–125). For more severe sleepiness, methylphenidate (5–10 mg b.i.d. or t.i.d., 100 mg/day) may be preferred (126,127). The last dose should not be taken after 6 P.M. to avoid insomnia. In nonresponsive patients, dextroamphetamine and methamphetamine (5–10 mg in the morning or b.i.d., 60 mg/day) can be used (128). Although side effects increase with higher doses, some patients obtain benefit from doses higher than the maximum dosage indicated. Headaches, nervousness, akathisia, irritability, tremor, insomnia, anorexia, gastrointestinal complaints, and palpitations are the most common side effects. Tolerance develops in up to 30% of cases, more commonly at high doses. Drug holidays of 1–2 days/week with lower doses or no medication appear to benefit some patients. Hypertension, myocardial ischemia, and stroke are rare in patients without cardiovascular risk factors (122). Hepatotoxicity has been reported with pemoline. Addiction and psychosis (<1–3% of cases) are more common in patients on high doses of stimulants or with underlying psychiatric disease. The use of moderate doses of stimulants seems to be safe in children, whereas it should be avoided when possible in pregnancy. In patients with intolerable side effects and those at high risk for stimulant abuse, selegiline (129), L-dopa (75), or protriptyline can be tried.

Cataplexy The anticataplectic effect of tricyclic agents is probably mainly related to an inhibition of the reuptake of norepinephrine. Imipramine (start with 50 mg/day), clomipramine (start with 20 mg/day), or proptriptyline (start with 5 mg/day) are often tried first. Alternatively, fluoxetine (start with 20 mg/day) can be used (73). Tolerance to tricyclics can develop, and their abrupt discontinuation can lead to nearly continuous cataplexy (status cataplecticus). Improvement of EDS can sometimes have positive effects on cataplexy.

Insomnia/parasomnias Short-acting benzodiazepines may be helpful for patients with insomnia. Clonazepam (start with 0.5 mg at bedtime) or L-dopa/carbidopa (start with 25–100 mg at bedtime) and pergolide (start with 0.05 mg at bedtime) can be helpful if PLMS contribute to insomnia. Gamma-hydroxybutyrate has been claimed to improve nocturnal sleep and, as a consequence, daytime symptoms in narcoleptics, but its usefulness in clinical practice remains controversial. RSBD responds to clonazepam (start with 0.5 mg at bedtime).

IDIOPATHIC HYPERSOMNIA

Historical Introduction

The existence of idiopathic hypersomnia (IH) was first suggested by Bedrich Roth in the 1950s (33), although functional hypersomnia without cataplexy has probably been recognized since the beginning of the 19th century (130). In the 1960s, after the discovery of SOREMPs in narcolepsy, IH was conceptualized as a non-REM-sleep hypersomnia and differentiated from narcolepsy, considered a REM-sleep hypersomnia (33,131,132). In a series of papers in the 1970s, Roth stressed the differences between narcolepsy and IH, emphasizing prolonged and deep sleep as well as sleep drunkenness as hallmarks of IH (133,134–140). The recognition of the existence of monosymptomatic forms of narcolepsy, overlapping features of narcolepsy and IH (93), and "new causes" of hypersomnia without cataplexy, including sleep apnea, PLMS, and insufficient-sleep syndrome, has cast doubt on the existence of IH.

Epidemiology

The narcolepsy:IH ratio has progressively decreased from the original series reported by Roth (226:174) (135) to the most recent ones of Billiard et al. (308:21) (136), and Bassetti and Aldrich (258:42) (16). Idiopathic hypersomnia probably represents only about 1% of patients seen in a sleep clinic (16). The estimated prevalence of IH is about 2–5 per 100,000. Narcolepsy and IH rarely occur in members of the same family.

Clinical Features

Excessive Daytime Sleepiness

Idiopathic hypersomnia is characterized by continuous, nonimperative EDS with long and unrefreshing naps lasting up to 8 hours. Roth differentiated a monosymptomatic and a polysymptomatic ("classic") form of IH. *Monosymptomatic IH* is defined by EDS with no abnormalities of night sleep and awakening (135). A few patients with IH report a narcolepsy-like hypersomnia with overwhelming sleepiness and short, refreshing naps (16,135). This form of IH may be identical to the non-REM variant of monosymptomatic narcolepsy. *Polysymptomatic IH* [40–60% of cases (135)] also includes prolonged nighttime sleep as well as difficulty awakening. Sleep is most frequently deep and undisturbed, although sleep-onset insomnia and increased awakenings are occasionally reported (16,40,135). Some patients may report a sleep time exceeding 15 hours per day.

Sleep Drunkenness

Sleep drunkenness—*Schlaftrunkenheit* in German (137), *ivresse du sommeil* or *Elpénor syndrome* in French (138)—refers to a severe problem in awakening experienced by 20–60% of patients with IH and accompanied by nonsense or slurred speech, gait difficulties, and amnesia. Clinical examination during sleep drunkenness reveals reduced performance on psychometric testing, gait ataxia, hypo-areflexia, and orthostatic and vestibular signs (139). Patients report the need to use several alarm clocks or to be awakened by others. The time to "get going" in the morning may exceed 1 hour.

Other Disturbances

Other disturbances include depressed mood in up to over 25% of patients (16,42) and neurovegetative symptoms such as orthostatic disturbances, fainting spells, headache, and Raynaud-like symptoms. Automatic behavior was originally thought to be a specific feature of IH (24), a suggestion that was later contradicted (93). Occasionally, patients with IH report hypnagogic hallucinations and, in 13–43% of cases, sleep paralysis (5,16,93,114).

Evolution

Idiopathic hypersomnia usually starts in the second or third decade of life. As with narcolepsy, hypersomnia can first appear after abrupt changes in sleep–wake schedule, severe insomnia, viral illness (41), anesthesia, or minor head trauma, and can be enhanced by meals, a warm environment, and alcohol. The disease frequently presents first with difficulty awakening, subacute onset of hypersomnia, and stable course. Fluctuations of IH may be present in about 10% of cases (16,135). In a few patients, IH improves (135) or even disappears over years (41). A viral illness is implicated in some cases of IH (16). In some patients with initial diagnosis of IH, definite cataplexy may subsequently appear.

Pathophysiology

Neurophysiology

The pathophysiology of IH is unknown but may be related to a diencephalic dysfunction leading to a facilitation of non-REM sleep. A lesion of ascending activating noradrenergic pathways leads to continuous hypersomnia in cats (140). Sleep drunkenness occurs when patients with IH are awakened from deep (slow-wave) non-REM sleep and corresponds, on EEG recordings, to episodes of "microsleep" (139).

Neurochemistry

Cerebrospinal fluid analysis studies in IH have revealed increased levels of monoamine metabolites (141).

Etiology

A positive family history in 30–40% of cases (16) points to the contribution of genetic factors in IH (135). No specific association with the HLA-DR15 haplotype was found—not even in patients with the "narcoleptic-type" IH—in most reported IH series (16,142,143). Montplaisir and Poirier (144) suggested a higher prevalence of HLA-DR5 and HLA-Cw2. In some patients, a positive family history for diabetes mellitus, as described in narcolepsy, is found (16).

Diagnosis

In the absence of a gold standard, idiopathic hypersomnia remains a diagnosis of exclusion. The classic (polysymptomatic) form of *idiopathic hypersomnia* should be considered in patients with nonimperative EDS of unknown origin with long and nonrefreshing naps, prolonged nighttime sleep, sleep drunkenness, and positive family history of EDS.

Nocturnal Polysomnography

Results of nocturnal PSG are usually unremarkable. Occasionally, increased amounts of slow-wave sleep or some sleep fragmentation can be observed. Sleep drunkenness may be less common in the sleep laboratory than at home. Prolonged (e.g., 24-hour) polysomnographic monitoring may be helpful in documenting the facilitation of non-REM sleep in IH with >12 hours of sleep per day (136).

Multiple Sleep Latency Test

Daytime naps in IH are characterized by reduced sleep latencies (usually 5–10 minutes), absence of SOREMPs, and presence of slow-wave sleep. Exceptionally, SOREMPs may be observed in patients with polysymptomatic IH (16,135,143).

Genetic Studies

No genetic testing can be suggested at present time to diagnose or rule out IH.

Differential Diagnosis

Idiopathic hypersomnia must be differentiated from other causes of (non-REM) *hypersomnia without cataplexy* and without SOREMPs (Table 3). History, physical examination, and PSG usually reveal the syndromes of upper-airway resistance, chronic sleep insufficiency, PLMS, and organic causes of hypersomnias related to, for example, neurological diseases.

Differentiation among the possible causes of functional hypersomnias without cataplexy may be more difficult because of a significant overlap between these entities. This is particularly true for narcolepsy and IH (41,93,143). Clinically, the only specific feature distinguishing IH from narcolepsy is the absence of cataplexy. Overwhelming sleepiness (''sleep attacks''), daily or almost-daily napping, cataplexy-like episodes, SP, hypnagogic hallucinations, MSLT with decreased sleep latencies and SOREMPs, and HLA-DR2 are suggestive of *monosymptomatic narcolepsy*. However, up to one in five patients with IH may have clinical features similar to those of classic narcolepsy, including clinical REM-sleep phenomena (hallucinations, SP) in the absence of abnormal REM sleep (16). Overlapping clinical features, including onset in young age, depressed mood, and neurovegetative symptoms, are also present between IH and depression with hypersomnia (16). *Depression with hypersomnia* is typically characterized by mood disturbances paralleling the course of EDS, clinophilia (tendency to maintain a reclining position), eating disturbances, and borderline or only mildly abnormal MSLT results (145). A few patients with depression may have ''true hypersomnia'' with increased sleep over 24 hours and abnormal MSLT results (145–147). *Postviral hypersomnia* is a condition in which EDS appears in the course of a viral syndrome (e.g., Epstein-Barr infection) and usually resolves, occasionally only after several months to years (148). *Posttraumatic hypersomnia* is a poorly known condition that may complicate severe as well as mild head trauma (149). In many cases, the causal relationship between hypersomnia and viral infection or (minor) head trauma is unclear, and, at least in some patients, the two conditions may only represent factors contributing to or exacerbating an underlying EDS (16).

Sleep drunkenness, first described in the psychiatric literature at the beginning of the century (137), is characteristic but not specific of IH. It may be found in patients with symptomatic hypersomnias, narcolepsy [16% in Roth's experience (139)], alcohol abuse, and other sleep disorders, and in normal subjects when awakened from slow-wave sleep.

Treatment

Roth (135) emphasized the poor response to treatment of patients with IH. Recent studies, however, suggest that a significant percentage of patients with IH may respond to stimulants, including modafinil (16,150). Patients with classic IH may respond better to antidepressants than to stimulants. Improvement of sleepiness following prolonged sleep over several days, as suggested by Roth, appears—even when feasible—to be mostly ineffective.

KLEINE-LEVIN SYNDROME AND OTHER PERIODIC HYPERSOMNIAS

Historical Introduction

Kleine, in 1925 (151), and shortly thereafter Levin, in 1929 (152), offered the first descriptions of a syndrome characterized by periodic hypersomnia and hyper- (mega-)phagia (overeating). In 1935, Kaplinsky and Schulman first reported a case of periodic hypersomnia related to menstruation (153). In 1942, McDonald Critchley proposed the the eponym Kleine-Levin syndrome (KLS) and in 1962, based on the description of 26 patients published in the literature, suggested the diagnostic criteria: male gender, onset in adolescence, periodic hypersomnia, megaphagia, and spontaneous remission) (154).

Epidemiology

About 200 case reports of KLS have been published. Bedrich Roth found only two patients with KLS in a series of 642 patients with hypersomnia (155). Billiard reported in his series a narcolepsy:KLS ratio of 308:18 (156). Most patients with KLS appear to have an incomplete (atypical) form of the syndrome. Only a few females with KLS have been reported (157,158).

Clinical Features

Viral infection, minor head trauma, physical or emotional stress, seasickness, menstruation, and pregnancy may trigger the onset of KLS. The hypersomnolent episodes are occasionally preceded by a depressed mood. The onset of hypersomnia is usually rapid, within hours or days. During attacks, patients may sleep up to 20 hours per day, awakening only to eat and void. The patient may present with overeating (particularly of sweets), which can lead to weight gain at the end of the episode. Mental changes include irritability, confusional state, occasionally of hallucinatory character, and hypersexuality with inadequate sexual advances. Polydipsia, water retention, and increased sweating are occasionally observed (134). The episodes may last from 1 day to several weeks (usually 3–4 days) and occasionally end in association with a short phase (e.g., a single night) of insomnia.

Whether recurrent hypersomnia without mental changes and megaphagia (so-called *monosymptomatic Kleine-Levin syndrome*) and *periodic hypersomnia related to menstruation* belong to the spectrum of KLS remains controversial (159–161).

KLS typically starts in adolescence, although onset in childhood and adulthood has been reported (162). Relapses may occur at intervals of a few months to up to 20 years, although in most patients severity and frequency of hypersomnolent episodes decrease over time (154).

Pathophysiology

The pathophysiology of KLS is unknown but may be related to (homeostatic?) changes in sleep needs similar to those experienced by patients with bipolar mood disorder. The clinical picture and a few endocrinological studies, documenting a disturbed hypothalamic-pituitary axis in some but by far not all patients, suggest a hypothalamic dysfunction (163).

Etiology

The etiology of KLS is unknown. Clinical and polygraphic features of KLS have some similarities with those in patients with hypersomnolent depression (atypical depression) and idiopathic hypersomnia (16), including a good response to lithium (164). In a few cases, a focal diencephalic encephalitis may be responsible (165,166). Cerebrospinal fluid in KLS, however, is typically normal. Traumatic or vascular brain lesions have been implicated in a very few cases of KLS (167,168). There are no reports of familial cases of KLS; however, a positive family history of depression is occasionally found (154).

Diagnosis

The diagnosis of KLS relies on the clinical criteria defined by Critchley. In atypical/incomplete forms of KLS, symptomatic and psychiatric forms of hypersomnia should be excluded first. The EEG of patients with KLS can be normal or show a slowing of background activity.

Nocturnal Polysomnography

The PSG findings of KLS are variable and include normal architecture, increase or decrease of slow-wave sleep, and appearance of SOREMPs (156,169,170). Prolonged (e.g., 24-hour) polysomnographic (or actigraphic) monitoring can document an increased amount of sleep per day (169).

Multiple Sleep Latency Test

The results of the MSLT in KLS may be normal or document decreased sleep latency and SOREMPs (171).

Genetic Studies

No specific genetic marker of KLS has yet been recognized. Six of seven patients with periodc hypersomnia reported by Harada et al. (143) were HLA-DR2-negative.

Differential Diagnosis

The most important differential signs of KLS are psychiatric conditions including depression, bipolar mood disorders, and psychogenic hypersomnia (170,172–174). Less common causes of periodic hypersomnia are brain neoplasia (cranipharyngioma, third and fourth ventricle, hypothalamic tumor, pinealoma) (175), encephalitis (176), and drug (benzodiazepine) intoxications.

Treatment

The rarity of cases of KLS and the tendency of the syndrome to have a spontaneous resolution limit assessment of treatment efficacy. During hypersomnolent episodes, stimulants can be tried, usually with limited effects. Lithium and carbamazepine have been found in isolated cases to prevent recurrent episodes of hypersomnia (164).

REFERENCES

1. Gélineau JBE. De la narcolepsie. Gaz Hôp 1880; 53, 54:626–628, 635–637.
2. Lennox WG. Thomas Willis on narcolepsy. Arch Neurol Psychiatry 1939; 41:348–351.
3. Westphal C. Eigentümliche mit Einschlafen verbundene Anfälle. Arch Psychiat Nervenkr 1877; 7:631–635.
4. Mitchell SW. Some disorders of sleep. Am J Med Sci 1890; 100:109–127.
5. Wilder J. Narkolepsie. In: Bumke O, Foerster O, eds. Handbuch der Neurologie. Berlin: Springer, 1935. 17:87–140.
6. Wilson SA. The narcolepsies. Brain 1928; 51:63–109.
7. Löwenfeld L. Ueber Narkolepsie. Münchner Medizinische Wochenschrift 1902; 49:1041–1045.
8. Adie WJ. Idiopathic narcolepsy: a disease sui generis: with remarks on the mechanism of sleep. Brain 1926; 49:257–306.
9. Redlich E. Epilegomena zur Narkolepsiefrage. Zeitschrift für Gesundheit Psychiatrie und Neurologie 1931; 129–173.
10. Daniels LE. Narcolepsy. Medicine 1934; 13:1–122.
11. Yoss RE, Daly DD. Criteria for the diagnosis of the narcoleptic syndrome. Mayo Clin Proc 1957; 32:320–328.
12. Vogel G. Studies in psychophysiology of dreams. III. The dream of narcolepsy. Arch Gen Psychiatry 1960; 3:421–428.
13. Honda Y, Asaka A, Tanaka Y, Juji T. Discrimination of narcolepsy by using genetic markers and HLA. Sleep Res 1983; 12:254.
14. Hublin C, Partinen M, Kaprio J, Koskenvuo M, Guilleminault C. Epidemiology of narcolepsy. Sleep 1994; 17:S7–S12.
15. Hublin S, Kaprio J, Partinen M, Heikkila K, Kskimies S, Guilleminault C. The prevalence of narcolepsy: an epidemiological study of the Finnish twin cohort. Ann Neurol 1994; 35:709–716.

16. Bassetti C, Aldrich M. Idiopathic hypersomnia: a study of 42 patients. Brain 1997; 120:1432–1435.
17. Guilleminault C, Mignot E, Grumet FC. Familial patterns of narcolepsy. Lancet 1989; 335:1376–1379.
18. Billiard M, Pasquié-Magnetto V, Heckmann M, et al. Family studies in narcolepsy. Sleep 1994; 17:S54–S59.
19. Hayduk R, Flodman P, Spence MA, Erman MK, Mitler MM. HLA haplotypes, polysomnography, and pedigrees in a case series of patients with narcolepsy. Sleep 1997; 20:850–857.
20. Nevsimalova S, Mignot E, Sonka K, Arrigoni JL. Familial aspects of narcolepsy–cataplexy in the Czech republic. Sleep 1997; 20:1021–1026.
21. Yoss RE, Daly DD. Narcolepsy. Med Clin North Am 1960; 44:955–968.
22. Rüther E, Meier–Ewert K, Gallitz A. Zur Symptomatologie des narkoleptischen Syndroms. Nervenarzt 1972; 43:640–643.
23. Mullington J, Broughton R. Daytime sleep inertia in narcolepsy-cataplexy. Sleep 1994; 17:69–76.
24. Guilleminault C, Philipps R, Dement WC. A syndrome of hypersomnia with automatic behaviour. Electroencephalogr Clin Neurophysiol 1975; 38:408–413.
25. Honda Y. Clinical features of narcolepsy: Japanese experiences. In: Honda Y, Juji T, eds. HLA in Narcolepsy. Berlin: Springer-Verlag, 1988:24–57.
26. Rosenthal C. Ueber das Auftreten von halluzinatorisch-kataplektischen Angstsyndrom, Wachanfällen und ähnlichen Störungen bei Schizophrenen. Mschr Psychiat Neurol 1939; 102:11–38.
27. Guilleminault C. Cataplexy. In: Guilleminault C, Dement WC, Passouant P, eds. Narcolepsy. Proceedings of the First International Symposium on Narcolepsy. Montpellier, France: Spectrum Publications, 1976:125–143.
28. Meier-Evert K, Schöpfer B, Rüther E. Drei narkoleptische Syndrome. Katamnestische und polygraphische Ergebnisse. Nervenarzt 1975; 46:624–635.
29. Parkes JD, Chen SY, Clift SJ, Dahlitz MJ, Dunn G. The clinical diagnosis of the narcoleptic syndrome. J Sleep Res 1998; 7:41–52.
30. Mignot E, Hajduk R, Black J, Grumet FC, Guillemiaault C. HLA DQB1*0602 is associated with cataplexy in 509 narcoleptic patients. Sleep 1997; 20:1012–1020.
31. Lascelles RF, Mohr PD, Peart J. Unilateral cataplexy associated with systemic lupus erythematodes. J Neurol Neurosurg Psychiatry 1976; 39:1023–1026.
32. Meier-Ewert K. Tagesschläfrigkeit. Ursachen, Differentialdiagnose, Therapie. betz–Druck gmbH, 1989.
33. Roth B. Narkolepsie und Hypersomnie. In: Roth B, ed. Narkolepsie und Hypersomnie. Berlin: VEB Verlag, 1962.
34. Vgontzas AN, Sollenberger SE, Kales A, Bixler EO, Vela-Bueno A. Narcolepsy–cataplexy and loss of sphincter control. Postgrad Med J 1996; 72:493–494.
35. Hishikawa Y, Shimizu T. Physiology of REM sleep, cataplexy, and sleep paralysis. In: Hallet M, Lüders HO, Marsden CD, eds. Negative Motor Phenomena. Philadelphia: Lippincott-Raven, 1995:245–271.
36. Passouant P, Billiard M. The evolution of narcolepsy with age. In: Guilleminault C, Dement WC, Passouant P, eds. Narcolepsy. New York: Spectrum Publications, 1976:179–200.

37. Ribstein M. Hypnagogic hallucinations. In: Guilleminault C, Dement WC, Passouant P, eds. Narcolepsy. Proceedings of the First International Symposium on Narcolepsy. Montpellier, France: Spectrum Publications, 1976:145–160.
38. Mayer G, Meier-Ewert K. Motor dyscontrol in sleep in narcoleptic patients (a life–long development?). J Sleep Res 1993; 2:143–148.
39. Schenck CH, Mahowald MW. Motor dyscontrol in narcolepsy: rapid-eye-movement (rem) sleep without atonia and rem sleep behavior disorder. Ann Neurol 1992; 32:3–10.
40. Roth B. Narcolepsy and hypersomnia. Basel: Karger Libri, 1980.
41. Bruck D, Parkes JD. A comparison of idiopathic hypersomnia and narcolepsy-cataplexy using self report measures and sleep diary data. J Neurol Neurosurg Psychiatry 1996; 60:576–578.
42. Roth B, Nevsimalova S. Depression in narcolepsy and hypersomnia. Schweizer Archiv für Neurologie und Psychiatrie 1975; 116:291–300.
43. Roberts HJ. Obesity due to the syndrome of narcolepsy and diabetogenic hyperinsulinism: clinical and therapeutic observations on 252 patients. J Am Geriatr Soc 1967; 15:721–743.
44. Honda Y, Doi Y, Ninomiya C, Ninomiya O. Increased frequency of non-insulin dependent diabetes mellitus among narcoleptics. Sleep 1986; 9:254–259.
45. Parkes JD, Baraitser M, Marsden CD, Asselman P. Natural history, symptoms and treatment of the narcoleptic syndrome. Acta Neurol Scand 1975; 52.
46. Billiard M, Besset A, Cadilhac J. The clinical and polygraphic development of narcolepsy. In: Guilleminault C, Lugaresi E, eds. Sleep/Wake Disorders: Natural History, Epidemiology, and Long–Term Evolution. New York: Raven Press, 1983:171–185.
47. Orellana C, Villemin E, Tafti M, Carlander B, Besset A, Billiard M. Life events in the year preceding the onset of narcolepsy. Sleep 1994; 17:S50–S53.
48. Montplaisir J, Billiard M, Takahashi S, Bell IR, Guilleminault C, Dement WC. Twenty-four-hour recording in REM-narcoleptics with special reference to nocturnal sleep disruption. Biolog Psychiatry 1978; 13:73–89.
49. Broughton R, Dunham W, Newman J, Lutley K, Duchesne P, Rivers M. Ambulatory 24 hour sleep-wake monitoring in narcolepsy-cataplexy compared to matched controls. Electroencephalogr Clin Neurophysiol 1988; 70:473–481.
50. Passouant P, Halberg F, Genicot R, Popoviciu L, Baldy-Moulinier M. La periodicité des accès narcoleptiques et le rhythme ultradien du sommeil rapide. Rev Neurol 1969; 121:155–164.
51. Broughton R, Valley V, Aguirre M, Roberts J, Suwalski W, Dunham W. Excessive daytime sleepiness and the pathophysiology of narcolepsy–cataplexy: a laboratory perspective. Sleep 1986; 9:205–215.
52. Besset A, Tafti M, Nobile L, Billiard M. Homeostasis and narcolepsy. Sleep 1994; 17:S29–S34.
53. Broughton R, Mullington J. Chronobiological aspects of narcolepsy. Sleep 1994; 17:S35–S44.
54. Broughton R. Performance and evoked potential measures of various states of daytime sleepiness. Sleep 1982; 5:135–146.
55. Broughton R, Dunham W, Weisskopf M, Rivers M. Night sleep does not predict day sleep in narcoleptics. Electroencephalogr Clin Neurophysiol 1994; 91:67–70.

56. Tafti M, Villemin E, Carlander B, Besset A, Billiard M. Sleep onset rapid–eye movement episodes in narcolepsy: REM sleep pressure or nonREM-REM sleep dysregulation. J Sleep Res 1992; 1:245–250.
57. Broughton RJ, Aguirre M. Differences between REM and NREM sleepiness measured by event-related potentials (P300, CNV), MSLT and subjective estimate in narcolepsy-cataplexy. Electroencephalogr Clin Neurophysiol 1987; 67:317–326.
58. Benbadis SR, Wolgamuth BR, Perry MC, et al. Dreams and rapid eye movement sleep in the multiple sleep latency test. Sleep 1985; 18:105–108.
59. Reese NB, Garcia-Rill E, Skinner RD. The pedunculopontine nucleus-auditory input, arousal and pathophysiology. Progress Neurobiol 1995; 42:105–133.
60. Angrilli A, Mauri A, Palomba D, et al. Startle reflex and emotion modulation impairment after a right amygdala lesion. Brain 1996; 119:1991–2000.
61. Calvo JM, Simon-Arceo K, Fernando-Mas R. Prolonged enhancement of REM sleep produced by carbachol microinjection into the amygdala. Neuroreport 1996; 7:577–580.
62. Nishino S, Tafti M, Reid SM, et al. Cholinergic stimulation in the basal forebrain ellicits cataplexy in narcoleptic canines. J Neurosci 1995; 15:4806–4814.
63. Siegel JM, Ninhuis R, Fahringer HM, et al. Neuronal-activity in narcolepsy: identification of cataplexy-related cells in the medial medulla. Science 1991; 252:1315–1318.
64. Wu MF, Gulyani A, Phan B, Siegel JM. Activity of ventrolateral preoptic neurons during cataplexy in the narcoleptic dog. Sleep 1998; 21(suppl):19.
65. Gulyani SA, Wu MF, Phan B, Siegel JM. Activity of amygdala neurons during cataplexy in the narcoleptic dog. Sleep 1998; 21(suppl):19.
66. Hishikawa Y. Sleep paralysis. In: Guilleminault C, Dement WC, Passouant P, eds. Narcolepsy. Proceedings of the First International Symposium on Narcolepsy. Montpellier, France: Spectrum Publications, 1976:97–125.
67. Hishikawa Y, Kaneko Z. Electroencephalographic study on narcolepsy. Electroencephalogr Clin Neurophysiol 1965; 18:249–258.
68. Vogel G, Foulkes D, Trosman H. Ego functions and dreaming during sleep onset. Arch Gen Psychiatry 1966; 14:238–248.
69. Baghdoyan HA, Lydic R, Callaway CW, Hobson JA. Neuropsychopharmacology 1989; 2:67–69.
70. Nitz D, Andersen A, Fahringer H, Nienhuis R, Mignot E, Siegel J. Altered distribution of cholinergic cells in the narcoleptic dog. Neuroreport 1995; 6:1521–1524.
71. Aldrich M, Rogers AE. Exacerbation of human cataplexy by prazosin. Sleep 1989; 12:254–256.
72. Aldrich MS, Prokopowicz G, Ockert K, Hollingsworth Z, Penney JB, Albin RL. Neurochemical studies of human narcolepsy: alpha-adrenergic receptor autoradiography of human narcoleptic brain and brainstem. Sleep 1994; 17:598–608.
73. Langdon N, Bandak S, Shindler J, Parkes JD. Fluoxetine in the treatment of cataplexy. Sleep 1986; 9:371–372.
74. Reid MS, Tafti M, Nishino S, Samapthkumaran R, Siegel J, Mignot E. Local administration of dopaminergic drugs into the ventral tegmental area modulates cataplexy in the narcoleptic canine. Brain Res 1996; 733:83–100.
75. Boivin D, Montplaisir J. The effects of L-dopa on excessive daytime sleepiness in narcolepsy. Neurology 1991; 41:1267–1269.

76. Aldrich MS, Holligsworth Z, Penney JB. Dopamine-receptor autoradiography of human narcoleptic brain. Neurology 1992; 42:410–413.
77. Kish SJ, Mamelak M, Slimovitch C, et al. Brain neurotransmitter changes in human narcolepsy. Neurology 1992; 42:229–234.
78. Khan N, Antonini A, Parkes D, et al. Striatal dopamine D2 receptors in patients with narcolepsy measured with PET and ^{11}C-raclopride. Neurology 1994; 44:2101–2104.
79. Rinne JO, Hublin C, Partinen M, et al. Positron emission tomography study of human narcolepsy: no increase in striatal dopamine D2 receptors. Neurology 1995; 45:1735–1738.
80. Mignot E. Genetic and familial aspects of narcolepsy. Neurology 1998; 50(suppl 1):S16–S22.
81. Tafti M, Nishino S, Aldrich MS, Liao W, Dement WC, Mignot E. Major histocompatibility class II molecules in the CNS: increased microglial expression at the onset of narcolepsy in a canine model. J Neurosci 1996; 16:4588–1595.
82. Siegel JM, et al. Neuronal degeneration in canine narcolepsy. J Neurosci 1999; 248–257.
83. Mignot E, Lin X, Arrigoni J, et al. DQB1*0602 and DQA1*0102 (DQ1) are better markers than DR2 for narcolepsy in Caucasian and black Americans. Sleep 1994; 17:60–67.
84. Mignot E, Lin X, Kalil E, et al. DQB1-0602 (DQw1) is not present in most nonDR2 Caucasian narcoleptics. Sleep 1992; 15:415–422.
85. Kaprio J, Hublin C, Partinen M, Heikkilä K, Koskenvuo M. Narcolepsy-like symptoms among adult twins. J Sleep Res 1996; 5:55–60.
86. Autret A, Lucas B, Henry-Lebras H, de Toffol B. Symptomatic narcolepsies. Sleep 1994; 17:21–24.
87. Bonduelle M, Degos C. Symptomatic narcolepsies: a critical study. In: Guilleminault C, Dement WC, Passouant P, eds. Narcolepsy. Proceedings of the First International Symposium on Narcolepsy. Montpellier, France: Spectrum Publications, 1976:313–332.
88. Challamel MJ, Mazzola ME, Nevsimalova S, Cannard C, Louis J, Revol M. Narcolepsy in children. Sleep 1994; 17:17–20.
89. Kandt RS, Emerson RG, Singer HS, Valle DL, Moser HW. Cataplexy in variant forms of Niemann-Pick disease. Ann Neurol 1982; 12:284–288.
90. Melberg A, Hetta J, Dahl N, Nennesmo I, et al. Autosomal dominant cerebellar ataxia deafness and narcolepsy. J Neurol Sci 1995; 134:119–129.
91. Ekbom K. Familial multiple sclerosis associated with narcolepsy. Arch Neurol 1966; 15:337–344.
92. Bassetti C, Aldrich MS, Quint DJ. MRI findings in idiopathic narcolepsy. Sleep 1997; 20:630–631.
93. Aldrich M. The clinical spectrum of narcolepsy and idiopathic hypersomnia. Neurology 1996; 46:393–401.
94. Tafti M, Rondouin G, Besset A, Billiard M. Sleep deprivation in narcoleptic subjects: effect on sleep stages and EEG power density. Electroencephalogr Clin Neurophysiol 1992; 83:339–349.
95. Rogers AE, Aldrich MS, Caruso CC. Patterns of sleep and wakefulness in treated narcoleptic subjects. Sleep 1994; 17:590–597.

96. Billiard M, Salwa MQ, De Koninck J, Besset A, Touchon J, Cadilhac J. Daytime sleep characteristics and their relationship with night sleep in the narcoleptic patient. Sleep 1986; 9:167–174.
97. Aldrich MS, Chervin RD, Malow BA. Value of the multiple sleep latency test (MSLT) for the diagnosis of narcolepsy. Sleep 1997; 20:620–629.
98. Guilleminault C, Mignot E, Partinen M. Controversies in the diagnosis of narcolepsy. Sleep 1994; 17:S1–S6.
99. Moscowitch A, Partinen M, Guilleminault C. The positive diagnosis of narcolepsy and narcolepsy's borderland. Neurology 1993; 43:55–60.
100. Mignot E, Young T, Lin L, Finn L, Palta M. Reduction of REM sleep latency associated with HLA-DQB1*0602 in normal adults. Lancet 1998; 351:727.
101. D'Alessandro R, Rinaldi R, Cristina E, Gamberini G, Lugaresi E. Prevalence of excessive daytime sleepiness: an open epidemiological problem. Sleep 1995; 18: 389–391.
102. Billiard M, Alperovitch A, Perot C, Jammes A. Excessive daytime somnolence in young men: prevalence and contributing factors. Sleep 1987; 10:297–305.
103. Gelardi JAM, Brown JW. Hereditary cataplexy. J Neurol Neurosurg Psychiatry 1967; 30:455–457.
104. Vossler DG, Wyler AR, Wilkus RJ, et al. Cataplexy and monoamine oxidase deficiency in Norrie disease. Neurology 1996; 46:1258–1261.
105. Fernandez JM, Sadaba F, Villaverde FJ, Alvaro LC, Cortina C. Cataplexy associated with midbrain lesion. Neurology 1995; 45:393–394.
106. Stahl SM, Layzer RB, Aminoff MJ, Townsend JJ, Feldon S. Continuous cataplexy in a patient with a midbrain tumor: the limp man syndrome. Neurology 1980; 30: 1115–1118.
107. Schwartz WJ, Stakes JW, Hobson JA. Transient cataplexy after removal of a craniopharyngioma. Neurology 1984; 34:1372–1375.
108. Munari C, Kahane P, Francione S, et al. Role of the hypothalamic hamartoma in the genesis of gelastic fits (a video-stereo–EEG study). Electroencephalogr Clin Neurophysiol 1995; 95:154–160.
109. Kirstein L, Silfverskiold BP. A family with emotionally precipitated "drop seizures." Acta Psychiatrica and Neurologica Scandinavica 1958; 33:471–476.
110. Brown P, Rothwell JC, Thompson PD, Britton TC, Day BL, Marsden CD. The hyperkplexias and their relationship to the normal startle reflex. Brain 1991; 114: 1903–1928.
111. Oppenheim H. Ueber Lachschlag. Mschr Psychiat Neurol 1902; 11:242.
112. Roth B, Bruhova S, Berkova L. Familial sleep paralysis. Schweizer Archiv für Neurologie und Psychiatrie 1968; 102:321–330.
113. Ohayon M, Priest RG, Caulet M, Guilleminault C. Hypnagogic and hypnopompic hallucinations: pathological phenomena. Br J Psychiatry 1996; 169:459–467.
114. Bassetti C, Sturzenegger C, Gugger M, Mathis J. The clinical spectrum of narcolepsy with cataplexy, monosymptomatic narcolepsy, and idiopathic hypersomnia. Sleep 1998; 21(suppl):177.
115. Vihvelin H. On the differentation of some typical forms of hypnagogic hallucinations. Acta Psych Neurol Scan 1948; 23:359–389.

116. Lhermitte MJ. Syndrome de la calotte du pédoncule cérébral: les troubles psychosensoriels dans les lésions mésocéphaliques. Rev Neurol 1922; 29:1359–1365.
117. Teunisse RJ, Cruysberg JR, Hoefnagels WH, Verbek AL, Zitman FG. Visual hallucinations in psychologically normal people: Charles Bonnet's syndrome. Lancet 1996; 347:794–797.
118. Broughton R, Ghanem Q. The impact of compound narcolepsy on the life of the patient. In: Guilleminault C, Dement W, Passouant P, eds. Narcolepsy. New York: Spectrum Publications, 1976:201–219.
119. Douglas NJ. The psychosocial aspects of narcolepsy. Neurology 1998; 50(suppl 1):S27–S30.
120. Fry JM. Treatment modalities for narcolepsy. Neurology 1998; 50(suppl 1):S43–S48.
121. Séréville JE, Boer C, Rambert FA, Duteil J. Lack pf pre-synaptic dopaminergic involvement in modafinil in anaesthetized mice: in vivo voltammetry studies. Neuropharmacology 1994; 33:755–761.
122. Mitler M, Aldrich MS, Koob GF, Zarcone VP. Narcolepsy and its treatment with stimulants. Sleep 1994; 17:352–371.
123. Billiard M, Besset A, Montplaisir J, et al. Modafinil: a double-blind multicentric study. Sleep 1994; 17:S107–S112.
124. U.S. Modafinil in Narcolepsy Study G. Randomized trial of modafinil for the treatment of pathological somnolence in narcolepsy. Ann Neurol 1998; 43:88–97.
125. Broughton R, Fleming JAE, George CFP, Hill JD, et al. Randomized, double-blind, placebo-controlled crossover trial of modafinil in the treatment of excessive daytime sleepiness in narcolepsy. Neurology 1997; 49:444–451.
126. Yoss RE, Daly D. Treatment of narcolepsy with ritalin. Neurology 1959; 9:171–173.
127. Honda Y, Hishikawa Y, Takahashi Y. Long-term treatment of narcolepsy with methylphenidate. Curr Ther Res 1979; 25:288–298.
128. Mitler MM, Hajdukovic R, Erman MK. Treatment of narcolepsy with methamphetamine. Sleep 1993; 16:306–317.
129. Hublin C, Partinen M, Heinonen EH, Puukka P, Salmi T. Selegiline in the treatment of narcolepsy. Neurology 1994; 44:2095–2101.
130. Furukawa T. Heinrich Bruno Schindler's description of narcolepsy in 1829. Neurology 1987; 37:146.
131. Dement W, Rechtschaffen A, Gulevich G. The nature of the narcoleptic sleep attack. Neurology 1966; 16:18–33.
132. Roth B, Bruhovà S. A clinical and polygraphic study of dreams in narcolepsy and hypersomnia. Activitas Nervosa Superior 1969; 11:223–228.
133. Roth B, Nevsímalovà S, Rechtschaffen A. Hypersomnia with "sleep drunkenness." Arch Gen Psychiatry 1972; 26:456–462.
134. Roth B. Narcolepsy and hypersomnia: review and classification of 642 personally observed cases. Archives Suisses de Neurologie, Neurochirugie et de Psychiatrie 1976; 119:31–41.
135. Roth B. Idiopathic hypersomnia: a study of 187 personally oberved cases. Int J Neurol 1981; 15:108–118.
136. Billiard M. Idiopathic hypersomnia. Neurol Clin 1996; 14:573–582.

137. Gudden H. Die physiologische und pathologische Schlaftrunkenheit. Arch Psychiat Nervenkr 1905; 40:989–1015.
138. Carrot JVeR. Syndrome d'Elpénor. Vol 55. Presse Médicale 1947:573.
139. Roth B, Nevsimalova S, Sagova V, Paroubkova D, Horakova A. Neurological, psychological, and polygraphic findings in sleep drunkenness. Schweizer Archiv für Neurologie und Psychiatrie 1981; 129:209–222.
140. Petitjean F, Jouvet M. Hypersomnie et augmentation de l'acide 5-hydroxy-indolacétique cérébral par lésion isthmique chez le chat. Can Roy Soc Biol 1970; 164: 2288–2293.
141. Faull KF, Guilleminault C, Berger PA, Barchas JD. Cerebrospinal fluid monoamine metabolites in narcolepsy and hypersomnia. Ann Neurol 1983; 13:258–263.
142. Honda Y, Juji T, Matsuki K, et al. HLA-DR2 and Dw2 in narcolepsy and other disorders of excessive somnolence without cataplexy. Sleep 1986; 9:133–142.
143. Harada S, Matsuki K, Honda Y, Someya T. Disorders of excessive daytime sleepiness without cataplexy, and their relationship with HLA in Japan. In: Honda Y, Juji T, eds. HLA in Narcolepsy. Berlin: Springer-Verlag, 1988:172–185.
144. Montplaisir J, Poirier G. HLA in disorders of excessive daytime sleepiness without cataplexy in Canada. In: Honda Y, Juji T, eds. HLA in Narcolepsy. Berlin: Springer-Verlag, 1988:186–190.
145. Billiard M, Dolenc C, Aldaz C, Ondze B, Besset A. Hypersomnia associated with mood disorders:a new perspective. J Psychosom Res 1994; 38(suppl 1):41–47.
146. van den Hoed J, Kraemer H, Guilleminault C, et al. Disorders of excessive daytime somnolence: polygraphic and clinical data for 100 patients. Sleep 1981; 4:23–37.
147. Hawkins DR, Taub JM, Van de Castle L. Extended sleep (hypersomnia) in young depressed patients. Am J Psychiatry 1985; 142:905–910.
148. Guilleminault C, Mondini C. Mononucleosis and chronic daytime sleepiness: a long-term follow-up study. Arch Intern Med 1986; 146:1333–1335.
149. Guilleminault C, Faull KF, Miles L, van den Hoed J. Posttraumatic excessive daytime sleepiness: a review of 20 patients. Neurology 1983; 33:1584–9.
150. Bastuji H, Jouvet M. Successful treatment of idiopathic hypersomnia and narcolepsy with modafinil. Prog Neuro-Psychopharmacol Biolog Psychiatry 1988; 12: 695–700.
151. Kleine W. Periodische Schlafsucht. Monatschrift der Psychiatrie und Neurologie 1925; 57:285–320.
152. Levin M. Narcolepsy (Gélineau syndrome) and other varieties of morbid somnolence. Arch Neurol Psychiatry 1929; 22:1172–1200.
153. Kaplinsky MS, Schulmann ED. Periodische Schlafsucht. Acta Medica Scandinavica 1935; 85:107–128.
154. Critchley M. Periodic hypersomnia and megaphagia in adolescent males. Brain 1962; 85:627–656.
155. Roth B. Functional hypersomnia. In: Guilleminault C, Dement WC, Passouant P, eds. Narcolepsy. Proceedings of the First International Symposium on Narcolepsy. Montpellier, France: Spectrum Publications, 1976:333–349.
156. Billiard M, Carlander B. Troubles de l'éveil: Première partie. Troubles primaires de l'éveil. Rev Neurol 1998; 154:11–129.

157. Gallinek A. The syndrome of episodes of hypersomnia, bulimia and abnormal mental state. JAMA 1954; 154:1081–1083.
158. Duffy JP, Davison K. A female case of the Kleine-Levin syndrome. Br J Psychiatry 1968; 114:77–84.
159. Bamford CR. Menstrual-associated sleep disorder: an unusual hypersomniac variant associated with both menstruation and amenorrhea with a possible link to prolactin and metoclopramide. Sleep 1993; 16:484–486.
160. Billiard M, Guilleminault C, Dement WC. A menstruation-linked periodic hypersomnia. Neurology 1975; 25:436–443.
161. Lhermitte J, Dubois E. Crises d'hypersomnie prolongées rhythmées par les règles chez une jeune fille. Rev Neurol 1941; 73:608–609.
162. Nevsimalova S, Roth B, Zouhar A, Zemanovà H. The occurence of narcolepsy-cataplexy and periodic hypersomnia in infancy and early childhood. In: Koella WP, Obal F, Schultz H, Visser P, eds. Sleep '86. Stuttgart: Gustav Fischer, 1988:399–401.
163. Fernandez JM, Lara J, Gila L, O'Neill of Tyrone A, Tovar J, Gimeno A. Disturbed hypothalamic-pituitary axis in idiopathic recurring hypersomnia syndrome. Acta Neurol Scan 1990; 82:361–363.
164. Hart EJ. Kleine-Levin syndrome: normal CSF monoamines and response to lithium therapy. Neurology 1985; 35:1395–1396.
165. Merriam AE. Kleine-Levin syndrome following acute viral encephalitis. Biolog Psychiatry 1986; 21:1301–1304.
166. Carpenter S, Yassa R, Ochs R. A pathological basis for Kleine-Levin syndrome. Arch Neurol 1982; 39:25–28.
167. Drake ME. Kleine-Levine syndrome after multiple cerebral infarctions. Psychosomatics 1987; 28:329–33o.
168. Will RG, Young JP, Thomas JD. Kleine-Levin syndrome. Br J Med 1988; 152: 410–412.
169. Mayer G, Nakajima T, Leonhard E, Pawelzik M, Meier-Ewert K. Kleine-Levin syndrome: polygraphic, actimetric and neuroendocrinological findings in three male patients. J Sleep Res 1996; 5(suppl 1):138.
170. Reynolds CF, Black RS, Coble PA, et al. Similarities in EEG sleep findings for Kleine-Levin syndrome and unipolar depression. Am J Psychiatry 1980; 137:116–118.
171. Reynolds CF, Kupfer DJ, Christiansen CL, et al. Multiple sleep latency test findings in Kleine-Levin syndrome. J Nerv Ment Disorders 1980; 172:41–44.
172. Godenne GD. Report of a case of recurrent hysterical pseudostupors. J Ment Disorders 1966; 141:670–677.
173. Jeffries JJ, Lefebvre A. Depression and mania associated with Kleine-Levin-Critchley syndrome. Can Psychiatr Assoc J 1973; 18:439–444.
174. Billiard M, Cadhilac J. Les hypersomnies récurrentes. Rev Neurol 1988; 144:249–258.
175. Guillain G, Bertrand I, Perisson J. Etude anatomo-clinique d'une tumeure du troisième ventricle. Rev Neurol 1925; 41:467–473.
176. Gordon A. Encéphalite léthargique des centres végétatifs: syndrome de somnolence périodique avec polyphagie et polydipsie. Revue Neurologique 1939; 71:411–416.

17

Headache Disorders and Sleep

Antonio Culebras
Veterans Affairs Medical Center
State University of New York
and Community General Hospital
Syracuse, New York

INTRODUCTION

There is an intimate relationship between headache disorders and sleep that is complex and difficult to sort out. Both excessive and insufficient sleep may trigger headaches, and patients with headaches may suffer sleep disorders in a mutual relationship with common reinforcements. In a review of sleep and headache syndromes, Sahota and Drexter (1) categorized the relationship as follows: 1) headaches ocurring during or after sleep, 2) sleep-stage-related headaches, 3) excess, lack, or disruption of sleep causing headaches, 4) headaches relieved by sleep, 5) headaches associated with sleep disorders, 6) effect of headaches on sleep, and 7) dreams and headaches. Migraineurs are more prone to develop parasomnias, and statistically there is a correlation between migraine and narcolepsy. Cluster headaches may exhibit a specific correlation with stages of sleep such as REM-sleep-locked headache, which appears during REM sleep. Headaches caused by brain tumors have a tendency to appear during sleep, although, owing to the low prevalence of brain tumors, most headaches that occur during sleep have another origin. Headaches on awakening are idiosyncratic and have traditionally been linked with the sleep apnea syndrome, but not all patients with sleep apnea develop headache. Patients with chronic headache commonly complain of daytime fatigue and insomnia. Therapeutic modification of sleep deprivation or of a sleep disorder reduces the incidence and intensity of headache.

Historically, Freud was aware of the relationship between headaches and sleep, mentioning "headache-dreams" and giving a psychodynamic interpretation of their occurrence (2). Headaches on awakening or morning headaches were described as early as 1945 by Bing (cited in Ref. 1), and more recently Gans wrote about treating migraines with sleep-rationing (3). Dexter and Weitzman (4) reported the relationship between headaches and sleep-stage patterns, and Lance and colleagues (5) provided a neurophysiological account of the relationship between the nucleus locus coeruleus and mechanisms underlying migraine. The intriguing association between paroxysmal hemicrania and REM sleep (6) has attracted attention to the circadian sleep rhythms and their influence in triggering headaches.

The International Classification of Sleep Disorders (7) recognizes the following headache disorders in association with sleep: classic migraine, migraine with aura, common migraine, migraine without aura, cluster headaches, chronic patroxysmal hemicrania, nocturnal migraine, vascular headaches, early-morning headaches, and tension-type headache. The diagnostic criteria require: 1) a complaint of headaches during sleep, 2) more than 75% of headache episodes occurring during sleep, 3) a diagnosis of one or more types of headache, and 4) polysomnographic recordings that demonstrate an awakening associated with a complaint of headache or onset of headache in sleep, typically REM sleep. In addition: 5) the headaches may be associated with other medical disorders and 6) other sleep disorders may be present.

EPIDEMIOLOGY

Surveys of headache patients indicate a high prevalence of nocturnal or sleep-related headaches. Paiva et al. (8) reported that 17% of patients attending a headache clinic suffered headaches during the nocturnal period or early in the morning (before final awakening). In the headache subgroup, 55% of patients had a specific sleep disorder identifiable by polysomnography in a sleep center.

The prevalence of migraine in the general population is 10% for men and 16% for women (9). Cluster headache, occurring in 0.4% of men and 0.08% of women (10), is predominantly a nocturnal disorder, since 75% of cluster headaches appear between 9 P.M. and 10 A.M. (11), and half of them are associated with REM sleep (12). Headache on awakening occurs in one-third of patients with sleep apnea (13), and although headache is unrelated to severity of obstructive sleep apnea syndrome, patients with sleep apnea had more headaches than control subjects (14).

Children with migraine have a higher incidence of disturbed sleep and parasomnias (15), night terrors, and enuresis (16). As many as 30% of children with migraine report episodes of somnambulism (17). Prolonged deep sleep is a risk factor for development of sleep terrors and somnambulism, as well as for migraine attacks in susceptible patients (18), a phenomenon that suggests shared pathogenetic mechanisms.

HEADACHE SYNDROMES AND SLEEP

Certain types of headaches may be associated with specific stages of sleep and thereby lead to sleep disruption. Migraine attacks have been described in association with sleep stages 3, 4, and REM. Cluster headaches and chronic paroxysmal hemicrania have been linked with REM sleep. Sleep-related migraine attacks, similar to daytime episodes, are characterized by unilateral throbbing head pain associated with nausea and vomiting, scotomata, visual-field defects, photophobia, paresthesias, and sometimes hemiparesis or aphasia. Migraines are highly idiosyncratic and not all symptoms are present. Attacks may last from several hours to a few days.

Cluster headaches commonly occur during sleep and are characterized by severe unilateral, periorbital, malar, and temporal pain with lacrimation, nasal engorgement, rhinorrhea, sweating forehead, and flushing of the malar area. Attacks last less than 2 hours and may appear several times daily, sometimes at the same time of the day or night, commencing and terminating abruptly. Spontaneous remissions lasting several months characterize the syndrome. Situational insomnia of a transient nature in association with cluster headache resolves after the headache syndrome subsides (19).

Chronic paroxysmal hemicrania is characterized by attacks of severe pain associated with conjunctival hyperemia, rhinorrhea, and, rarely, Horner's syndrome. Events are shorter than in cluster headache but more frequent; they may occur predominantly at night, generally at the same hour, and do not remit spontaneously. *REM-sleep-locked headache* refers to a specific form of paroxysmal hemicrania that shows a close linkage to REM sleep.

Sleep-related migraine, cluster headache, and chronic paroxysmal hemicrania are benign conditions that do not alter the lifespan of the individual. Work incapacity may occur during severe attacks, and global incapacity may occur if attacks are severe and frequent. In women, attacks may cease after menopause.

Headaches occurring on awakening appear in conjunction with a variety of disorders. Although common in children with brain tumors, they occur in only 5% of adults with brain tumors. In the sleep apnea syndrome, patients complain of diffuse headache in the morning localized to the frontal region, with a frequency that is independent of the severity of the disease (14). The pain is mild to moderate and tends to disappear within 30 minutes after getting out of bed. The following mechanisms have been implicated in headaches on awakening in patients with sleep apnea syndrome: hypoxemia, hypercapnia, altered cerebral blood flow, excessive neck movements, and sleep disturbance caused by depression. In patients with sleep apnea syndrome, prolonged afternoon naps may be followed by headache. Morning headaches, although seemingly independent of the severity of sleep apnea syndrome, respond to the successful treatment of the nocturnal respiratory disturbance. Significant improvement of chronic headache is observed in 30% of treated patients (20). Headaches on awakening are not the exclusive province of the sleep apnea syndrome. Morning headaches are also observed in relation to bruxism, systemic hypertension, depression, muscle-contraction headache, alcohol intoxication, and sinus inflammation.

Hypnic headache is a benign headache disorder of the elderly characterized by regular awakenings from sleep at a constant time of night (21). The headache is diffuse, lasts 30 to 60 minutes, and is sometimes associated with a dream. The hypnic headache syndrome has been linked to an abnormality of the circadian clock based on the regularity of events, but scientific proof is lacking. The association with dream content suggests linkage to REM sleep.

The exploding-head syndrome is a peculiar condition characterized by flashing lights and sounds during the night that terrify patients (22). Polysomnographic studies have shown that the attacks take place during awakenings, without evidence of epileptogenic discharges (21).

Chronic insomnia and headaches form the core of the postconcussion syndrome that develops following head trauma in some individuals. Symptoms appear in conjunction with memory deficit, depression, anxiety, and irritability, along with judgment and personality disorder in susceptible patients. Polysomnographic studies immediately following severe head trauma have shown alpha-wave intrusion, increased amount of sleep spindles, decreased REM density, and enhanced muscle tone in REM sleep, while individual sleep stages become less distinct. Weeks to months following recovery of consciousness, stages 3, 4, and REM are decreased along with total sleep time (23). Sleep spindles are reduced and the polysomnogram is punctuated with numerous arousals and awakenings. The postconcussion syndrome appears within hours to days following head trauma and may persist for as long as 2 years thereafter.

Psychogenic headache occurs after awakening, as suggested by early polysomnographic studies performed by Dexter and Weitzman (4). This observation suggests that polysomnographic evaluation may be useful to differentiate genuine sleep-related headaches and psychogenic headache.

SLEEP DISORDERS AND HEADACHE

Snoring has been associated with headache (odds ratio 1.5, with a 95% confidence interval) independently of other potential confounders, in a study of 3323 middle-aged and elderly men in Denmark (24). Although obstructive sleep apnea could underlie such an association, lack of nocturnal measurements precluded the evaluation of that hypothesis.

Clenching and grinding of teeth during sleep, or bruxism, occurs predominantly in stage 2 of sleep, although it has also been noted in REM sleep. Hundreds of events occurring during the night may lead to abnormal wear of the teeth, temporomandibular joint disorder, and jaw pain (25). Some patients with bruxism have associated muscle-contraction headaches. Headaches associated with bruxism are presumed to be secondary to the muscle activity or the temporomandibular joint stress.

There appears to be an association between somnambulism and migraine headaches. In a controlled study of 100 patients with migraine, Dexter (16) found that 71% of the subjects had pavor nocturnus, 55% somnambulism, and 41% enuresis, indicating a higher incidence than in control subjects. Other authors (17,26) have corroborated these associations, in particular with somnambulism.

Insomnia and daytime fatigue are common complaints in patients with chronic headache. A recent study of the prevalence and intensity of fatigue in chronic headache sufferers (27) has shown that these patients feel more tired, especially the women, and do not sleep as well at night, especially the men.

Dreams loaded with anxiety and terror may culminate in migraine, as reported by Levitan (28), who offered a psychodynamic hypothesis to explain the association that fails to satisfy modern concepts of headache mechanism.

ETIOPATHOGENESIS

The cause of migraine, cluster headaches, and chronic paroxysmal hemicrania remains unknown, and the interaction between headaches and sleep is poorly understood. In rare instances, intracranial tumors cause severe headaches that awaken the patient at night. Meningitis causes insomnia because of head pain.

Migraine headaches may be triggered by sleep, but the most common association is for sleep to follow a migraine attack. Current theories of migraine suggest that neural stimuli originating in the hypothalamus or brainstem cause changes in cerebral and extracranial circulation. Stimulation of the noradrenergic locus coeruleus decreases regional cerebral blood flow (5), whereas stimulation of the serotonergic raphe nuclei increases cerebral blood flow (29). The "therapeutic" need for sleep (30) in some patients having an attack of migraine may be related to disorders of serotonin metabolism in migraine but proof is lacking. Calcitonin gene-related peptide elevation in the jugular venous blood of migraineurs during the attack (29) has led to the hypothesis of involvement of the trigeminovascular system that promotes vasodilation and release of calcitonin gene-related peptide and substance P (31).

Serotonin (5-HT) is released from platelets during migraine headaches, and 5-hydroxyindolacetic acid, the main metabolite of serotonin, is excreted in excess in the urine following a migraine attack (32). Sumatriptan—an agonist of the 5-

HT1 receptor found in cerebral arteries, where it has an inhibitory effect—aborts the migraine headache. Methysergide—an antagonist of the 5-HT2 receptor found mainly in temporal arteries, where it has an excitatory effect—also terminates migraines. Serotonin, implicated in mechanisms of non-REM sleep, is a possible neurotransmitter link between migraine and sleep.

Cluster headache shows a remarkable periodicity in its occurrence, suggesting a linkage to the circadian rhythm. The neurovascular hypothesis suggests excitation of autonomic fibers of the greater superficial petrosal nerve that would be responsible not only for lacrimation and conjunctival injection but also for edema of the wall of the internal carotid artery with pain and ipsilateral Horner's syndrome. The association between migraine attacks, cluster headache, chronic paroxysmal hemicrania, and REM sleep remains unexplained. Chronic paroxysmal hemicrania is considered a variant of cluster headache, however, with sufficient individual traits to be listed separately. In this condition, attacks of pain are more frequent but of shorter duration than in typical cluster headache, and the therapeutic response to indomethacin is quasi-specific.

DIFFERENTIAL DIAGNOSIS

Migraine and cluster headaches occurring at night need to be differentiated from other acute severe headaches, such as those associated with intracranial brain tumors, ruptured aneurysm, and meningitis. Patients with intracranial tumors may be awakened at night by headache that improves upon getting out of bed. Headaches on awakening, as observed in sleep apnea patients, are also seen in patients with severe hypertension, depression, intracranial tumor, muscle-contraction headache, alcohol intoxication, and craniofacial sinus disease. Causes for concern are first or worst-ever headache, associated neurological symptoms or signs, progressive worsening of headache over days or weeks, intractable nausea or vomiting, fever, lethargy, confusion, and stiff neck. Hypnic headaches differ from cluster headaches and chronic paroxysmal hemicrania in their lack of unilateral pain with autonomic symptoms and their older age of onset.

Neurological consultation, neuroimaging studies, and lumbar puncture are indicated in patients who exhibit causes for concern. The sleep apnea syndrome is investigated with nocturnal polysomnography using the sleep apnea protocol followed by a multiple sleep latency test. Minimal criteria for the diagnosis of sleep apnea syndrome are the presence of five or more episodes of respiratory interruption of more than 10 seconds duration per hour of sleep, associated with excessive sleepiness, loud snoring, morning headaches, and dry mouth on awakening. Parasomnias are studied with nocturnal polysomnography that includes a seizure protocol and videotaping. Somnambulism and sleep terrors are associated with stages 3 and 4 of sleep. Patients with migraine, cluster headache, and hypnic headache may wake up with an acute attack more frequently during REM sleep than during other stages of sleep, and those with cluster headache may suffer the attack at the same time every night.

The use of polysomnography has been recommended by Paiva and coworkers (33) in patients complaining of morning and nocturnal headaches. In a study of 25 patients with headache, disturbed sleep was found in 21. The clinical diagnosis was reassessed after polysomnography in 13 patients on account of the finding of obstructive sleep apnea, periodic limb movements, alpha-delta sleep, and insomnia.

MANAGEMENT

Proper sleep hygiene is paramount in the prevention of sleep-related headaches. Patients with migraine, cluster headaches, and chronic paroxysmal hemicrania should be instructed to follow good sleep hygiene and to avoid potential precipitating factors such as sleep deprivation, excessive sleep, stress, trauma, and ingestion of certain idiosyncratic foods, including alcohol.

Migraine attacks that occur more than twice a month or are prolonged and refractory to acute therapy warrant daily administration of preventive therapy. All effective headache medications interact with the serotonergic system and thus will likely have some corollary effect on sleep. Preventive treatment of migraine includes β-blockers; calcium-channel blockers; serotonin receptor antagonists (methysergide, for a period not to exceed 4 weeks), and 5-HT2 antagonists cyproheptadine and methylergonovine; antidepressants that interact with serotonergic receptors such as tricyclics, MAO inhibitors, and serotonin-reuptake inhibitors (fluoxetine and sertraline); anticonvulsants, particularly in children with abnormal EEG; and nonsteroidal anti-inflammatory agents (34). Sumatriptan, a 5-HT1-selective agonist, administered via subcutaneous injection (6 mg, may repeat after 1 hour, limit two injections in 24 hours) is a new and effective medication for migraine attacks. Other abortive medications include ergotamine derivatives, acetaminophen, corticosteroids, and nonsteroidal anti-inflammatory derivatives. Symptomatic treatment for migraine attacks includes non-steroidal anti-inflammatory derivatives, mixed barbiturate and analgesics, antiemetics (promethazine 50 mg), and, in special circumstances of severity, meperidine (50 mg) or codeine sulfate (30 mg).

Cluster headaches are prevented by avoiding triggering factors, foremost of which is alcohol consumption. Sleeping late in the morning has been cited as a precipitating factor that should be avoided by patients with cluster headache. Cluster headaches are arrested with ergotamine derivatives at bedtime (1 to 3 mg sublingual), amitriptyline (150 mg daily), methysergide (6 to 8 mg daily), prednisone (40 mg daily), and lithium carbonate (initial dose 250 mg). An acute attack may be terminated with inhalation of oxygen. Chronic paroxysmal hemicrania responds specifically to indomethacin (50 mg at bedtime or 25 mg three times a day). Hypnic headaches respond to the administration of lithium (300 to 600 mg) at bedtime (21). Dodick et al. (37) reported that successful prophylaxis was achieved by drinking coffee at bedtime; with ergotamine tartrate 0.6 mg, phenobarbital 40 mg, and belladona 0.2 mg at bedtime; with atenolol 25 mg at bedtime; and with aspirin 325 mg and caffeine 40 mg at bedtime. Reassurance and administration of clomipramine are curative in most instances of exploding-head syndrome. Bruxism is treated with stress management, a mouthguard, or an intraoral occlusal splint (35). For short-term management, diazepam (5 mg) given at bedtime will reduce the tooth-grinding activity.

The symptoms of postconcussional syndrome may respond to the administration of tricyclic antidepressants. Good to excellent relief of symptoms has also been obtained with the administration of intravenous dihydroergotamine and metoclopramide (36).

Successful treatment of sleep apnea syndrome with nasal CPAP, Bi-PAP, or tracheostomy will eliminate associated headaches on awakening.

Remissions of migraine attacks and cluster headaches are common during pregnancy. Preventive medications should be discontinued during pregnancy. Ergotamine and its derivatives are to be avoided during pregnancy.

REFERENCES

1. Sahota PK, Dexter JD. Sleep and headache syndromes: a clinical review. Headache 1990; 30:80–84.
2. Freud S. The Interpretation of Dreams. Birmingham, AL: Classics of Medicine Library, Gryphon Editions, 1988:189.
3. Gans M. Part II. Treating migraine by "sleep-rationing." J Nerv Ment Dis 1951; 113:405–429.
4. Dexter JD, Weitzman ED. the relationship of nocturnal headaches to sleep stage patterns. Neurology 1970; 20:513–518.
5. Lance JW, Lambert GA, Goadsby PJ, Duckworth JW. Brainstem influences on the cephalic circulation: experimental data from cat and monkey of relevance to the mechanisms of migraine. Headache 1983; 23:258–265.
6. Kayed K, Goadtlibsen OB, Sjaastad O. Chronic paroxysmal hemicrania. IV. "REM sleep locked" nocturnal headache attacks. Sleep 1978; 1:91–95.
7. Diagnostic Classification Steering Committee, Thorpy MJ, Chairman. International Classification of Sleep Disorders: Diagnostic and Coding Manual. Rochester, MN: American Sleep Disorders Association, 1990.
8. Paiva T, Farinha A, Martins A, Batista A, Guilleminault C. Chronic headache and sleep disorders. Arch Intern Med 1977; 157:1701–1705.
9. Green J. A survey of migraine in England 1975–76. Headache 1977; 17:67–68.
10. Kudrow LL. Cluster Headache: Mechanisms and Management. New York: Oxford University Press, 1980.

11. Russell D. Cluster headache: severity and temporal profile of attacks and patient activity prior to and during attacks. Cephalalgia 1981; 1:209–219.
12. Pfaffenrath V, Pollmmman W, Ruther E, Lund R, Hajak G. Onset of nocturnal attacks of chronic cluster headache in relation to sleep stages. Acta Neurol Scand 1986; 73; 403–407.
13. Guilleminault C, Hold J, Mitler MM. Clinical overview of the sleep apnea syndromes. In: Guilleminault C, Dement WC, eds. Sleep Apnea Syndromes. New York: Alan R Liss, 1978:1–12.
14. Aldrich MS, Chauncey JB. Are morning headaches part of obstructive sleep apnea syndrome? Arch Intern Med 1990; 150:1265–1267.
15. Bruni D, Fabrizzi P, Ottaviano S, Cortesi F, Giannotti F, Guidetti V. Prevalence of sleep disorders in childhood and adolescence with headache: a case-control study. Cephalalgia 1997; 17:492–498.
16. Dexter JD. The relationship between disorders of arousal from sleep and migraine. Headache 1986; 26:322.
17. Barabas G, Ferrari M, Matthews WS. Childhood migraine and somnambulism. Neurology 1983; 33:948–949.
18. Dalessio DJ. Diagnosing the severe headache. Neurology 1994; 44(suppl 3): S6-12.
19. Sahota PK, Dexter JD. Transient recurrent situational insomnia associated with cluster headache. Sleep 1993; 16:255–257.
20. Poceta JS, Dalessio DJ. Identification and treatment of sleep apnea in patients with chronic headache. Headache 1995; 35:586–589.
21. Raskin NH. The hypnic headache syndrome. Headache 1988; 28:534–536.
22. Pearce JMS. Exploding head syndrome. Lancet 1988; ii:270–271.
23. Ron S, Algom D, Hary D, Cohen M. Time-related changes in the distribution of sleep stages in brain-injured patients. Electroencephalogr Clin Neurophysiol 1980; 48:432–441.
24. Jennum P, Hein HO, Suadicani P, Gyntelberg F. Headache and cognitive dysfunctions in snorers. Arch Neurol 1994; 51:937–942.
25. Rugh JD, Harlan J. Nocturnal bruxism and temporo-mandibular disorders. In: Jankovic J, Tolosa E, eds. Advances in Neurology. Vol 49. Facial Dyskinesias. New York: Raven Press, 1988.
26. Giroud M, D'Aghis PH, Guard O, Dumas R. Migraine et somnambulisme: une enquete portant sur 122 migraineux. Rev Neurol (Paris) 1986; 1:42–46.
27. Spierings EL, van Hoof MJ. Fatigue and sleep in chronic headache sufferers: an age- and sex-controlled questionnaire study. Headache 1997; 37:549–552.
28. Levitan H. Dreams which culminate in migraine headaches. Psychother Psychosom 1984; 41:161.
29. Goadsby PJ, Lance JW. Brainstem effects on intra- and extra-cerebral circulations: relation to migraine and cluster headache. In: Olesen J, Edvinsson L, eds. Basic Mechanisms of Headache. Amsterdam: Elsevier, 1988:413–427.
30. Dexter JD. Headaches and sleep. Headache 1988; 28:671–672.
31. Moskowitz MA, Buzzi MG, Linnik M, Sakas D. Pain mechanisms underlying vascular headaches: progress report. Rev Neurol 1989; 145:181–193.

32. Sicuteri F, Testi A, Anselmi B. Biomedical investigations in headache: increase in hydroxyindoleacetic acid excretion during migraine attacks. Int Arch Allergy 1961; 19:55–58.
33. Paiva T, Batista A, Martinns P, Martins A. The relationship between headaches and sleep disturbances. Headache 1995; 35:590–596.
34. Baumel B. Migraine: a pharmacologic review with newer options and delivery modalities. Neurology 1994; 44(suppl 3):S13–S17.
35. Holmgren K, Sheikholeslam A, Riise C. Effect of full arch maxillary occlusal splint on parafunctional activity during sleep in patients with nocturnal bruxism and signs and symptoms of craniomandibular disorders. J Prosthet Dent 1993; 69:293–297.
36. McBeath JG, Nanda A. Use of dihydroergotamine in patients with postconcussion syndrome. Headache 1994; 34:148–151.
37. Dodick DW, Mosek AC, Campbell JK. The hypnic (''alarm clock'') headache syndrome. Cephalalgia 1998; 18:152–156.

18

Sleep in Traumatic Brain Injury and Other Acquired CNS Conditions

Mark W. Mahowald
Hennepin County Medical Center and
University of Minnesota Medical School
Minneapolis, Minnesota

INTRODUCTION

Sleep is an active and integral component of the central nervous system (CNS), and may be one of its most important functions. Sleep is generated exclusively by the brain, and the brain is the sole benefactor of sleep: there is little evidence that any other organ system requires or benefits from sleep. All elements of wake–sleep function (the biological clock and the generators of all three states of being: wakefulness, non-REM, and REM sleep) reside in the brain. That given, it would be expected that any condition that affects the CNS could result in abnormalities of wake–sleep functioning. The ostensible purpose of this chapter is to review the effects of acquired brain dysfunction on wakefulness and sleep. The true purposes of this chapter are to underscore the fact that there is a massive void of knowledge in this most important area and to encourage further study, the results of which will add immeasurably to our knowledge of brain function and of the wake–sleep process.

ACQUIRED CNS CONDITIONS AND THEIR EFFECTS ON SLEEP AND WAKEFULNESS

Traumatic Brain Injury

Of the acquired CNS lesions, traumatic brain injury (TBI) is the most (but still very inadequately) studied. TBI may result in substantial abnormalities of sleep–wake function. The importance of this is revealed by the numbers: head trauma results in the hospitalization of 500,000 individuals in the United States annually and permanent disability in 90,000, with severe, complicated, and often devastating social, medical, and personal consequences (1,2). The prevalence of mild TBI is much greater, affecting approximately 1.5 million individuals (3). Despite the incredible prevalence of TBI, its effects on sleep–wake functioning are mentioned only briefly, if at all, in recent textbooks on sleep medicine, neurology, and rehabilitation medicine.

Normal sleep mechanisms are extensively reviewed elsewhere in this volume, as is the clinical and laboratory evaluation of wake–sleep complaints. It must be remembered that sleep disorders are extremely prevalent in the general population. A pre-TBI sleep disorder could have been causative in the TBI, and certainly would be expected to persist following the TBI. Given the role of the CNS wake–sleep functioning, clearly the prevalence of sleep–wake disorders is much higher in the TBI population.

Actigraphy as a means of studying wake–sleep functioning in the TBI population deserves special emphasis. Prolonged sleep–wake diaries completed by the patient or observer may give an at-a-glance overview of wake–sleep patterns not obviously apparent by clinical history. If the sleep–wake disturbance is bothersome and cannot be diagnosed by history alone, procedures to obtain objective information regarding the quality, quantity, and/or timing of sleep should be performed. Actigraphy is an underutilized tool for the evaluation of sleep–wake complaints, and may be of particular value in the evaluation of the TBI population. In many cases, analysis of sleep diaries may be insufficient to verify a tentative diagnosis in patients with suspected wake–sleep-cycle abnormalities. In such cases, definitive objective data may be obtained by actigraphy, a recently developed technique to record activity during wake and sleep that supplements the subjective sleep log. An actigraph is a small wrist-mounted device that records the activity plotted against time, usually for a week or two. The principles of the different models of actigraphs are reviewed elsewhere (4,5). When data collection has been completed, the results are transferred into a personal computer, where software displays activity versus time. The actigraphic reports shown in Figures 1 and 2 demonstrate how the rest–activity pattern is apparent at a glance. There is direct correlation between the rest–activity recorded by the actigraph and the wake–sleep pattern as determined by polysomnography (PSG) (6,7). Actigraphy

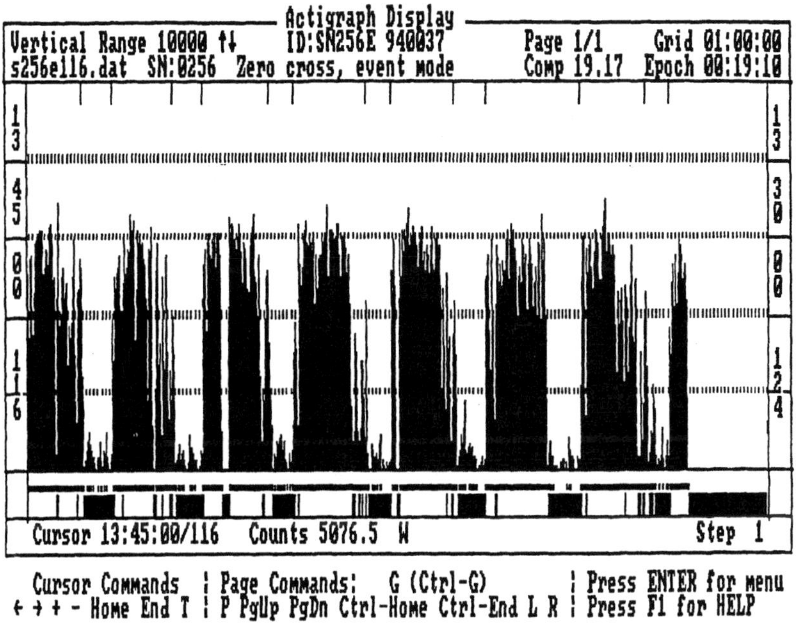

Figure 1 Typical actigraphic report. The vertical bars represent activity levels plotted over seven consecutive 24-hour periods, permitting rapid assessment of objective rest/activity patterns, which correlate highly with sleep–wake patterns. The overall wake–sleep pattern appears normal.

is particularly valuable in two settings: 1) confirming or refuting a bizarre sleep–wake complaint (such as ''I sleep only 2 hours per night'' or ''I am sleeping 18 hours a day'') and 2) in the setting of circadian rhythm abnormalities. Correct diagnosis and proper treatment of such conditions may be impossible without actigraphic information (8).

Effect of TBI on Wake–Sleep Function

Neuropathology of TBI The mechanisms of brain injury are very complex. Direct blows to the head are not necessary: severe TBI may occur simply from cranial acceleration/deceleration injuries. Shearing injuries in direct and indirect TBI produce pathological changes that are often very diffuse, affecting multiple portions of the CNS, including the brainstem (9). Since sleep–wake generation is dependent on the proper, simultaneous functioning of multiple levels of the nervous system, particularly the brainstem, basal forebrain, and hypothalamus,

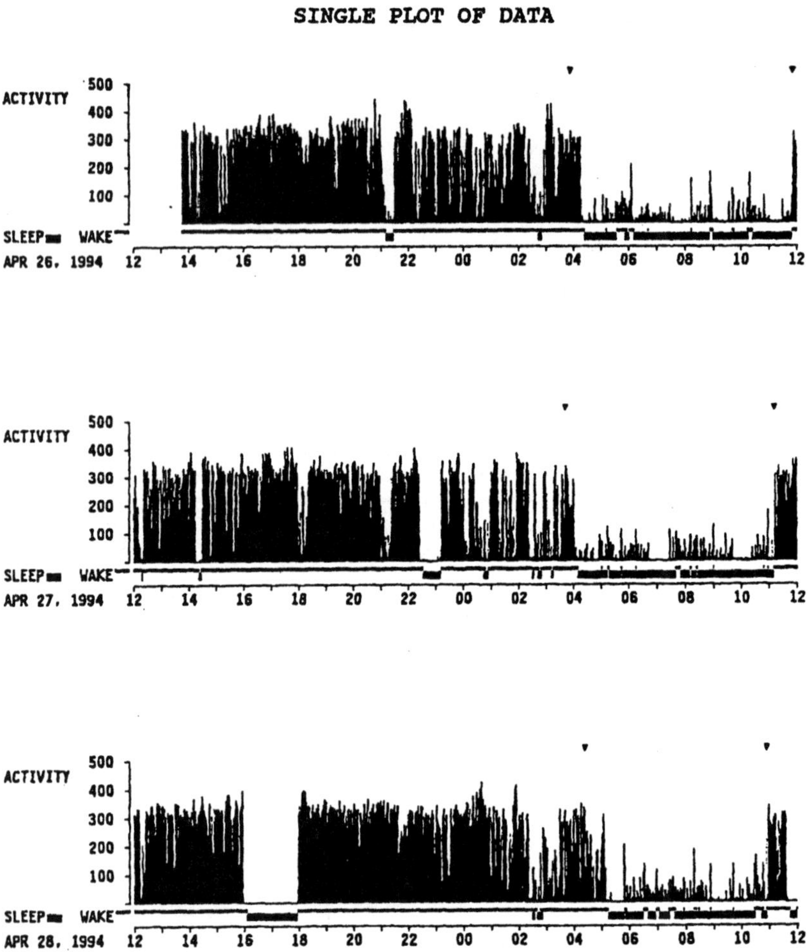

Figure 2 An expanded display of the 24-hour periods of the actigraphic study shown in Figure 1. It is now readily apparent that although the overall wake–sleep pattern is normal, the timing of the sleep period is very abnormal, with sleep onset not possible until approximately 4 A.M. This study confirms a severe delayed-sleep-phase syndrome and would be of intense value in the management of a patient in rehabilitation following TBI. Actigraphy is the only practical and reliable means of obtaining this clinically invaluable information.

severe TBI could be expected to involve at least some of the structures involved in sleep–wake declaration and function.

TBI-induced increased intracranial pressure Intracranial pressure (ICP) normally has circadian or sleep-state determinants, being increased during sleep. The ICP increase noted to occur during REM sleep (10–14) was formerly attributed to sleep-related CO_2 retention. The change in ICP is now thought to be related to a diurnal increase in blood volume. The increased ICP during sleep may be further exaggerated in patients whose ICP is already elevated (15–20). Cerebral blood flow, which may be compromised in the setting of increased ICP, may be monitored by the transcranial Doppler ultrasound technique (21,22). In TBI patients with nocturnal decompensation of ICP, severe bradycardia and systemic arterial hypertension were inaccurate surrogate predictors of the increased ICP (23).

Secondary CNS injury in TBI Acute TBI may be associated with apnea and systemic hypotension, which may individually result in additional secondary CNS damage, further increasing morbidity and mortality (24). It must be remembered that sleep-disordered breathing identified following TBI may have been present prior to the TBI, may have resulted from the neurological injury, or may be due to associated nonneurological (cervical spine, thoracic cage, cardiopulmonary) injuries. It is important to detect and treat obstructive sleep apnea (OSA) because it causes severe sleep fragmentation, sleep-related hypoxia, and/or hypercapnia, which may impede recovery from TBI. Another important reason to identify and treat OSA is that there may be marked episodic increases in ICP during the apneic episodes (25–28). This is particularly relevant for TBI patients who may already have increased ICP from their head injury.

Sleep Studies in Severe TBI

There have been numerous reports of the presence or absence of normal polygraphic sleep patterns as an indicator of the extent or severity of brain injury, and as a predictors of recovery from TBI. Given the fact that multiple levels of the CNS are necessary to generate and orchestrate the sleep–wake cycle, it should follow that the more abnormal the sleep–wake patterns are in a TBI patient, the more extensive the damage to the CNS. Conversely, the more normal the sleep–wake cycle, the more likely it is that the integrity of the CNS has been maintained, and perhaps the better the outcome. Many of the commonly cited studies are thoroughly reviewed in Ref. 29.

Analysis of the existing studies is difficult. The reporting of sleep is variable with subjective report, limited EEG monitoring, and variable formal polysomnographic recording. There is no objective confirmation of insomnia or excessive daytime sleepiness in studies reporting those complaints. It is difficult to compare these studies because the selection criteria, methods of monitoring, and outcome measures are quite variable, as was the severity of TBI and the interval between TBI and study. By definition, there are no behavioral manifestations of sleep–wake cycling in comatose patients; however, electrophysiological evidence of sleep–wake is seen as various stages of non-REM sleep reappear, followed by episodes of REM sleep. It may be tentatively concluded that the early appearance of wake–sleep cycling generally, but not uniformly, indicates a better prognosis. The same may be said for the correlation (again, incomplete) between the preservation or reappearance of REM sleep and cognitive recovery. Although it has been suggested that this supports the postulated role of REM sleep in memory, it could just as reasonably indicate that the better the return of brain function, the better the memory.

Several studies have employed neurophysiological measures other than sleep as prognosticators in TBI. One of the most comprehensive is that of Rae-Grant et al. (30), who found a high correlation between Glasgow outcome score and a number of EEG criteria, including sleep spindles and EEG reactivity and variability. EEG reactivity was also found to be prognostically significant in other studies (31–33).

All objective sleep-EEG studies in TBI performed to date have been performed on patients with severe TBI, and the outcome variables have been generally gross. Given the broad spectrum of EEG changes attendant with acute severe TBI and the variable rate of recovery, it is questionable whether further sleep-EEG study of this acute and severely affected population will be fruitful. Although there may be some general predictive value of acute sleep-EEG studies on outcome in severe TBI, the degree of overlap among the various groups provides little, if any, meaningful value in individual cases (34). These studies are very expensive, in terms of both time and money. Attention may be better directed at evaluation of wake–sleep functioning in the patient who has recovered sufficiently from TBI to participate in a rehabilitation program.

Despite the importance of nighttime sleep and daytime alertness on daytime function and performance, studies of psychosocial outcome of severe head injury have made no mention of sleep, either objective or subjective (35). In discharged TBI patients with sleep complaints, neurobehavioral impairments and occupational outcome were worse than in those without sleep complaints (36). Further objective study is obviously of the utmost importance.

Sleep–Wake Functioning Following Minor Head Injury

The situation is even bleaker in studies of wake–sleep function in minor head-injury patients. In one subjective questionnaire study, Levin et al. (37) listed "sleep disturbance" as a subscale of the "emotional disturbance" category. In a questionnaire survey of 75 patients following minor head injury, sleep interruption and impaired sleep quality were reported. The percentage experiencing sleep–wake complaints was not stated, and no objective studies were performed

(38). In another study of minor head injury, about 20% of patients reported subjective "dysfunction of sleep and rest" (39). Indicating that minor head injuries may result in long-term wake–sleep sequelae, one (subjective) study of 39 patients with the "postconcussion" syndrome indicated a much higher frequency of long-term wake–sleep complaints (both insomnia and daytime hypersomnia) than in a matched group of noncerebral trauma patients (40). It is likely that insomnia is a much more common complaint following mild head injury than the complaint of hypersomnia (41). One preliminary report of objective PSG study in a group of 15 patients with mild TBI found impressive circadian rhythm and sleep-architecture abnormalities in all patients (42). Clearly, larger and more rigorous objective studies are needed.

Regrettably, objective study of wake–sleep functioning and cycling in patients who have regained consciousness and who are candidates for rehabilitation has never been undertaken. It is clear that insomnia, excessive daytime sleepiness, and shifts in the timing of the wake–sleep cycle are common following TBI and should be expected to pose severe impediments to rehabilitation programs. There is some clinical suggestion (without objective verification) that the complaint of disturbed sleep and impaired attention during wakefulness may change as the patient progresses (43). These complaints may be confounded or exacerbated by the routines employed in most rehabilitation and chronic care facilities. For instance, the practice of putting patients to bed at the same time, usually very early, is more for the convenience of the staff than in the best interest of the patients (or with respect for their biological clocks). Imposing such constraints on a patient's sleep–wake cycle may result in sleep-onset "insomnia" or early-morning awakenings, leading to unnecessary administration of medication. Such practices could be expected to exacerbate circadian abnormalities.

Chronopharmacology

The circadian timing of administration of a wide variety of (and perhaps all) medications and other therapies such as x-ray irradiation may have profound effects on their efficacy and toxicity (44–47). There is compelling evidence of the importance of considering circadian cycle in drug administration in other conditions such as cancer chemotherapy, use of anesthetics and antiepileptic drugs, and steroid administration (48). There have been no studies to date on the circadian considerations of drugs utilized in the setting of TBI. It is likely that chronopharmacological considerations will prove to be of importance in TBI.

Sleep Disorders Associated with TBI

Hypersomnia Obstructive sleep apnea (OSA) is prevalent in the general population; therefore, 4% of female and 9% of male patients on the rehabilitation service could be expected to have pre-existing OSA (49). TBI may cause OSA by altering respiratory control systems (50). Furthermore, many patients with

TBI have also sustained noncerebral injuries that would predispose to OSA. OSA may result from injury, burns, or surgery to the upper airway (51,52). OSA may also result from simple nasal obstruction (53) or nasal packing used for treatment of upper-airway problems commonly seen in conjunction with TBI (54). Sleep-disordered breathing is particularly prevalent in patients with cervical spinal-cord lesions, which may be associated with some degree of loss of central respiratory muscle control. The prevalence of sleep disordered breathing in this population is clearly underappreciated. In one series, 10 of 22 unselected adult patients with stable spinal-cord injury were found to have sleep apnea (55). Another study showed significant sleep-disordered breathing in a group of quadriplegic patients in whom there was a low clinical suspicion for sleep-disordered breathing (56). Persistence of sleep-disordered breathing in patients with traumatic tetraplegia has been documented in a longitudinal study (57). This has obvious therapeutic implications. In addition, many medications frequently administered on rehabilitation services (sedative/hypnotics, myorelaxants, and analgesics) may exacerbate sleep-disordered breathing (58). To make matters worse, many patients who are relatively immobile tend to gain weight, a known risk factor for the development of OSA.

Sleep-disordered breathing is readily diagnosed and easily treated. Regrettably, the diagnosis is often simply not suspected.

Narcolepsy and idiopathic CNS hypersomnia are two conditions characterized by excessive daytime sleepiness in the absence of sleep deprivation or other identifiable abnormality during sleep such as obstructive sleep apnea (59,60). Documented narcolepsy or idiopathic CNS hypersomnia following head injury is very uncommon (61). The lack of documentation relates to the fact that many older reports were based on clinical criteria and have not utilized objective studies, such as formal sleep studies, or HLA typing. Clearly, narcolepsy may, albeit rarely, develop as a consequence of acquired CNS lesions (62). The relationship between narcolepsy and TBI requires systematic study. In some reported cases, narcolepsy was probably a pre-existing condition (63). Others suggest that narcolepsy may be induced by TBI, or that TBI may be a triggering factor in unmasking a genetic predisposition for narcolepsy (64,65). A single case of TBI resulting in cataplexy (without objective studies) has been reported (66). Careful study of 20 patients with objectively evaluated posttraumatic hypersomnia revealed multiple causes, including sleep-disordered breathing, nonspecific objective hypersomnia, and two cases with subjective, but not objective, hypersomnia (67). The multiple etiologies identified mandate objective study of the complaint or observation of hypersomnia in TBI. Clearly, there are numerous possible causes of post-TBI hypersomnia that require accurate diagnosis by objective PSG and multiple sleep latency test (MSLT), as the treatments are diagnosis-specific. The hypersomnia of narcolepsy and idiopathic CNS hypersomnia usually respond satisfactorily to stimulant medication (68,69).

The *Kleine-Levin syndrome* is characterized by recurring hypersomnia lasting days to weeks, occurring at intervals of days to years, with intervening normal wake–sleep function and alertness. The classic form is idiopathic and seen in adolescent males, but it may affect both sexes and all age groups. The periodic hypersomnia may be associated with hyperphagia and hypersexuality, and likely represents recurrent hypothalamic dysfunction. Many cases are not associated with hyperphagia or hypersexuality (70). A posttraumatic form responsive to lithium has been reported (71).

Wake–sleep cycle abnormalities The wake–sleep cycle in mammals is determined by the suprachiasmatic nucleus (SCN), entrained by the environmental light–dark cycle. Given the fact that the SCN is a brain structure, it would be expected that TBI affecting the SCN may result in severe abnormalities of the wake–sleep cycle. Although circadian dysrhythmias have most important rehabilitation implications, they have been virtually ignored in TBI research. A single case of delayed-sleep-phase syndrome following a minor head injury (5-minute loss of consciousness) has been reported. There were no subjective (behavioral ratings or sleep logs) or objective confirmatory studies (72). In one study of severely head-injured patients, Billiard et al. (73) found that in seven of nine there was a reversal of the normal circadian rhythmicity. In another study, a large percentage of comatose TBI patients demonstrated a persistent 24-hour temperature cycle, which was advanced or delayed from the usual wake–sleep cycle by a number of hours. This study suggested that the biological clock is resilient but may become ''reset'' relative to the environment following TBI (74). Chronobiological abnormalities are undoubtedly far more common in TBI patients than generally appreciated (42). Identification of cycle abnormalities is most important, as these disorders could be expected to severely impede rehabilitation, and a number of effective treatment options are available.

Visual dysfunction may occur in patients with TBI, and when the injury is severe, blindness may ensue. The majority of blinded individuals have abnormal wake–sleep cycles (75,76). Therefore, some patients who have pregeniculate (lesions anterior to the SCN) blindness as a result of a TBI could be expected to develop abnormalities of the wake–sleep cycle.

There is a striking relationship between circadian rhythms and certain psychiatric disorders, particularly seasonal affective disorder, primary depression, and bipolar affective disorder (77–80). Localized brain damage has been implicated in the development of posttraumatic mania (81). Appreciation of this relationship may be relevant in the rehabilitation of TBI patients with major neuropsychological problems, either premorbid or posttraumatic. It is also likely that there is a high incidence of premorbid psychosocial disorders in patients with TBI resulting from high-risk behaviors such as recklessness and abuse of alcohol or illicit drugs.

Consideration and identification of circadian dysrhythmias in the TBI population are of more than academic interest. Untreated, these disorders may severely interfere with rehabilitation efforts. Importantly, these conditions are diagnosable and treatable.

Insomnia No studies specifically address the association between TBI and insomnia. Insomnia—a symptom of many different conditions and not a disorder in and of itself—is a common complaint following TBI (82). Insomnia-promoting factors such as pain, anxiety, medications, or adverse sleep environment are present in many TBI patients during the period of rehabilitation. It should also be remembered that persistent insomnia affects 30% of the adult population, and therefore will be a pre-existing condition in many TBI patients, hardly being expected to improve following TBI. Once the factors contributing to insomnia are identified in a given case, specific effective behavioral and/or pharmacological therapies may be undertaken.

Parasomnias Parasomnias are undesirable motor or behavioral events that occur exclusively or predominately during the sleeping state. These may result in potentially injurious and violent behaviors, or disruption to caregivers or wardmates (83,84). They may even present in the hospital/intensive care setting (85). Many conditions may present with such bothersome or injurious sleep-period-related behaviors: disorders of arousal, REM-sleep behavior disorder (RSBD), and nocturnal seizures among others. These conditions are undoubtedly present in the TBI population, but virtually no systematic studies are available to indicate whether they are more common following TBI than in the population at large. There are no studies addressing TBI and disorders of arousal. In some cases, the TBI may have resulted from a pre-existing disorder of arousal that led to the injurious behavior (e.g., frenzied sleepwalking or driving a motor vehicle during a ''sleep-driving'' episode). It is probable that RSBD and nocturnal seizures result from TBI, although neither anecdotal nor systematic studies are available.

Psychiatric conditions A number of ''psychiatric'' conditions may occur predominately during the sleep period, including nocturnal panic, posttraumatic stress disorder, and psychogenic dissociative states. The current concept that these conditions probably have a psychobiological basis and may be triggered by emotional or physical trauma indicate that they must occur in the TBI population (86). Virtually no studies are available in this most important area.

Psychogenic dissociative states No reports of posttraumatic psychogenic dissociative states could be found. It is likely that fugue states may result in TBI. There is a single report of a TBI patient who was not progressing as expected. She was found to have had long-standing, but previously undiagnosed, multiple-personality disorder that antedated the TBI. Her lack of improvement had been incorrectly attributed to cognitive defects acquired from the TBI (87). It must be remembered that failure to recover as expected from TBI may be the manifestation of a pre-existing condition.

Dreaming The cessation of dreaming has been reported following TBI. This alteration in oneiric (dreaming) activity may be related to impairment of visual memory (88). In one study of 10 patients reporting decreased or absent dreaming following head injury, there was no correlation between the dream-change complaint and the amount of time spent in REM sleep (89). This may reflect the fact that much dream mentation occurs during non-REM sleep (90). Another study questioned the common belief that dream recall is reduced following severe head injury. It found, rather, a change in the content (more threatening, fewer with sexually manifest content) but not in the overall incidence (91). More studies of larger numbers of subjects are needed.

Hallucinations In many cases, apparent ''hallucinations'' simply represent the release of dreaming (either REM or non-REM) into wakefulness, a manifestation of state dissociation. Clearly, waking hallucinations do not necessarily indicate major psychiatric disorders (90), and treatment of organic hallucinations with haloperidol is often effective (92).

Sleep Disorders as a Cause of TBI

Sleep disorders not only may result from TBI but may actually cause it. The true consequence of sleep disorders and sleepiness—with particular reference to accidents on the highway and in the workplace—is now known, and the figures are alarming. In the United States alone in 1990, it is estimated that 200,000 motor vehicle accidents were due to falling asleep at the wheel (93). Statistics on motor vehicle accidents clearly indicate that fall-asleep accidents are more prevalent in patients with untreated obstructive sleep apnea and narcolepsy (94–97). This undoubtedly holds true for other sleepy populations such as shift workers and volitionally sleep-deprived individuals. Frequent episodes of falling asleep on the job have been well documented in night-shift workers (98), including pilots while ''at the stick'' (99). The potential for TBI in this setting is obvious. Violent parasomnias, particularly sleepwalking, sleep terrors, and RSBD, have resulted in significant injury, and it is likely that TBI may result (100–102).

Just as in the multiple-personality-disorder case cited above, it must be remembered that any sleep disorder following TBI may have pre-existed, and may, in fact, have even caused the TBI. Given the known consequences of sleepiness due to sleep disorders and sleep deprivation, the American public, employers, and policymakers must consider these conditions a significant *cause* of TBI. Sleepiness and sleep disorders can no longer be discounted as ''minor annoyances.''

Sleep Disorders and TBI: Summary and Directions for the Future

Review of available literature indicates that, although much is known about the nature of sleep and wake–sleep cycling, there is a striking lack of specific information regarding sleep and sleep–wake disorders in patients (both as cause and consequence) with TBI. Given the huge numbers of TBI patients, and the prevalent and incapacitating nature of sleep–wake disorders, much work needs to be done. Most sleep disorders can be readily diagnosed, with effective therapeutic implications. Their identification and treatment in the TBI population will have important and exciting rehabilitation ramifications. There are critical scientific lessons to be learned from this population, and, more significantly, there are substantial therapeutic implications.

CNS Tumors

There have been no systematic studies of wake–sleep function associated with brain or spinal cord tumors. As with TBI, it should be obvious that CNS tumors and their treatment may result in wake–sleep abnormalities. The literature in this area is composed primarily of anecdotal case reports or very small series.

Postcerebral Irradiation Somnolence

A postcerebral radiation somnolence syndrome, which may be an early indicator of long-term neurological sequelae, has been well described, but few formal sleep studies are available (103–105). As a possible explanation for the commonly observed growth retardation in children following cranial irradiation, there is some evidence that there is a reduction in the amount of growth hormone released during sleep, but no effect on the sleep-related timing of the release (106,107).

Circadian Dysrhythmias

Tumors involving the pineal region or its environs should be expected to result in circadian dysrhythmias. For instance, craniopharyngiomas may result in severe sleep-maintenance insomnia and daytime hypersomnia (108). Melatonin replacement in patients with circadian rhythm irregularities due to abnormalities of melatonin secretion secondary to pineal tumors may restore the wake–sleep cycle (109).

Narcolepsy and RSBD

Neoplastic structural lesions of the CNS may very rarely result in narcolepsy or RSBD (62,110).

Sleep-Disordered Breathing

Obstructive sleep apnea may result from CNS tumors (111,112). Central hypoventilation has been reported associated with a paraspinal ganglioneuroblastoma.

The mechanism of the hypoventilation was unclear (113). Central sleep apnea may be associated with syringobulbo-myelia associated with a spinal extramedullary tumor (114). Obstructive sleep apnea may result from acromegaly (115). The high prevalence of sleep-disordered breathing associated with high cervical spinal-cord lesions is discussed above in the section on TBI.

Periodic Limb Movements of Sleep and Propriospinal Myoclonus

Spinal-cord mass lesions have been associated with periodic leg movements in sleep. The suspected mechanism is disinhibition of spinal-cord locomotor pattern generators (116). Propriospinal myoclonus is a spinal-cord-mediated movement disorder, which is in the differential diagnosis of restless-legs syndrome and which may shed light on the pathophysiology of restless-legs syndrome and periodic limb movement disorder (117–125). The concept of spinal-cord locomotor centers that persist intact following CNS lesions should be of intense interest, from both a scientific and a rehabilitation standpoint (126,127).

Cerebrovascular Disorders

There appears to be a very high prevalence of clinically significant sleep-disordered breathing, both central and obstructive sleep apnea, following cerebrovascular accidents (CVAs). It is suspected that sleep-disordered breathing may be a risk factor for the occurrence of CVAs (128). In one of the rare large studies of the occurrence of sleep-disordered breathing following CVAs, the prevalence of sleep-disordered breathing was very high. There was no correlation with age, body-mass index, pre-CVA history of snoring or hypersomnia, or stroke topography between subjects with and without sleep-disordered breathing (129). This would suggest that, in this particular study population, the sleep-disordered breathing was not a predisposing condition. The complex nature of the relationship between sleep-disordered breathing and the development of CVAs, and between sleep-disordered breathing caused by CVAs, warrants aggressive study because the identification of sleep-disordered breathing, either before or following the appearance of CVAs, has important therapeutic implications (130). The potential impediment to rehabilitation of unsuspected and untreated obstructive sleep apnea in a stroke patient is obvious.

CNS Infections

Virtually no studies have addressed the acute effects of CNS infections on wake–sleep function. Scattered studies indicate that some CNS infections may result in hypersomnia. Although encephalitis lethargica is often thought of as a thing of the past, having occurred in the 1914 to 1930 pandemic, it should be remembered that sporadic cases still occur (131). One fascinating fact is that in the case of "African sleeping sickness" there is good evidence that, except in the terminal stages, the primary abnormality is in the wake–sleep cycle. Affected individuals do not sleep more per 24-hour period but, rather, experience a disintegration of the circadian pacemaker function. The brunt of the pathology appears to involve the suprachiasmatic nucleus (132,133).

The widespread neurological dysfunction following encephalitis of any type would indicate that wake–sleep disorders should be common in this patient population, again with important therapeutic and rehabilitation implications. Virtually no studies are available.

SUMMARY AND IMPERATIVES FOR FUTURE OPPORTUNITIES

Over the past few decades, much has been learned about wake–sleep function. As amply documented in this chapter, there remains a woeful and massive void of knowledge regarding the effects of most neurological conditions on wakefulness and sleep. Inasmuch as one of the most important functions of the brain is the generation of sleep, wakefulness, and consciousness, systematic study of these functions in a wide variety of neurological conditions should yield invaluable information about both functioning of the CNS and the nature of wakefulness, sleep, and even consciousness (134). Recent advances in technology (polysomnography, actigraphy, functional neuroimaging techniques, and sophisticated neurophysiological monitoring at the cellular level) have provided us with exciting and powerful tools. In the realm of CNS function (and dysfunction) and wakefulness, sleep, and consciousness, there exist nearly limitless opportunities for the close collaboration of basic sleep and neurophysiology researchers with their clinical counterparts to advance our knowledge of both normal and abnormal brain function.

REFERENCES

1. Goldstein M. Traumatic brain injury. Ann Neurol 1990; 27:327.
2. Gennarelli TA, Champion HR, Sacco WJ, Copes WS, Alves WA. Mortality of patients with head injury and extracranial injury treated in trauma center. J Trauma 1989; 29:1193–1201.
3. Sosin DM, Sniezek JE, Thurman DJ. Incidence of mild and moderate brain injury in the United States. Brain Injury 1996; 10:47–54.
4. Tryon WK. Activity Measurement in Psychology and Medicine. New York: Plenum Press, 1991.
5. Mahowald MW, Ettinger MG. Circadian rhythm disorders. In: Chokroverty S, ed. Sleep Disorders Medicine: Basic Science, Technical Considerations, and Clinical Aspects. Boston: Butterworth-Heinemann, 1998.
6. Brown A, Smolensky M, D'Alonzo G, Redmond D, Conrad E, Hsi B. Circadian rhythm in human activity objectively quantified by actigraphy. In: Hays DK, ed.

Chronobiology: its Role in Clinical Medicine, General Biology, and Agriculture. Part A. New York: John Wiley and Sons, 1990:77–83.

7. Brown AC, Smolensky M, D'Alonzo GE, Redman DP. Actigraphy: a means of assessing circadian patterns in human activity. Chronobiol Int 1990; 7:125–133.
8. Mahowald MW. Sleep disorders. In: Evans R, ed. Diagnostic Testing in Neurology. 1998.
9. Adams JH. Head injury. In: Adams JH, Duchen LW, eds. Greenfield's Neuropathology. New York: Oxford University Press, 1992:106–152.
10. Pierre-Kahn A, Gabersek V, Hirsch J-F. Intracranial pressure and rapid eye movement sleep in hydrocephalus. Child's Brain 1976; 2:156–166.
11. Renier D, Sainte-Rose C, Marchac D, Hirsch J-F. Intracranial pressure in craniostenosis. J Neurosurg 1982; 57:370–377.
12. Hirsch JC, Pierre-Kahn A, Hirsch J-F. Experimental study of intracranial pressure during rapid eye movement sleep in the chronic cat. Neurosci Lett 1978; 7:245–249.
13. Di Rocco C, McLone DG, Shimoji T, Raimondi AJ. Continuous intraventricular cerebrospinal pressure recording in hydrocephalic children during wakefulness and sleep. J Neurosurg 1975; 42:683–689.
14. Gucer G, Vierstein LJ. Intracranial pressure in the normal monkey while awake and asleep. J Neurosurg 1979; 51:206–210.
15. Ueno H, Shima K, Chigasaki H, Ishii S. Oscillation of intracranial pressure and sleep. Clin Neurol Neurosurg 1986; 88:163–168.
16. Yokota A, Matsuoka S, Ishikawa T, Koshi K, Kajiwara H. Overnight recordings of intracranial pressure and electroencephalography in neurosurgical patients. Part I. Intracranial pressure waves and their clinical correlations. J UOEH 1989; 11: 371–381.
17. Yokota A, Matsuoka S, Ishikawa T, Koshi K, Kajiwara H. Overnight recordings of intracranial pressure and electroencephalography in neurosurgical patients. Part II. Changes in intracranial pressure during sleep. J UOEH 1989; 11:383–391.
18. Cooper R, Hulme A. Changes of the EEG, intracranial pressure and other variables during sleep in patients with intracranial lesions. EEG Clin Neurophysiol 1969; 27:12–22.
19. Munari C, Calbucci F. Correlations between intracranial pressure and EEG during coma and sleep. EEG Clin Neurophysiol 1981; 51:170–176.
20. Furuse M, Ikeyama A, Mabe H, Hasuo M, Kuchiwaki H, Nakaya T, Toyama K, Teraoka M, Jagai H, Kageyama N. Relationship between rapid variations in intracranial pressure and changes in respiratory pattern during postoperative monitoring. Neurol Med Chir 1979; 19:9–16.
21. Goh D, Minns RA, Pye SD, Steers AJW. Cerebral blood flow velocity and intermittent intracranial pressure elevation during sleep in hydrocephalic children. Developmental Med Child Neurol 1992; 34:676–689.
22. Newell DW, Aaslid R, Stooss R, Reulen HJ. The relationship of blood flow velocity fluctuations to intracranial pressure B waves. J Neurosurg 1992; 76:415–421.
23. Marshall LF, Smith RW, Shapiro HM. The influence of diurnal rhythms in patients with intracranial hypertension: implications for management. Neurosurgery 1978; 2:100–102.

24. Chestnut RM, Marshall LF, Klauber MR, Blunt BA, Baldwin N, Eisenberg HM, Jane JA, Marmarou A, Foulkes MA. The role of secondary brain injury in determining outcome from severe head injury. J Trauma 1993; 34:216–222.
25. Sugita Y, Iijima S, Teshima Y, Shimizu T, Nishimura N, Tsutsumi T, Hayashi H, Kaneda H, Hishikawa Y. Marked episodic elevation of cerebrospinal fluid pressure during sleep in patients with sleep apnea hypersomnia syndrome. EEG Clin Neurophysiol 1985; 60:214–219.
26. Jennum P, Borgesen SE. Intracranial pressure and obstructive sleep apnea. Chest 1989; 95:279–283.
27. Doyle KJ, Tami TA. Increased intracranial pressure and blindness associated with obstructive sleep apnea. Otolaryngol Head Neck Surg 1991; 105:613–616.
28. Kuchiwaki H, Takada S, Ishiguri H, Kageyama N, Terashima M, Furuse M, Sugiura M. Pressure wave with apnea evaluated by sleep level in patient with ventricular dilation. Neurolog Res 1988; 10:105–111.
29. Mahowald MW, Mahowald ML. Sleep disorders. In: Rizzo M, Trandel D, eds. Head Injury and Postconcussive Syndrome. New York: Churchill-Livingstone, 1996:285–304.
30. Rae-Grant AD, Barbour PJ, Reed J. Development of a novel EEG rating scale for head injury using dichotomous variables. EEG Clin Neurophysiol 1991; 79:349–357.
31. Synek VM. Prognostically important EEG coma patterns in diffuse anoxic and traumatic encephalopathies in adults. J Clin Neurophysiol 1988; 5:161–174.
32. Gutling E, Gonser A, Imhof H-G, Landis T. EEG reactivity in the prognosis of severe head injury. Neurology 1995; 45:915–918.
33. Tsubokawa T, Yamamoto T, Katayama Y. Prediction of outcome of prolonged coma caused by brain damage. Brain Injury 1990; 4:329–337.
34. Evans BM, Bartlett JR. Prediction of outcome in severe head injury based on recognition of sleep related activity in the polygraphic electroencephalogram. J Neurol Neurosurg Psychiatry 1995; 59:17–25.
35. Bond MR. Outcome of severe damage to the central nervous system. In: Porter R, Fitzsimons DW, eds. Ciba Foundation Symposium 34 (new series). New York: Elsevier, 1975:141–157.
36. Cohen M, Oksenberg A, Snir D, Stern MJ, Groswasser Z. Temporally related changes of sleep complaints in traumatic brain injured patients. J Neurol Neurosurg Psychiatry 1992; 55:313–315.
37. Levin HS, Mattis S, Ruff RM, Eisenberg HM, Marshall LF, Tabaddor K, High WMJ, Frankowski RF. Neurobehavioral outcome following minor head injury: a three-center study. J Neurosurg 1987; 66:234–243.
38. Parsons LC, Ver Beek D. Sleep-awake patterns following cerebral concussion. Nursing Res 1982; 31:260–264.
39. Dikmen S, McLean A, Temkin N. Neuropsychological and psychosocial consequences of minor head injury. J Neurol Neurosurg Psychiatry 1986; 49:1227–1232.
40. Perlis ML, Artiola L, Giles DE. Sleep complaints in chronic postconcussion syndrome. Perceptual Motor Skills 1997; 84:595–599.
41. Segalowitz SJ, Lawson S. Subtle symptoms associated with self-reported mild head injury. J Learning Disabilities 1995; 28:309–319.

42. Schreiber S, Gur-Hartman T, Klag E, Gross Y, Pick CG. Polysomnographic and actigraphic findings of patients with minor traumatic brain injury [abstr]. J Neuropsychiatry 1997; 9:640.
43. Kowatch RA. Sleep and head injury. Psychiatr Med 1989; 7:37–41.
44. Halberg F. Chronobiology. Ann Rev Physiol 1969; 31:675–725.
45. Moore-Ede MC. Circadian rhythms of drug effectiveness and toxicity. Clin Pharmacol Ther 1973; 14:925–935.
46. Radzialowski RM, Bousquet WF. Daily rhythmic variation in hepatic drug metabolism in the rat and mouse. J Pharmacol Exp Ther 1968; 163:229–238.
47. Reinberg A. The hours of changing responsiveness or susceptibility. Perspect Biol Med 1967; 11:111–126.
48. Koren G, Ferrazzini G, Sohl H, Robieux I, Johnson D, Giesbrecht E. Chronopharmacology of methotrexate pharmacokinetics in childhood leukemia. Chronobiol Int 1992; 9:434–438.
49. Young T, Palta M, Dempsey J, Skatrud J, Weber S, Badr S. The occurrence of sleep-disordered breathing among middle-aged adults. N Engl J Med 1993; 328: 1230–1235.
50. Chokroverty S. Sleep, breathing, and neurological disorders. In: Chokroverty S, ed. Sleep Disorders Medicine. Boston: Butterworth-Heinemann, 1994:295–335.
51. Sher AE. The upper airway in obstructive sleep apnea syndrome: pathology and surgical management. In: Thorpy MJ, ed. Handbook of Sleep Disorders. New York: Marcel Dekker, 1990:311–335.
52. Robertson CF, Zuker R, Dabrowski B, Levison H. Obstructive sleep apnea: a complication of burns to the head and neck in children. J Burn Care Rehabil 1985; 6: 353–357.
53. Olsen KD, Kern EB, Westbrook PR. Sleep and breathing disturbance secondary to nasal obstruction. Otolaryngol Head Neck Surg 1981; 89:804–810.
54. Johannessen N, Jensen PF, Kristensen S, Juul A. Nasal packing and nocturnal oxygen desaturation. Acta Otolaryngol 1992; 492(suppl):6–8.
55. Short DJ, Stradling JR, Williams SJ. Prevalence of sleep apnoea in patients over 40 years of age with spinal cord lesions. J Neurol Neurosurg Psychiatry 1992; 55: 1032–1036.
56. Cahan C, Gothe B, Decker MJ, Arnold JL, Strohl KP. Arterial oxygen saturation over time and sleep studies in quadriplegic patients. Paraplegia 1993; 31:172–179.
57. Bach JR, Wang T-G. Pulmonary function and sleep disordered breathing in patients with traumatic tetraplegia: a longitudinal study. Arch Physical Med Rehabil 1994; 75:279–284.
58. Sanders MH. Medical therapy for sleep apnea. In: Kryger MH, Roth T, Dement WC, eds. Principles and Practice of Sleep Medicine. Philadelphia: WB Saunders, 1994:678–693.
59. Nishino S, Mignot E. Pharmacological aspects of human and canine narcolepsy. Progress Neurobiol 1997; 52:27–78.
60. Aldrich MS. The neurobiology of narcolepsy. Progress Neurobiol 1992; 41:538–541.
61. Billiard M, Carlander B, Ondze B, Besset A. Post-traumatic hypersomnia associated with cataplexy, hypnagogic hallucinations, sleep paralysis and disturbed noc-

turnal sleep but not with SOREM episodes and HLA DR2. Sleep Res 1993; 22: 171.
62. Aldrich MS, Naylor MW. Narcolepsy associated with lesions of the diencephalon. Neurology 1989; 39:1505–1508.
63. Good JL, Barry E, Fishman PS. Posttraumatic narcolepsy: the complete syndrome with tissue typing. J Neurosurg 1989; 71:765–767.
64. Maccario M, Ruggles KM, Meriwether MW. Post-traumatic narcolepsy. Military Med 1987; 152:370–371.
65. Lankford DA, Wellman JJ, O'Hara C. Posttraumatic narcolepsy in mild to moderate closed head injury. Sleep 1994; 17:S25–S28.
66. Sadowski S. Post-traumatic cataplexy. CMA J 1982; 126:1150–1151.
67. Guilleminault C, Faull KF, Miles L, van den Hoed J. Posttraumatic excessive daytime sleepiness: a review of 20 cases. Neurology 1983; 33:1584–1589.
68. American Sleep Disorders Association. Practice parameters for the use of stimulants in the treatment of narcolepsy. Sleep 1994; 17:348–351.
69. Guilleminault C. Idiopathic central nervous system hypersomnia. In: Kryger MH, Roth T, Dement WC, eds. Principles and Practice of Sleep Medicine. Philadelphia: WB Saunders, 1994:562–566.
70. Smolik P, Roth B. Kleine-Levin syndrome: etiopathogenesis and treatment. Acta Univ Carol Med Monographia 1988; CXXVIII:1–94.
71. Gill RG, Young JPR, Thomas DJ. Kleine-Levin syndrome: report of two cases with onset of symptoms precipitated by head trauma. Br J Psychiatry 1988; 152:410–412.
72. Patten SB, Lauderdale WM. Delayed sleep phase disorder after traumatic brain injury. J Am Acad Child Adolesc Psychiatry 1992; 31:100–102.
73. Billiard M, Negri C, Baldy-Moulinier M, Roquefeuil B, Passouant P. Organisation du sommeil chez les sujets atteints d'inconscience post-traumatique chronique. Rev EEG Neurophysiol 1979; 9:149–152.
74. Alster J, Pratt H, Feinsod M. Density spectral array, evoked potentials, and temperature rhythms in the evaluation and prognosis of the comatose patient. Brain Injury 1993; 7:191–208.
75. Sack RL, Lewy AJ, Blood ML, Keith LD, Nakagawa H. Circadian rhythm abnormalities in totally blind people; incidence and clinical significance. J Clin Endocrinol Metab 1992; 75:127–134.
76. Sack RL, Lewy AJ. Human circadian rhythms: lessons from the blind. Ann Med 1993; 25:303–305.
77. Rosenthal NE, Sack DA, Gillin JC, Lewy AF, Goodwin FK, Davenport Y, Mueller PS, Newsome DA, Wehr TA. Seasonal affective disorder: a description of the syndrome and preliminary findings with light therapy. Arch Gen Psychiatry 1984; 41: 72–89.
78. Rosenthal NE, Joseph-Vanderpool JR, Levendosky AA, Johnson SH, Allen R, Kelly KA, Souetre E, Schultz PM, Starz KE. Phase-shifting effects of bright morning light as treatment for delayed sleep phase syndrome. Sleep 1990; 13:354–361.
79. Wehr TA. Effects of wakefulness and sleep on depression and mania. In: Montplaisir J, Godbout R, eds. Sleep and Biological Rhythms: Basic Mechanisms and Applications to Psychiatry. New York: Oxford University Press, 1990:42–86.

80. Kupfer DJ, Monk TH, Barchas JD. Biological Rhythms and Mental Disorders. New York: Guilford Press, 1988:357.
81. Starkstein SE, Mayberg HS, Berthier ML, Fedoroff P, Price TR, Dannals RF, Wagner HN, Leiguardia R, Robinson RG. Mania after brain injury: neuroradiological and metabolic findings. Ann Neurol 1990; 27:652–659.
82. Beetar JT, Guilmette TJ, Sparadeo FR. Sleep and pain complaints in symptomatic traumatic brain injury and neurologic populations. Arch Physical Med Rehab 1996; 77:1298–1302.
83. Schenck CH, Mahowald MW. REM parasomnias. Neurol Clinics 1996; 14:697–720.
84. Mahowald MW, Schenck CH. NREM parasomnias. Neurol Clinics 1996; 14:675–696.
85. Schenck CH, Mahowald MW. Injurious sleep behavior disorders (parasomnias) affecting patients on intensive care units. Intensive Care Med 1991; 17:219–224.
86. Mahowald MW, Schenck CH. Parasomnia purgatory: the epileptic/non-epileptic interface. In: Rowan AJ, Gates JR, eds. Non-Epileptic Seizures. Boston: Butterworth-Heinemann, 1993:123–139.
87. Sandel ME, Weiss B, Ivker B. Multiple personality disorder: diagnosis after a traumatic brain injury. Arch Physical Med Rehab 1990; 71:523–525.
88. Humphrey ME, Zangwill OL. Cessation of dreaming after brain injury. J Neurol Neurosurg Psychiatry 1951; 14:322–325.
89. Prigatano GP, L SM, Orr WC, Zeiner HK. Sleep and dreaming disturbances in closed head injury patients. J Neurol Neurosurg Psychiatry 1982; 45:78–80.
90. Mahowald MW, Woods SR, Schenck CH. Sleeping dreams, waking hallucinations, and the central nervous system. Dreaming 1998; 8:89–102.
91. Benyaker M, Tadir M, Groswasser Z, Stern MJ. Dreams in head-injured patients. Brain Injury 1988; 2:351–356.
92. Horvath TB, Siever LJ, Mohs RC, Davis K. Organic mental syndromes and disorders. In: Kaplan HI, Sadock BJ, eds. Comprehensive Textbook of Psychiatry. Vol 1. Baltimore: Williams & Wilkins, 1989:635.
93. National Commission on Sleep Disorders Research. Report of the National Commission on Sleep Disorders Research. Washington, DC: Research DHHS Pub. Supplier of Documents, US Government Printing Office, 1992.
94. Findley L, Unverzagt M, Guchu R, Fabrizio M, Buckner J, Suratt P. Vigilance and automobile accidents in patients with sleep apnea or narcolepsy. Chest 1995; 108: 619–624.
95. Findley LJ, Weiss JW, Jabour R. Drivers with untreated sleep apnea: a cause of death and serious injury. Arch Intern Med 1991; 151:1451–1452.
96. Haraldsson P-O, Carenfelt C, Tingvall C. Sleep apnea syndrome symptoms and automobile driving in a general population. J Clin Epidemiol 1992; 45:821–825.
97. Broughton R, Ghanem Q, Hishikawa Y, Sugita Y, Nevsimalova S, Roth B. Life effects of narcolepsy: relationships to geographic origin (North American, Asian, or European) and to other patient and illness variables. Can J Neurol Sci 1983; 10: 100–104.
98. Akerstedt T. Sleepiness at work: effects of irregular hours. In: Monk TH, ed. Sleep,

Sleepiness and Performance. Chichester, England: John Wiley and Sons, 1991: 129–152.
99. Moore-Ede M. The Twenty-Four-Hour Society. Reading, MA: Addison-Wesley, 1993:81–96.
100. Schenck CH, Hurwitz TD, Bundlie SR, Mahowald MW. Sleep-related injury in 100 adult patients: a polysomnographic and clinical report. Am J Psychiatry 1989; 146:1166–1173.
101. Dyken ME, Lin-Dyken DC, Seaba P, Yamada T. Violent sleep-related behavior leading to subdural hemorrhage. Arch Neurol 1995; 52:318–321.
102. Gross PT. REM sleep behavior disorder causing bilateral subdural hematomas. Sleep Res 1992; 21:204.
103. Ch'ien LT, Aur RJA, Stagner S, Cavallo K, Wood A, Goff J, Pitner S, Husto HO, Seifert MJ, Somone JV. Long-term neurological implications of somnolence syndrome in children with acute lymphocytic leukemia. Neurology 1980; 8:273–277.
104. Berg RA, Ch'ien LT, Lancaster W, Williams S, Cummins J. Neuropsychological sequelae of postradiation somnolence syndrome. Develop Behav Pediatr 1983; 4: 103–107.
105. Littman P, Rosenstock J, Gale G, Krisch RE, Meadows A, Sather H, Coccia P, DeCamargo B. The somnolence syndrome in leukemic children following reduced daily dose fractions of cranial radiation. Int J Radiation Oncol Biol Phys 1984; 10: 1851–1853.
106. Fagioli I, Brauner R, Rappaport R. Polygraphic sleep patterns and growth hormone secretion in children after cranial irradiation. Eur J Pediatr 1991; 150:200–204.
107. Ahmed SR, Shalet SM, Beardwell CG. The effects of cranial irradiation on growth hormone secretion. Acta Pediatr Scand 1986; 75:255–260.
108. Palm L, Nordin V, Elmquist D, Blennow G, Persson E, Westgren U. Sleep and wakefulness after treatment for craniopharyngioma in childhood: influence on the quality and maturation of sleep. Neuropediatrics 1992; 23:39–45.
109. Etzioni A, Luboshitzky R, Tiosano D, Ben-Harush M, Goldsher D, Lavie P. Melatonin replacement corrects sleep disturbances in a child with pineal tumor. Neurology 1996; 46:261–263.
110. Matsuoka S, Yokota A, Yasukouchi H, Harada A, Kadoya C, Wada S-I, Ishikawa T, Okuda S. Clival chordoma associated with pathological laughter. J Neurosurg 1993; 79:428–433.
111. Ito K, Murofushi T, Mizuno M, Semba T. Pediatric brain stem gliomas with predominant symptom of sleep apnea. Int J Pediatr Otorhinolaryngol 1996; 37:53–64.
112. Garcia-Rio F, Prados C, Racionero MA, Serrano S, Pino JM, Villamor J. Nocturnal arterial oxygen desaturation secondary to a sphenoidal meningioma. Respiration 1997; 64:229–232.
113. Diez Garcia R, Carrillo A, Bartolome M, Casanova A, Prieto M. Central hypoventilation syndrome associated with ganglioneuroblastoma. Eur J Pediatr Surg 1995; 5:292–294.
114. Tokoro K, Chiba Y, Yagishita S, Kunimi Y. Cordectomy for syringobulbo-myelia with sleep apnea secondary to a spinal extramedullary tumor: case report. Neurosurgery 1989; 24:118–124.

115. Mickelson SA, Rosenthal LD, Rock JP, Senior BA, Friduss ME. Obstructive sleep apnea syndrome and acromegaly. Otolaryngol Head Neck Surg 1994; 111.
116. Lee MS, Choi YC, Lee SH, Lee SB. Sleep-related periodic leg movements associated with spinal cord lesions. Movement Disord 1996; 11.
117. Brown P, Thompson PD, Rothwell JC, Day BL, Marsden CD. Axial myoclonus of propriospinal origin. Brain 1991; 114:197–214.
118. Brown P, Rothwell JC, Thompson PD, Marsden CD. Propriospinal myoclonus: evidence for spinal ''pattern'' generators in humans. Movement Disord 1994; 9: 571–576.
119. Nishiyama K, Ugawa Y, Takeda K, Sakuta M. Axial myoclonus mediated by the propriospinal tract: a case report. Eur Neurol 1994; 34:48–50.
120. Chokroverty S, Walters A, Zimmerman T, Picone M. Propriospinal myoclonus: a neurophysiologic analysis. Neurology 1992; 42:1591–1595.
121. Kapoor R, Brown P, Thompson PD, Miller DH. Propriospinal myoclonus in multiple sclerosis. J Neurol Neurosurg Psychiatry 1992; 55:1086–1088.
122. Fouillet N, Wiart L, Arne P, Alaoui P, Petit H, Barat M. Propriospinal myoclonus in tetraplegic patients: clinical, electrophysiological and therapeutic aspects. Paraplegia 1995; 33:678–681.
123. Plazzi G, Provini F, Ligouri R, Lugaresi E, Montagna P. Propriospinal myoclonus at the transition from wake to sleep. Sleep Res 1996; 26:438.
124. Trenkwalder C, Walters AS, Hening W. Periodic limb movements and restless legs syndrome. Neurolog Clinics 1996; 14:629–650.
125. Yokota T, Hirose K, Tanabe H, Tsukagoshi H. Sleep-related periodic leg movements (nocturnal myoclonus) due to spinal cord lesion. J Neurolog Sci 1991; 104: 13–18.
126. Rossignol S, Dubuc R. Spinal pattern generation. Curr Opin Neurol 1994; 4:894–902.
127. Rossignol S, Chau C, Brustein E, Belanger M, Barbeau H, Drew T. Locomotor capacities after complete and partial lesions of the spinal cord. Acta Neurobiol Exp 1995; 56:449–463.
128. Caplan HJ, Peterson DD. Transient ischemic attacks and minor stroke during sleep: relationship to obstructive sleep apnea syndrome. Stroke 1995; 2361–2365.
129. Bassetti C, Aldrich MS, Quint D. Sleep-disordered breathing in patients with supra- and infratentorial strokes: a prospective study of 39 patients. Stroke 1997; 28:1765–1772.
130. Dyken ME, Somers VK, Yamada T, Ren ZY, Zimmerman MB. Investigating the relationship between stroke and obstructive sleep apnea. Stroke 1996; 27:401–407.
131. Blunt SB, Lane RJM, Turjanski N, Perkin GD. Clinical features and management of two cases of encephalitis lethargica. Movement Disord 1997; 12:354–359.
132. Bentivoglio M, Grassi-Zucconi G, Olsson T, Kristensson K. Trypanosoma brucei and the nervous system. TINS 1994; 17:325–329.
133. Buguet A, Bert J, Tapie P, Tabaraud F, Doua F, Lonsdorfer J, Bogui P, Dumas M. Sleep-wake cycle in human African trypanosomiasis. J Clin Neurophysiol 1993; 10:190–196.
134. Mahowald MW. Synchrony, sleep, dreams, and consciousness: clues from K-complexes. Neurology 1997; 49:909–911.

19

Sleep Disorders Associated with Multiple Sclerosis

Antonio Culebras
Veterans Affairs Medical Center
State University of New York
and Community General Hospital
Syracuse, New York

INTRODUCTION

Fatigue is one of the most prominent symptoms in patients with multiple sclerosis. It may take the form of mental tiredness, physical exhaustion, or excessive somnolence. Inappropriate daytime sleepiness and nocturnal sleeplessness, together or independent of each other, are common complaints in multiple sclerosis. The mechanism is multivariate, suggesting causes that range from depression to brain-lesion site, and its investigation is a cost-effective clinical exercise that may help determine corrective therapy. Descriptions of cases of multiple sclerosis associated with sleep attacks, variously termed narcolepsy, drowsiness, and deep sleep, have appeared in the neurological literature since the first half of the 20th century (1–3). A specific linkage of multiple sclerosis with narcolepsy was the focus of attention of various studies after a description of cases and reviews that appeared in 1949 (4). Later, cases of narcolepsy-cataplexy and multiple sclerosis (5) and of familial multiple sclerosis with narcolepsy-cataplexy were reported (6), including a citation of the presence of the DR2 histocompatibility antigen in two patients with narcolepsy and multiple sclerosis, which triggered the suggestion of a common inheritance for both conditions (7). Other authors (8,9) have indicated that sleep disturbance is relatively common in multiple sclerosis and the etiology multifactorial.

CLINICAL MANIFESTATIONS

Excessive somnolence and inappropriate daytime sleep can occur in patients with multiple sclerosis. In some individuals, excessive daytime sleepiness and sleep attacks appear in conjunction with cataplexy, sleep paralysis, and hypnagogic hallucinations, leading to a diagnosis of narcolepsy. Excessive somnolence and other narcoleptic symptoms may appear before (10) or after (11) the onset of multiple sclerosis, with the age of presentation varying widely. Laboratory confirmation of narcolepsy is lacking in older reports, or, if present, has failed to confirm a diagnosis of narcolepsy (12). The common complaint of chronic fatigue in multiple sclerosis may confound the interpretation of sleep disturbances. In a study by Ekbom (6) of families with concurrent multiple sclerosis and narcolepsy-cataplexy, two members had narcolepsy appearing shortly after the onset of multiple sclerosis, and one had narcolepsy as the putative initial symptom of multiple sclerosis. In Berg and Hanley's two cases with concurrent diseases (5), narcolepsy was the initial symptom of multiple sclerosis. Schrader et al. (11) described the case of a woman with definite multiple sclerosis who developed typical symptoms of incapacitating narcolepsy-cataplexy at the age of 56 years, 25 years after onset of multiple sclerosis. The sleep disorder was confirmed polygraphically, and the authors argued that the unusually late onset of severe narcolepsy-cataplexy strongly favored a causal relationship between both conditions. Younger and colleagues' two patients had narcolepsy preceding and following, respectively, the onset of multiple sclerosis, and both had presence of the DR2 antigen (7).

Patients with multiple sclerosis also report difficulty falling asleep, restless sleep, nonrestorative sleep, and early-morning awakenings more frequently than control subjects (13). In a study of 28 consecutive patients with multiple sclerosis, 15 patients (54%) reported sleep-related problems (14), including difficulty initiating or maintaining sleep, frequent awakenings due to leg spasms, habitual snoring, and nocturia. Three patients showed episodes of nocturnal oxygen desaturation, and two had sleep apnea syndrome. Magnetic resonance imaging of the brain showed abnormalities in 20 of 22 cases studied. In another study of 10 patients with definite multiple sclerosis, Wunderlin et al. (15) used limited nocturnal polysomnography, fatigue and sleep questionnaires, and magnetic resonance imaging of the brain to investigate whether fatigue was the result of sleep apnea syndrome. None of the patients with abnormal fatigue or sleep scores had an abnormal sleep apnea index, suggesting that fatigue and sleepiness cannot be explained solely on the basis of sleep respiratory disturbances.

ETIOLOGY AND PATHOGENESIS

The association between multiple sclerosis and sleep disturbance is more intimate than expected by chance. In one series (9), the prevalence of nocturnal sleep difficulties assessed by the Minnesota Multiphasic Personality Inventory in patients with mild definite multiple sclerosis was 25.2%. In another series (12), the prevalence by questionnaire in 70 patients with multiple sclerosis of daytime sleep attacks was 77% and of cataplectic attacks 56%, without a difference between DR2-positive and -negative multiple sclerosis patients. Nine patients in this series were studied using polygraphic evaluation, but no objective evidence of narcolepsy or excessive sleepiness was obtained, indicating a major discordance between sleep symptoms and objective findings.

Patients with narcolepsy exhibit the highest known association with the HLA-DR2 and DQw1 antigens, estimated at 95% or above in most series (16–18). The susceptibility to multiple sclerosis is coded by genes at or close to the HLA-DR-DQ subregion (19). The coincidence of genetic susceptibility between multiple sclerosis and narcolepsy converging on the HLA-DR2 histocompatibility antigen has led some authors to postulate a common immunogenetic etiology that remains to be confirmed (7). In a study of DRB5 alleles in Dw2-positive patients with multiple sclerosis or narcolepsy, Fogdell et al. (20) found that the HLA-Dw2 haplotype in multiple sclerosis and narcolepsy patients extends to the DRB5 locus. Rumbach and coworkers (21) measured daytime sleep latencies in patients with multiple sclerosis, and failed to observe a clear difference between DR2-positive patients and controls, suggesting that, by themselves, the genes coding for HLA-DR2 and DQw1 are not sufficient to cause an early sleep onset in patients with multiple sclerosis.

The remitting course of sleep attacks (5) and the late onset in life of incapacitating narcolepsy-cataplexy (11) exhibited by some patients with multiple sclerosis have been interpreted as an indication that multiple sclerosis may cause symptomatic narcolepsy. This hypothesis received some impetus with the observation by Castaigne and Escourolle (22) of midbrain plaques in the hypothalamic periventricular region of a patient with sleep attacks and multiple sclerosis.

The observation of lesions in the supplementary motor area identified by magnetic resonance in patients with mild but definite multiple sclerosis led Clark and associates (9) to suggest that the motor lesions triggered periodic limb movements during sleep, resulting in sleep interruptions and depression, a correlation found in 25.2% of patients studied. Spasms or discomfort in the legs have also been cited as a mechanism of frequent arousal in patients with multiple sclerosis (14). Others (8) have found that patients engage in more daytime napping than control subjects (53% versus 21% of controls), perhaps as a result of nocturnal and early-morning awakenings caused by bladder problems. Intractable hiccups persisting for more than 48 hours and sleep apnea syndrome were associated in two patients with lesions detected by magnetic resonance imaging in the tegmentum of the medulla (23), suggesting a pathogenetic correlation between anatomical location and clinical manifestations. In the view of these authors, development of intractable hiccups should suggest the associated presence of sleep apnea syndrome.

To investigate whether fatigue and sleep disturbance in multiple sclerosis patients might be due to disrupted circadian sleep regulation, Taphoorn et al. (24) performed actigraphy and multiple sleep latency tests in 16 patients with prominent complaints of fatigue and sleep disorder. Sleep latency values were altered in some patients with multiple sclerosis, but actigraphy scores did not differ from control values, failing to provide evidence of circadian rhythm disturbance in patients with multiple sclerosis. Accumulation of cytokines in the cerebrospinal fluid of patients with active multiple sclerosis (25) may contribute to sleep changes since these substances intervene in sleep mechanisms.

DIFFERENTIAL DIAGNOSIS AND LABORATORY EVALUATION

Sleep disorders may be suspected by patient testimony, but confirmation in a sleep laboratory is recommended. Nocturnal polysomnography identifies sleep disruption, and daytime multiple latency tests measure daytime sleepiness. Narcolepsy is diagnosed when REM sleep appears in two or more segments of the multiple sleep latency test and the onset of daytime sleep demonstrates a latency of 10 minutes or less. Narcolepsy-cataplexy should be distinguished from other sleep disturbances in patients with multiple sclerosis. Fatigue is a common symptom in multiple sclerosis that may be confused with or contribute to disordered sleep. A variety of underlying physical and emotional factors (bladder problems, spasticity, muscle spasms, periodic leg movements, depression, and anxiety) that converge to disturb nocturnal sleep in patients with multiple sclerosis should be considered. Excessive daytime somnolence in multiple sclerosis may be secondary to nocturnal disruption and nonrestorative sleep perhaps amenable to proper management.

Sleep laboratory evaluations in patients with multiple sclerosis have underscored that sleep disturbance is common and its etiology multifactorial, involving both physical and psychological features (8,26). Polysomnographic studies of patients with definite multiple sclerosis have shown significantly reduced sleep efficiency and more awakenings during sleep (27). Periodic leg movements were found in 36% of patients compared to 8% in controls, and central sleep apnea was found in two patients. Magnetic resonance imaging of the brain showed a greater load of lesions in cerebellum and brainstem in patients with periodic leg movements.

The diagnostic criteria for multiple sclerosis serve to identify patients with this condition (28). Polysomnography and multiple sleep latency testing are required to distinguish narcolepsy from other causes of excessive daytime sleepiness while identifying possible causes of sleep disruption. Human leukocyte antigen typing demonstrates DR2 positivity in 95% of narcoleptic patients (16,18) and in 50 to 60% of multiple sclerosis patients (29).

MANAGEMENT

Sleep disturbance in multiple sclerosis is multifactorial, involving physical and emotional features (8). Bladder problems, spasticity, depression (8), periodic limb movements (26), and lesion sites that subserve supplementary motor areas (9) may cause or contribute to sleep disturbance in multiple sclerosis.

Antidepressant medication has been suggested for the treatment of sleep disorders in multiple sclerosis (13), while clonazepam has been advocated for the treatment of periodic limb movements and amantadine for chronic fatigue (26). Increased evening wakefulness has been reported by patients with multiple sclerosis treated with selegiline (30).

Narcolepsy-cataplexy should be treated conventionally. Anecdotal case reports suggest that symptoms respond to habitual treatment modalities, including methylphenidate to enhance alertness and clomipramine for alleviation of cataplectic attacks. Protryptiline should be used with caution in patients with spinal-cord disease who are prone to develop periodic limb movements.

There is one report of resolution of sleep paralysis in a patient with multiple sclerosis using transcranial electromagnetic field therapy (31). The patient was a 40-year-old woman with remitting-progressive multiple sclerosis. Episodes of sleep paralysis occurring once a week occurred on awakening in the morning and were enhanced by mental stress, fatigue, sleep deprivation, and exacerbation of multiple sclerosis. Experimental treatment with alternate-current-pulsed applications of picotesla-intensity electromagnetic fields of 5 Hz frequency were applied extracerebrally one or two times per week. Three weeks after initiation of treatment, sleep paralysis gradually abated and eventually disappeared and there was improvement in fatigue, memory, and other symptoms related to multiple sclerosis.

REFERENCES

1. Jacobsohn E. Fall von Narcolepsie. Klin Wochenschr 1926; 2:2188.
2. Guillain G, Alajouanine T. La somnolence dans la sclérose en plaques: les episodes aigus ou subaigus de la sclérose en plaques pouvant simuler l'encéphalite léthargique. Ann Med 1928; 24:111–118.
3. Grigioresco D. Contribution a l'étude des troubles du sommeil à des lésions des noyeaux gris centraux dans la sclérose en plaques. Rev Neurol II 1932; 27–45.
4. Drake FR. Narcolepsy: brief review and report of cases. Am J Med Sci 1949; 218: 101–114.
5. Berg O, Hanley J. Narcolepsy in two cases of multiple sclerosis. Acta Neurol Scand 1963; 39:252–257.
6. Ekbom K. Familial multiple sclerosis associated with narcolepsy. Arch Neurol 1966; 15:337–344.

7. Younger DS, Pedley TA, Thorpy MJ. Multiple sclerosis and narcolepsy: possible similar genetic susceptibility. Neurology 1991; 41:447–448.
8. Leo GJ, Rao M, Bernardin L. Sleep disturbances in multiple sclerosis. Neurology 1991; 41(suppl 1):320.
9. Clark CM, Fleming JA, Li D, Oger J, Klonoff H, Paty D. Sleep disturbance, depression, and lesion site in patients with multiple sclerosis. Arch Neurol 1992; 49:641–643.
10. Bonduelle M, Degos C. Symptomatic narcolepsies: a critical study. In: Guilleminault C, Dement WC, Passouant P, eds. Narcolepsy. New York: Spectrum, 1976:322–325.
11. Schrader H, Gotlibsen OB, Skomedal GN. Multiple sclerosis and narcolepsy/cataplexy in a monozygotic twin. Neurology 1980; 30:105–108.
12. Poirier G, Montplaisir J, Dumont M, Duquette P, Decary F, Pleines J, Lamoureux G. Clinical and sleep laboratory study of narcoleptic symptoms in multiple sclerosis. Neurology 1987; 37:693–695.
13. Saunders J, Whitham R, Schaumann B. Sleep disturbance, fatigue, and depression in multiple sclerosis. Neurology 1991; 41(suppl 1):320.
14. Tachibana N, Howard RS, Hirsch NP, Miller DH, Moseley IF, Fish D. Sleep problems in multiple sclerosis. Eur Neurol 1994; 34:320–323.
15. Wunderlin BW, Kesselring J, Ginzler H, Walser B, Kuhn M, Reinhart WH. Fatigue in multiple sclerosis is not due to sleep apnea. Eur J Neurol 1997; 4:72–78.
16. Langdon N, Welsh K, van Dam M, Vaughan RW, Parkes D. Genetic markers in narcolepsy. Lancet 1984; ii:1178–1180.
17. Marcadet A, Gebuhrer L, Betuel H, Seignalet J, Freidel AC, Confavreux C, Billiard M, Dausset J, Cohen P. DNA polymorphism related to HLA-DR2 Dw2 in patients with narcolepsy. Immunogenetics 1985; 22:679–683.
18. Honda Y. Clinical features of narcolepsy: Japanese experiences. In: Honda Y, Juji T, eds. HLA in Narcolepsy. Berlin: Springer, 1988:24–57.
19. Hillert J, Olerup O. Multiple sclerosis is associated with genes within or close to the HLA-DR-DQ subregion on a normal DR15, DQ6, Dw2 haplotype. Neurology 1993; 43:163–168.
20. Fogdell A, Hillert J, Sachs C, Olerup O. The multiple sclerosis- and narcolepsy-associated HLA class II haplotype includes DRB5*0101 allele. Tissue Antigens 1995; 46:333–336.
21. Rumbach L, Tongio MM, Warter JM, Collard M, Kurtz D. Multiple sclerosis, sleep latencies and HLA antigens. J Neurol 1989; 236:309–310.
22. Castaigne P, Escourolle R. Etude topographique des lesions anatomiques dans les hypersomnies. Rev Neurol 1967; 116:547–584.
23. Funakawa I, Hara K, Yasuda T, Terao A. Intractable hiccups and sleep apnea syndrome in multiple sclerosis: report of two cases. Acta Neurologica Scandinavica 1993; 88:401–405.
24. Taphoorn MJ, van Someren E, Snoek FJ, Stijers RL, Swaab DF, Visscher F, de Waal LP, et al. Fatigue, sleep disturbances and circadian rhythm in multiple sclerosis. J Neurol 1993; 240:446–448.
25. Hauser SL, Doolittle TH, Lincoln R, Brown RH, Dinarello CA. Cytokine accumulations in CSF of multiple sclerosis patients: frequent detection of interleukin-1

and tumor necrosis factor but not interleukin-6. Neurology 1990; 40(11):1735–1739.

26. Potolicchio SJ, Calderon ET, Richert J. Periodic limb movements of sleep and chronic fatigue in multiple sclerosis: correlations between diagnosis and treatment. Neurology 1991; 41(suppl 1):320.
27. Ferini-Strambi L, Filippi M, Martinelli V, Oldani A, Rovaris M, Zucconi M, Comi G, Smirne S. Nocturnal sleep study in multiple sclerosis: correlations with clinical and brain magnetic resonance imaging findings. J Neurol Sci 1994; 125(2):194–197.
28. Poser CM, Paty DW, Scheinberg L, McDonald WI, Davis FA, Ebers GC, Johnson KP, Sibley WA, Silberberg DH, Tourtellotte WW. New diagnostic criteria for multiple sclerosis: guidelines for research protocols. Ann Neurol 1983; 13:227–231.
29. Duquette P, Decary F, Pleines J, Boivin D, Lamoureux G, Cosgrove JB, Lapierre Y. Clinical sub-groups of multiple sclerosis in relation to HLA: DR alleles as possible markers of disease progression. Can J Neurol 1985; 12:106–110.
30. Desrouleaux R, Weinreb HJ. Fatigue in multiple sclerosis: pilot trial with selegiline. Neurology 1991; 41(suppl 1):321.
31. Sandyk R. Resolution of sleep paralysis by weak electromagnetic fields in a patient with multiple sclerosis. Int J Neurosci 1997; 90:145–157.

20

Sleep Disorders and Neuromuscular Disorders

Antonio Culebras
Veterans Affairs Medical Center
State University of New York
and Community General Hospital
Syracuse, New York

INTRODUCTION

Changes in the physiology of respiration in sleep increase the risk for the development of sleep-related respiratory alterations and respiratory failure. A variety of sleep-determined changes that converge in the sensory and effector mechanisms of the respiratory system may compromise the already challenged ability to breathe in patients with a neuromuscular disorder. Included under this heading are alterations of the lower motor neuron, the neuromuscular junction, and muscle. Diaphragmatic weakness, chest-wall weakness, restrictive lung disease, weakness of the pharyngeal wall, obesity, and nocturnal hypoventilation of central origin are the principal causes of sleep-related respiratory insufficiency in patients with a neuromuscular disorder.

Anatomy and Physiology of Respiration in Sleep

The control of breathing is of paramount importance while the animal or human being is asleep and unconscious and thus unable to introduce voluntary variations. During sleep, there are powerful mechanisms that control ventilation and ultimately awaken the animal should an overpowering impediment occur. The control of breathing is different in non-REM and REM sleep.

The respiratory muscle groups, which include the diaphragm, intercostal muscles, and upper respiratory dilator muscles, receive appropriate signals from a medullary respiratory center. Three types of stimuli modulate the activity of the medullary center: chemical, chest/lung mechanical, and behavioral. Chemical stimuli arise from chemoreceptors that are responsive to $PaCO_2$, PaO_2, and pH. $PaCO_2$ receptors are located in the carotid body and medulla and respond to increases in $PaCO_2$ by stimulating a hyperventilatory response. PaO_2 receptors located in the carotid body trigger a hyperventilatory response via the glossopharyngeal nerve when the PaO_2 descends below 60 mm Hg. Very low PaO_2 levels depress the respiratory center. Mechanical receptors in the chest wall and lungs respond to inflation and deflation. Signals are transmitted centrally via the vagus nerve, causing the respirations to become shallow and rapid. Behavioral control of breathing is exerted in the awake state and is involved with functions in which airflow is necessary, such as speaking, singing, crying, and laughing. Supramedullary signals originating in cerebral centers override chemical stimuli.

Both hypoxia and hypercapnia stimulate arousals independently, but when combined, hypoxia increases the sensitivity to arousals caused by PCO_2. Cough is suppressed during sleep and can occur only after an arousal. Laryngeal stimulation during sleep causes reflex apnea that is longer in REM than in non-REM sleep.

Non-REM Sleep

In light non-REM sleep, which includes stage 1 and early stage 2, respirations are dependent on stimuli originating in chemoreceptors responsive to PCO_2 and PaO_2, but the ventilatory response to hypoxia and to hypercapnia is decreased. Respirations are irregular, with periodic variations in amplitude, and thus the label of *periodic breathing* is applied by some authors. The wakefulness stimulus is of primary importance in sustaining breathing through changes in chemical stimulation or when obstructions to respiration occur in sleep. Both hypoxia and hypercapnia are arousal stimuli that contribute to the respiratory and sleep–wake instability early on.

For reasons that remain obscure, respiratory stability is achieved as stage 2 takes firmer control. Breathing becomes regular, both in amplitude and frequency, resulting in decreased minute ventilation that may be the consequence of a decrease in both respiratory rate and tidal volume. Overall, ventilation is lower during non-REM sleep, and this relationship progresses as non-REM sleep deepens. Electromyographic activity increases in intercostal muscles as the ventilatory rate decreases, suggesting increased upper-airway resistance that reflects a partial impediment to airflow. Detailed studies of pharyngeal EMG activity during non-REM sleep have shown a decrease in activity in dilator muscles that probably contributes importantly to the upper-airway resistance encountered in this stage.

REM Sleep

In REM sleep, respirations become faster and more irregular, with changes in amplitude and rate. The irregularity persists through hypoxia, hypercapnia, and metabolic alkalosis, suggesting a strong neural influence. As in non-REM sleep, there is an overall decrease in ventilation and in responsiveness to chemical stimuli, with minute ventilation being the lowest during phasic REM sleep. Muscle atonia in REM sleep reduces the activity of intercostal muscles without affecting diaphragmatic muscle tone, which may even be increased to compensate for the intercostal loss. Upper-airway resistance is also higher during REM sleep, contributing to a decreased efficiency of the ventilatory effort that results in mild hypoxemia.

Neuromuscular Disorders and Respiration

The physiological reduction of muscle tone in non-REM sleep and virtual loss of activity of intercostal muscles with preservation or enhancement of diaphragmatic drive in REM sleep create a unique series of circumstances. In patients with muscular disorders, the challenged ventilatory mechanism may exhibit diverse patterns as a result of the various clinical forms of muscular weakness. Focal deficit of diaphragmatic function, as in acid-maltase deficiency (1), is characterized by REM-sleep-related nocturnal breathlessness and respiratory failure even before limb weakness becomes symptomatic. Some generalized myopathies, such as Duchenne muscular dystrophy, present sleep-disordered breathing only in terminal stages of the disease. In general, patients with diaphragmatic weakness are particularly vulnerable to the development of hypoventilation in REM sleep. Sleep-related hypoxemia, nocturnal fragmentation of sleep, and decreased daytime function are potentially correctable in patients with muscular weakness, so their recognition and characterization become part of the work-up of a patient with a neuromuscular disorder.

Conditions associated with central neurological disease may yet show other patterns of involvement. Although sleep-disordered breathing is the principal sleep-related abnormality in most patients with a neuromuscular disorder, some sleep alterations cannot be explained solely on the basis of a mechanical respiratory disorder. Some patients with myotonic dystrophy have hypersomnia that is not corrected with ventilatory assistance or that appears without an obvious ventilatory impediment. These patients may have hypersomnia of central origin that remains poorly understood. In some cases of congenital myopathy, there is impairment of respiratory chemosensitivity with reduced sleep-related ventilatory drive independent of hypoxemia and hypercapnia, which suggests yet another form of central dysfunction and not a mere blunting of chemosensitivity.

FACTORS CAUSING SLEEP-DISORDERED BREATHING

In a recent study of 60 adult and pediatric patients with a variety of neuromuscular disorders, Labanowski et al. (2) found a high proportion of sleep-disordered breathing. The authors performed the study in a clinic population at an altitude of 1500 meters. They utilized a sleep–wake questionnaire, a disability index, pulmonary-function tests, and an EdenTrace II monitor for 1 night to measure oxygen saturation, total apneas, hypopneas, and respiratory disturbance index (RDI). They found that 42% of the population had an RDI >15, which is much higher than frequencies observed in general population surveys. The authors failed to find strong predictors of sleep-disordered breathing in the population tested but concluded that, given the high prevalence of respiratory disturbance, screen testing of patients with a neuromuscular disorder is warranted to identify early sleep-disordered breathing.

Diaphragmatic weakness is the major determinant of ventilatory compromise in patients with neuromuscular disease. The diaphragm may be weak in isolation or as part of a generalized muscle involvement. Diaphragmatic muscle weakness becomes specifically manifest during REM sleep, when the diaphragm is physiologically the only effective muscle pump. Diaphragmatic muscle weakness becomes apparent during REM sleep, particularly if the patient lies supine. Patients with diaphragmatic paralysis cannot breathe while supine even in the awake state. Individuals with neuromuscular disease and diaphragmatic involvement exhibit the greatest oxygen desaturations in REM sleep, so this stage becomes a test of diaphragmatic muscle function.

Patients with neuromuscular disease may have restrictive lung disorder as a consequence of chest-wall muscle weakness, scoliosis, and pulmonary microatelectases that result from chronic hypoventilation, repeated episodes of aspiration, and retained secretions. These changes may lead to perfusion of nonventilated lung, a phenomenon that contributes to hypoxemia.

Inspiratory upper-airway resistance and obstructive sleep apnea may affect patients with neuromuscular disorders (see Chapter 13 on sleep apnea), causing an additional burden on sleep-related ventilation. These conditions may develop as a result of weakness of pharyngeal muscle dilators, leading to increased upper-airway resistance and a tendency to collapse of the pharyngeal wall. The alteration is further aggravated by tonsillar hypertrophy, obesity, or craniofacial dysmorphias and micrognathia limiting the oropharyngeal lumen. Patients with congenital myopathies and muscular dystrophies commonly have poor development of facial bones and the mandible (3).

Scoliosis is a common occurrence in patients with neuromuscular disease. Mechanical alteration of the spine causes a disadvantage of intercostal muscles and diaphragmatic function that is translated into a less efficient inspiratory mechanism.

Sedentariness in patients with altered muscular function promotes obesity, another factor that burdens ventilatory efficiency during sleep. Accumulation of fat in oropharyngeal soft tissues may contribute to restriction of the oropharyngeal lumen. Obese patients also suffer mechanical reduction of intercostal muscle function, and subjects with abdominal obesity exhibit marked diaphragmatic dysfunction that is particularly evident during REM sleep. In a recent study with nocturnal polysomnography of patients with abdominal obesity (4), I observed identifiable REM-sleep-related episodes of desaturation (>15% drop) in patients with morbid obesity (>147 kg). Desaturations appeared in hypnograms (Figure 1B) as abrupt nadirs or as unique profound drops in oxygen-saturation levels occurring only in REM sleep. Episodes of heart-rhythm instability and clusters of arousals were observed in conjunction with segments of profound desaturation. The study pointed out that computer-assisted hypnograms are useful to identify REM-sleep-related diaphragmatic insufficiency in obese patients with mechanical

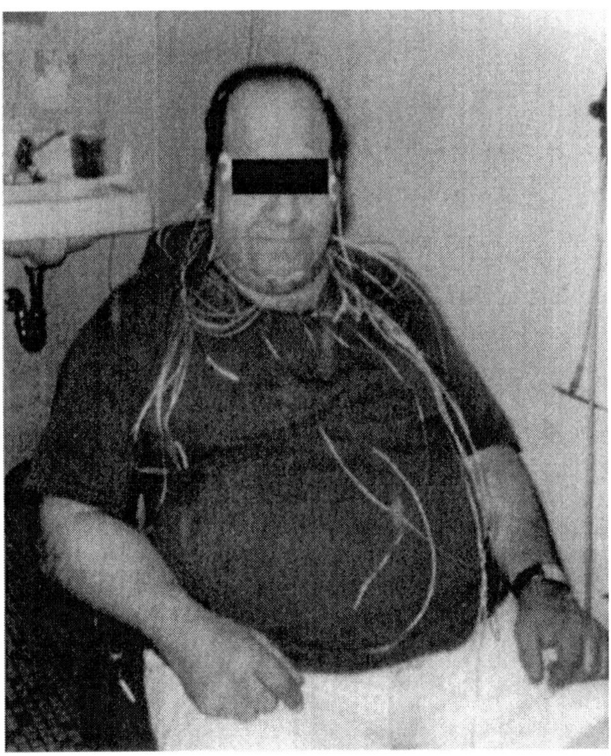

Figure 1A 56-year-old man with obesity (BMI = 40.3) and globular abdomen.

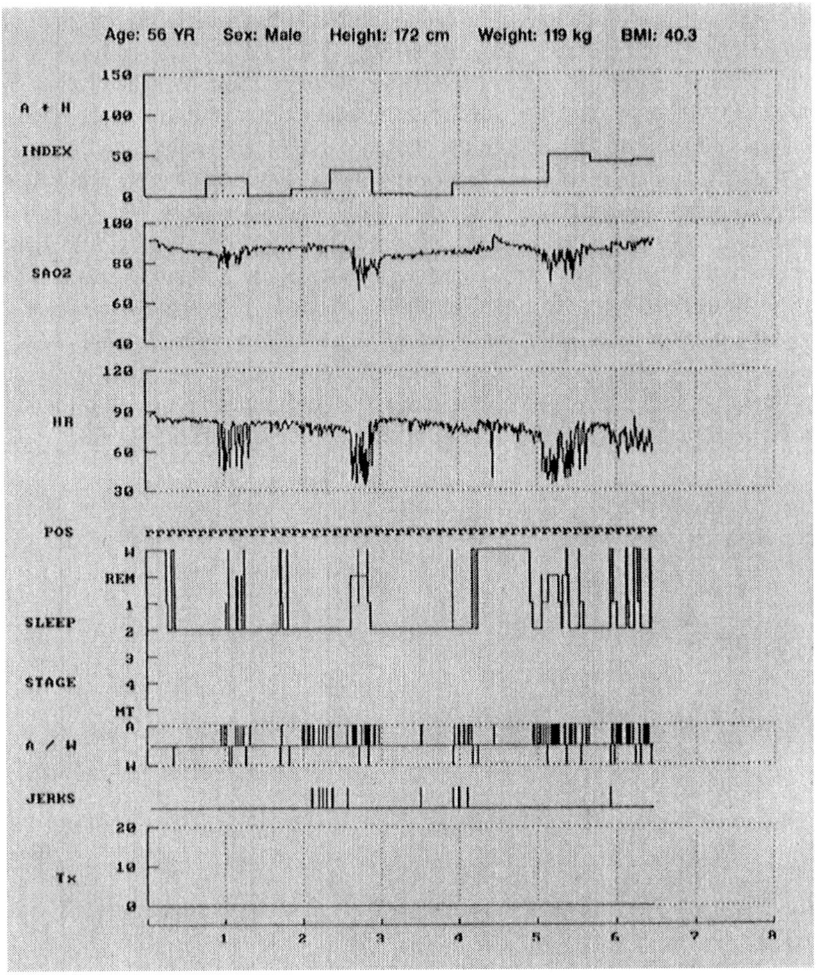

Figure 1B Hypnogram of patient in Figure 1A shows clusters of respiratory disturbance (A + H), desaturation events (SAO2), heart instability (HR), and arousals (A / W) in REM sleep as a result of mechanical disadvantage of the diaphragm. A + H index = apnea + hypopnea index; SAO2 = saturation of oxygen; HR = heart rate; POS = body position; A / W = arousals and awakenings; Tx = unused channel for CPAP pressures; 1, 2, 3, etc. = hours of nocturnal recording.

challenge of the diaphragm. Obese patients with a neuromuscular condition affecting the diaphragm are at even higher risk of developing REM-sleep-related disordered breathing.

Sleep-disordered breathing in patients with neuromuscular disease may cause nocturnal hypoxemia and episodes of desaturation associated with restlessness, partial arousals, and sleep fragmentation. Depending on the severity of the ventilatory deficit, patients may have continuous alveolar hypoventilation, even in the awake state, that in the most advanced circumstances becomes complicated with CO_2 retention. These patients exhibit secondary daytime excessive somnolence, a development that should prompt a thorough investigation of sleep-related ventilatory function, including polysomnography. Excessive daytime somnolence in very weak subjects could constitute a marker of preterminal muscular disease and herald pulmonary failure in the event of respiratory illness (5). Sitting positions in sleep, nocturnal cyanosis, morning drowsiness, headaches, and vomiting, and even cor pulmonale attributed to nocturnal hypoventilation have been reported in patients with advanced neuromuscular disease whose condition was reversed with appropriate ventilatory therapy (6).

Nocturnal hypoventilation with hypoxemia and hypercapnia, if not corrected, may lead to blunting of peripheral and central respiratory chemoreceptor responses that determine a state of chronic alveolar hypoventilation. However, in some forms of congenital myopathy, there is evidence of impairment of respiratory chemosensitivity that may be familial in nature (7). The combination of ventilatory muscle effector dysfunction and reduced central ventilatory drive is a high-risk situation.

PHRENIC NERVE AND DIAPHRAGMATIC PARALYSIS

The phrenic nerve originates in the phrenic nucleus which forms the ventral medial cell column of the cervical ventral gray horn, extending from the rostrocaudal extent of C3 to the caudal part of C5. Phrenic nerve damage resulting in diaphragmatic paralysis may be part of the spectrum of involvement in some diffuse neuropathies and in motor-neuron disease. Unilateral paralysis, sometimes observed as an elevation of the diaphragm in chest films, may be asymptomatic, but bilateral paralysis is invariably symptomatic and may be life-threatening; paresis or weakness with partial diaphragmatic dysfunction may cause exertional dyspnea and other manifestations of ventilatory insufficiency that, despite their typical character, may remain undiagnosed. If the diagnosis is not made early, repeated nocturnal desaturation events may precipitate cardiopulmonary morbidity. Bilateral paralysis causes orthopnea with striking severe inspiratory impairment that is out of proportion to the cardiopulmonary status. In the erect posture, the gravitational force improves the mechanical advantage of the respiratory muscles. However, patients complain of profound difficulty breathing when supine that reflects an increased inspiratory effort and is the result of a reduction in lung volume as the abdominal contents rise into the thorax. In severe or acute cases, patients present with nocturnal orthopnea, cyanosis, and fragmented sleep, followed by morning headaches, vomiting, and daytime lethargy. Polysomnography reveals hypoventilation that is particularly profound during REM sleep. As the desaturation event frequency increases in REM sleep, arousals and secondary daytime somnolence become increasingly prominent and the condition clinically resembles the sleep apnea syndrome. Undiagnosed bilateral diaphragmatic paralysis of any cause may lead to acute cardiopulmonary failure and death. Some reports describe unexplained failure to wean from a respirator as the presenting manifestation of diaphragmatic paralysis in patients with undiagnosed motor-neuron disease (9) or myopathies.

Phrenic nerve paralysis has been reported in patients with Charcot-Marie-Tooth disease (hereditary motor and sensory neuropathy) complicated with diabetes mellitus (10). Other conditions in which diaphragmatic paralysis has been observed include spinal-cord injury, poliomyelitis, Guillain-Barré syndrome, diabetes, diphtheric neuropathy, beriberi, alcoholic neuropathy, brachial plexus neuropathy, lead neuropathy, trauma, amyotrophic lateral sclerosis (ALS), myotonic dystrophy, Duchenne muscular dystrophy, paraneoplastic syndrome, and idiopathic conditions (9,10). In infantile muscular atrophy (Werdnig-Hoffmann disease) and adult motor-neuron disease, the diaphragm is rarely involved early in the disorder. There are reports, however, of chronic progressive motor-neuron disease presenting in acute respiratory failure as a result of bilateral diaphragmatic paralysis secondary to phrenic nerve nucleus involvement (9).

The diagnosis of diaphragmatic paralysis is suspected when paradoxical respirations are observed in the supine posture and when major discrepancies in vital capacity are detected between the erect and supine postures. Phrenic nerve stimulation studies, nerve conduction measurements, and EMG of selected muscles may aid in the diagnosis, along with fluoroscopy and computerized imaging studies of the chest. Nocturnal polysomnography is of critical importance to evaluate the presence and degree of sleep-disordered breathing in patients with suspected paralysis of the diaphragm. When the ventilatory muscle weakness is generalized, patients with the least diaphragmatic contribution to breathing are the most vulnerable to developing nocturnal oxygen desaturation (11). The severity of hypoventilation and the depth of oxygen desaturation in non-REM sleep are determined by the degree of involvement of chest-wall and accessory respiratory muscles.

NEUROMUSCULAR CONDITIONS WITH SLEEP DISORDER

Amyotrophic Lateral Sclerosis

The pattern of neuromuscular involvement in ALS, as a result of progressive degeneration of corticobulbar, corticospinal, and anterior horn cells, highlights this disorder as a prime target for sleep-related ventilatory abnormalities; however, severe sleep disruption has not been observed. Sleep-related respiratory dysfunction has been investigated in patients with ALS with the intention of searching for ventilatory alterations that are commonly observed in conditions in which muscle weakness predominates. Evaluation of the quality of sleep in one study (12) showed that only four of 12 patients described daily fatigue as an important symptom. In a prospective study of 21 patients with ALS to determine the relationship of pulmonary-function test abnormalities with quality of sleep and survival (13), the authors found that obstructive nocturnal events, although commonplace, were not accountable for nocturnal oxygen desaturation, while hypoventilation was found to be the primary explanation for the decline in oxygen saturation. Fasciculations were not reported to interfere with sleep, and affective depression was not evident. The group of patients had mild to moderate awake pulmonary-function deficits, and as a whole was not excessively somnolent as shown by the results of the multiple latency test, while the overall quality of sleep was surprisingly normal.

Patients with ALS may have dysfunction of the phrenic nerve, and, when paralysis of the diaphragm occurs, REM-sleep-related hypoventilation and oxygen desaturation are profound. This is exemplified in a case report (14) of a patient presenting with exertional dyspnea and hypersomnia followed several months later by respiratory failure that necessitated intubation. Neurological examination, electromyographic testing, and histological examination of the central nervous system confirmed a diagnosis of ALS with specific involvement of anterior horn cells from C3 to C7, a segment that includes the phrenic nuclei, where recognizable nerve cells could not be found.

Noninvasive respiratory support with CPAP or Bi-PAP apparatus may be indicated in patients with motor-neuron disease developing sleep-related respiratory disturbance, when diaphragmatic paralysis or bulbar involvement occurs. Elimination of nocturnal respiratory distress and restlessness, as well as alleviation of daytime somnolence and tiredness, improve the quality of life without altering the scheme for dignified survival.

Sleep and the Postpolio Syndrome

Some survivors of an acute attack of poliomyelitis have developed 20 to 30 years later a condition characterized by progressive fatigue, joint pains, and weakness in previously unaffected muscles. In this condition—appropriately termed the postpolio syndrome—central respiratory control and peripheral respiratory function may be altered, and it has been hypothesized that some of the postpolio symptoms are due to breathing disorders during sleep (15). In one study, 31% of 183 patients surveyed complained of sleep disturbances, even those without prior bulbar involvement (16). In this study, early-morning headache was the most common sleep-related complaint. Patients with kyphoscoliosis secondary to muscle atrophies often develop restrictive respiratory dysfunction, particularly if there is associated weakness of thoraco-abdominal and respiratory accessory muscles.

Sleep studies have shown central sleep apnea episodes in patients who had been weaned from respiratory support required by bulbar involvement (17). In another study with polysomnography of 13 postpolio patients with various degrees of involvement (15), most apneas observed were mixed or of the obstructive variety. The authors found that patients with obstructive and mixed apneas could often be treated with nasal CPAP, whereas those with hypoventilation and respiratory muscle weakness responded more favorably to the application of nasal-mask intermittent positive-pressure ventilation. They recommended that nocturnal polysomnography be performed in all postpolio patients complaining of sleep disturbance and respiratory manifestations since some of the complaints typically attributed to the postpolio syndrome, such as increasing fatigue, may be the result of nocturnal respiratory dysfunction and thus potentially correctable.

Myasthenia Gravis

Excessive fatigability and weakness of skeletal muscles are the cardinal manifestations in patients with myasthenia gravis. The disorder is caused when autoantibodies against muscle acetylcholine receptor attack the receptor at the neuromuscular junction. Typically, cranial nerve muscles are involved early in the disease, causing diplopia, ptosis of eyelids, facial weakness, difficulty chewing, and a speech impediment. In a large proportion of patients, the symptoms become generalized, affecting proximal limb muscles and involving the diaphragm and accessory respiratory muscles. Respiratory failure may occur in unmedicated, uncontrolled patients. Sleep-related complaints in some patients include waking up with a sensation of breathlessness, morning headaches, and daytime somnolence. Respiratory function may be altered during sleep, with respiratory failure and CO_2 retention serious enough to require ventilatory assistance (18). Polygraphic studies in treated patients show increased stage 1 and decreased stages 3, 4, and REM sleep. Patients also exhibit an increased sleep apnea index with predominantly mixed and obstructive sleep apnea episodes, along with oxygen desaturation of moderate severity. This is particularly evident during REM sleep, when the diaphragm is the only muscle that remains active in the exchange of air. Respiratory muscles may be focally affected in patients with myasthenia gravis (19).

In a study of 20 consecutive patients treated for myasthenia gravis, Quera-Salva et al. (18) evaluated body mass index, presence of upper-airway anatomical abnormalities, pulmonary function, presence of sleep-related complaints, and polygraphic measures during sleep. Results indicated that all patients had evidence of daytime diaphragmatic weakness, while older individuals with a higher body mass index and abnormal daytime blood-gas concentrations were primary candidates for the development of diaphragmatic sleep apneas and oxygen desaturation events during sleep, particularly during REM sleep.

Daytime somnolence in a patient with myasthenia gravis should suggest abnormal breathing during sleep, even in the absence of abnormal daytime functional activity. The dysfunction usually responds to the administration of slow-release pyridostigmine at night, although patients receiving appropriate treatment, with satisfactory daytime functional capacity may still have abnormal breathing during sleep.

Myotonic Dystrophy

Excessive daytime sleepiness and respiratory failure, both during wakefulness and in sleep, are commonly observed in patients with myotonic dystrophy. Hypersomnia is characterized by excessive daytime somnolence (20), with prolonged morning sleep inertia and sleepiness not relieved by naps, similar to the clinical picture observed in idiopathic hypersomnia. Occasionally, patients present features suggestive of narcolepsy, including sleep-onset REM periods (21,22). In a group of patients with myotonic dystrophy, Broughton et al. (23) found disrupted sleep with nocturnal fragmentation, short REM-sleep latencies, and reduced amounts of REM sleep. Hypersomnia may be aggravated by alveolar hypoventilation (24) and the sleep apnea syndrome, but it is not reversed entirely by CPAP applications (22), suggesting that hypersomnia is an intrinsic disorder related to central nervous system disease not caused by sleep apnea (25). Hypersomnia in myotonic dystrophy may respond successfully to the administration of methylphenidate (26).

Hypersomnia, apathy, mental decline, and "slow alpha" rhythms in subjects with moderately advanced disease have been linked to histological changes and dysfunction of the dorsomedial nuclei of the thalamus (27). In myotonic dystrophy, 10 to 30% of nerve cells of the dorsomedial nuclei contain eosinophilic cytoplasmic inclusion bodies that manifest neuronal damage. Eosinophilic bodies (28) are round, oval, or elongated, with smooth, sharply defined contours and an occasional peripheral halo ranging from 4 to 8 microns in diameter. Staining histological methods indicate that the bodies are acidophilic and composed of protein but not of amyloid. Ultrastructural studies have shown a fibrillar material within ribosome-bearing membranes, suggestive of a proteic nature. Inclusion bodies probably develop as the contents of expanding cisternae coalesce and become enclosed by condensing membranes. Eosinophilic inclusion bodies may represent the morphological expression of a block in the excretion or transport of a protein formed by the thalamic nerve cells, as well as a sign of neuronal degeneration.

As the disease advances, cognitive, sleep, EEG, and morphological brain changes worsen. Progressive enlargement of the third ventricle observed in some patients with myotonic dystrophy (29) may be the immediate consequence of progressive degeneration of the medial thalamus. Mental decline, psychosocial deterioration, apathy, inattention, and memory defect suggest a medial thalamic syndrome, while EEG changes characterized by slow alpha rhythms also suggest a diencephalic disorder (30). Testing has shown that the neuropsychological deficit cannot be attributed to the effect of sleep apnea or sleep disruption (23).

The sleep-related breathing disorder in myotonic dystrophy may be yet another manifestation of central alteration. Nonobstructive sleep apneas and sleep-related alveolar hypoventilation are common (24) and likely contribute to increased somnolence. Sleep-related breathing abnormalities are probably the result of central neuronal lesions and declining muscular function. In one study (31), obesity was found to correlate with levels of sleep hypoxemia, and body-mass index was significantly associated with the nadir of oxygen saturation, time spent at saturations below 85%, and the number of 4% drops in oxygen saturation. In a study comparing respiratory muscle weakness in patients with myotonic dystrophy and patients with nonmyotonic weakness (32), myotonic patients showed more frequent apnea and hypopnea events and more severe desaturation than the nonmyotonic group with muscle weakness. The study showed that abnormal breathing during sleep is common in myotonic dystrophy and suggested that sleep-related respiratory disturbance is not due solely to the direct effects of muscle weakness. Furthermore, somnolence was not clearly attributable to the sleep apnea/hypopnea syndrome or to the abnormal structure of nocturnal sleep.

Muscular weakness early in life in patients with myotonic dystrophy affects craniofacial and mandibular growth, contributing to the development of obstructive sleep apnea by increasing airway resistance in a stenotic oropharynx.

Muscular Dystrophies and Congenital and Metabolic Myopathies

Patients with Duchenne muscular dystrophy develop restrictive lung disease as muscle weakness progresses and ribcage deformities appear. A polysomnographic study of six patients with advanced Duchenne muscular dystrophy revealed nocturnal hypoventilation in all sleep stages with profound desaturation during REM sleep, despite normal awake minute ventilation (11). Five of the six patients had oxygen desaturation events exceeding 5% during REM sleep while breathing room air. The authors concluded that patients with diaphragmatic weakness are especially vulnerable to desaturation during REM sleep. Redding et al. (33) conducted another polysomnographic study of five subjects with severe restrictive lung disease and respiratory muscle weakness due to Duchenne muscular dystrophy without respiratory failure or cor pulmonale. The authors found abundant fragmentation of nocturnal sleep, many sleep-stage changes, and reduced REM sleep, but no evidence of nocturnal hypoxia. The authors further hypothesized that, in the absence of nocturnal hypoventilation, sleep abnormalities in patients with Duchenne muscular dystrophy might be inherent to the central neurological dysfunction observed in these patients.

Severe nocturnal respiratory failure has been described in two siblings with nemaline myopathy (34). This is a congenital myopathy with a relatively benign prognosis that affects all skeletal muscles including the diaphragm. Both patients developed marked sleep inertia in the morning with headaches, vomiting, and daytime lethargy. Subsequent medical evaluation disclosed marked hypoxia, hypercapnia, and cor pulmonale. Breathing at night was very irregular, with progressive hypercapnia as soon as they fell asleep. Nocturnal respiratory failure was attributed to a disturbance of central respiratory control with poor sensitivity to CO_2 inhalation, also detected in relatives. Nocturnal mechanical ventilation reversed respiratory failure in both siblings and permitted a return to daytime activities including school attendance.

Various combinations of nocturnal respiratory dysfunction have been described in patients with congenital fiber-type disproportion syndrome (10) and acid maltase deficiency (3,32). Hypersomnia was reported in a patient with bithalamic lesions and Kearns-Sayre syndrome (35). The nocturnal polysomnogram showed total absence of sleep spindles, and the authors hypothesized a thalamic dysfunction as a result of spongy degeneration, a commonly observed brain lesion in the Kearns-Sayre syndrome.

GENERAL APPROACH AND MANAGEMENT

Diaphragmatic weakness and failure are the most important determinants of sleep-related respiratory insufficiency in patients with a neuromuscular disorder. Hypoventilation becomes particularly severe in REM sleep when diaphragmatic function fails. Chest-wall weakness, along with restrictive lung disease, contributes to hypoventilation in all stages of sleep. Weakness of the pharyngeal wall compounded by obesity of sedentary origin and craniofacial maldevelopment facilitate the development of obstructive sleep apneas. Some patients with neuromuscular disorder exhibit nocturnal hypoventilation in the absence of airway obstruction or of major muscular weakness, suggesting an alteration of central respiratory drive.

Symptoms and signs that should alert the clinician to the presence of sleep-related ventilatory difficulty include nocturnal restlessness, frequent unexplained awakenings, loud snoring, and occasional episodes of awakening gasping for breath. Difficulty awakening in the morning and prolonged sleep inertia may interfere with morning activities. Daytime somnolence, fatigue, and inappropriate napping underlie failure to thrive in the very young and declining school grades or poor work performance at a later age. In advanced cases, patients develop nocturnal cyanosis, severe insomnia, morning lethargy, headaches, vomiting, and leg edema suggestive of acute respiratory failure and cor pulmonale.

Polysomnographic evaluation is necessary to distinguish among the different causes of sleep disturbance and to assess the severity of the disorder. Sometimes nocturnal disruption indicates nocturnal postural discomfort in a weak, incapacitated, or deformed patient. The daytime test may show excessive somnolence proportionate to the nocturnal alteration or, as in the case of myotonic dystrophy, may reveal excessive daytime somnolence that is not explained by the nocturnal findings. This suggests an intrinsic form of hypersomnia that in some cases has been associated with REM-sleep abnormalities.

Therapeutic goals are directed at elimination of excessive daytime somnolence, improvement of nocturnal desaturation, restoration of sleep architecture, and correction of respiratory and heart failure. Nocturnal application of CPAP and Bi-PAP can correct most nocturnal ventilatory abnormalities found in patients with neuromuscular disorder and should be considered whenever a sleep-related ventilatory deficit exists. Positive-pressure breathing eliminates obstructive sleep apnea, improves hypoventilation, and assists diaphragmatic failure. Supplemental oxygen bled into the mask is recommended when positive-air-pressure therapy is insufficient to overcome mean levels of hypoventilation of 85% or less. Bi-PAP is better tolerated by patients with weak chest walls and poor diaphragmatic function who cannot overcome expiratory forces. Supplemental oxygen via a nasal cannula may be sufficient in some cases to correct REM-sleep-related desaturations.

Patients with advanced restrictive lung disease, severe chest-wall muscle weakness, loss of sleep-related respiratory drive, and diaphragmatic paralysis pose special problems. Tracheostomy may be indicated in a few cases, but dependence, social disruption, and medical complications have to be weighed against the benefits obtained. Because children under the age of 6 years poorly tolerate nasal ventilation (36), other therapeutic measures may have to be considered, including temporal use of tracheostomy.

Protriptyline at bedtime slightly increases muscle tone in sleep and is of some value in patients with modest obstructive sleep apnea in which a weak pharyngeal wall is a component. It may also be useful to reduce REM sleep in patients with REM-sleep-related hypoventilation. Methylphenidate is of value in patients with myotonic dystrophy and hypersomnia who do not respond to the application of CPAP.

REFERENCES

1. Guilleminault C, Stoohs R, Quera-Salva MA. Sleep-related obstructive and nonobstructive apneas and neurologic disorders. Neurology 1992; 42(suppl 6):53.
2. Labanowski M, Schmidt-Nowara W, Guilleminault C. Sleep and neuromuscular disease: frequency of sleep-disordered breathing in a neuromuscular disease clinic population. Neurology 1996; 47:1173–1180.

3. Vargervik K. Experiments on the interaction between orofacial function and morphology. Ear Nose Throat J 1987; 66:201.
4. Culebras A. REM-sleep related diaphragmatic insufficiency. Neurology 1998; 50(suppl 4):393–394.
5. Smith PEM, Edwards RHT, Calverley PMA. Mechanisms of sleep-disordered breathing in chronic neuromuscular disease: implications for management. Quart J Med 1991; 296:961.
6. Heckmatt JZ, Loh L, Dubowitz V. Nocturnal hypoventilation in children with nonprogressive neuromuscular disease. Pediatrics 1989; 83:250.
7. Carroll JE, Zwillich C, Weil JV, et al. Depressed ventilatory response in oculocraniosomatic neuromuscular disease. Neurology 1976; 26:140–146.
8. Wilson DO. Sanders MH, Dauber JH. Abnormal ventilatory chemosensitivity and congenital myopathy. Arch Intern Med 1987; 147:1773.
9. Parhad IM, Clark AW, Barron KD, et al. Diaphragmatic paralysis in motor neuron disease. Neurology 1978; 28:18.
10. Chan CK, Mohsenin V, Loke J, et al. Diaphragmatic dysfunction in siblings with hereditary motor and sensory neuropathy. (Charcot-Marie-Tooth disease). Chest 1987; 91:567.
11. Smith PEM, Edwards RHT, Calverly PMA. Ventilation and breathing pattern during sleep in Duchenne muscular dystrophy. Chest 1989; 96:1346.
12. Minz M, Autret A, Laffont F, et al. A study on sleep in amyotrophic lateral sclerosis, Biomedicine 1979; 30:40.
13. Gay PC, Westbrook PR, Daube JR, et al. Effects of alterations in pulmonary function and sleep variables on survival in patients with amyotrophic lateral sclerosis. Mayo Clin Proc. 1991; 66: 686.
14. Meyrignac C, Poirier J, Degos JD. Amyotrophic lateral sclerosis with respiratory insufficiency as the primary complaint. Eur Neurol 1985; 24:115.
15. Steljes DG, Kryger MH, Kirk BW, Millar TW. Sleep in post-polio syndrome. Chest 1990; 98:133.
16. Cosgrove JL, Alexander MA, Kitts EL, Swan BE, et al. Late effects of poliomyelitis. Arch Phys Med Rehabil 1987; 68:4.
17. Guilleminault C, Motta J. Sleep apnea syndrome as long term sequel of poliomyelitis. In: Guilleminault C, Dement WC, eds. Sleep Apnea Syndromes. New York: Alan R Liss, 1978: 309–315.
18. Quera-Salva MA, Guilleminault C, Chevret S, Troche G, Fromageot C, McCann CC, et al. Breathing disorders during sleep in myasthenia gravis. Ann Neurol 1992; 31:186.
19. Mier-Jedrejowicz A, Brophy C, Green M. Respiratory muscle function in myasthenia gravis. Am Rev Respir Dis 1988; 138:867.
20. Phemister JC, Small JM. Hypersomnia in dystrophia myotonica. J Neurol Neurosurg Psychiatry 1961; 24:173.
21. Coccagna G, Marinelli P, Lugaresi E. Sleep and alveolar hypoventilation in myotonic dystrophy. Acta Neurol Belg 1982; 82:185.
22. Park YD, Radtke RA. Hypersomnolence in myotonic dystrophy. Neurology 1992; 42(suppl 3):352.
23. Broughton R, Stuss D, Kates M, Roberts J, Dunham W. Neuropsychological deficits and sleep in myotonic dystrophy. Can J Neurol Sci 1990; 17:410.

24. Hansotia P, Frens D. Hypersomnia associated with alveolar hypoventilation in myotonic dystrophy. Neurology 1981; 31:1336.
25. Meché FGA, Bogaard JM, Berg B. Treatment of hypersomnolence in myotonic dystrophy with a CNS stimulant. Muscle & Nerve 1986; 9:341.
26. Meché FGA, Bogaard JM, Sluys JCM, Schimsheimer RJ, Ververs CCM, Busch HFM. Daytime sleep in myotonic dystrophy is not caused by sleep apnea. J Neurol Neurosurg Psychiatry 1994; 57:626.
27. Culebras A, Feldman RG, Merk FB. Cytoplasmic inclusion bodies within neurons of the thalamus in myotonic dystrophy: a light and electron microscopy study. J Neurol Sci 1973; 19:319.
28. Culebras A, Segarra JM, Feldman RG. Eosinophilic bodies within neurons in the human thalamus: an age-related histological feature. J Neurol Sci. 1972; 16:177.
29. Glantz RH, Wright RB, Huckman MS, Garron DC, Siegel IM. Central nervous system magnetic resonance imaging findings in myotonic dystrophy. Arch Neurol 1988; 45:36.
30. Friedlander WJ, Bittenbender JB. EEG findings in myotonia dystrophica. Electroenceph Clin Neurophysiol 1964; 17:564.
31. Finnimore AJ, Jackson RV, Morton A, Lynch E. Sleep hypoxia in myotonic dystrophy and its correlation with awake respiratory function. Thorax 1994; 49:66.
32. Gilmartin JJ. Cooper BG, Griffiths CJ, et al. Breathing during sleep in patients with myotonic dystrophy and non-myotonic respiratory muscle weakness. Quart J Med 1991; 78:21.
33. Redding GJ. Okamoto GA, Guthrie RD, et al. Sleep patterns in non-ambulatory boys with Duchenne muscular dystrophy. Arch Phys Med Rehabil 1985; 66:818.
34. Maayan CH, Springer C, Armon Y, et al. Nemaline myopathy as a cause of sleep hypoventilation. Pediatrics 1986; 77:390.
35. Kotagal S, Archer CR, Walsh JK, et al. Hypersomnia, bithalamic lesions, and altered sleep architecture in Kearns-Sayre syndrome. Neurology 1985; 35:574.
36. Heckmatt JZ, Loh L, Dubowitz V. Night-time nasal ventilation in neuromuscular disease. Lancet 1990; 335:579.

Index

About the Editor

Antonio Culebras is Senior Neurologist at the Veterans Affairs Medical Center in Syracuse, New York; Professor of Neurology, Health Science Center, State University of New York, Syracuse; and Consultant at the Sleep Center of Community General Hospital, Syracuse, New York. The author or coauthor of 135 professional publications and the author or editor of four books, Dr. Culebras is a Councilor of the American Board of Sleep Medicine. He received the M.D. degree (1963) from the University of Madrid, Spain.